Biomedical Insights that Inform the Diagnosis of ME/CFS

Special Issue Editors

Brett A. Lidbury
Paul R. Fisher

MDPI • Basel • Beijing • Wuhan • Barcelona • Belgrade • Manchester • Tokyo • Cluj • Tianjin

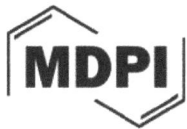

Special Issue Editors
Brett A. Lidbury
The Australian National University
Australia

Paul R. Fisher
La Trobe University
Australia

Editorial Office
MDPI
St. Alban-Anlage 66
4052 Basel, Switzerland

This is a reprint of articles from the Special Issue published online in the open access journal *Diagnostics* (ISSN 2075-4418) (available at: https://www.mdpi.com/journal/diagnostics/special_issues/ME_CFS).

For citation purposes, cite each article independently as indicated on the article page online and as indicated below:

LastName, A.A.; LastName, B.B.; LastName, C.C. Article Title. *Journal Name* **Year**, *Article Number*, Page Range.

ISBN 978-3-03928-390-3 (Pbk)
ISBN 978-3-03928-391-0 (PDF)

© 2020 by the authors. Articles in this book are Open Access and distributed under the Creative Commons Attribution (CC BY) license, which allows users to download, copy and build upon published articles, as long as the author and publisher are properly credited, which ensures maximum dissemination and a wider impact of our publications.

The book as a whole is distributed by MDPI under the terms and conditions of the Creative Commons license CC BY-NC-ND.

Biomedical Insights that Inform the Diagnosis of ME/CFS

Contents

About the Special Issue Editors vii

Brett A. Lidbury and Paul R. Fisher
Biomedical Insights that Inform the Diagnosis of ME/CFS
Reprinted from: *Diagnostics* **2020**, *10*, 92, doi:10.3390/diagnostics10020092 1

Mateo Cortes Rivera, Claudio Mastronardi, Claudia T. Silva-Aldana, Mauricio Arcos-Burgos and Brett A. Lidbury
Myalgic Encephalomyelitis/Chronic Fatigue Syndrome: A Comprehensive Review
Reprinted from: *Diagnostics* **2019**, *9*, 91, doi:10.3390/diagnostics9030091 5

Daniel Missailidis, Sarah J. Annesley and Paul R. Fisher
Pathological Mechanisms Underlying Myalgic Encephalomyelitis/Chronic Fatigue Syndrome
Reprinted from: *Diagnostics* **2019**, *9*, 80, doi:10.3390/diagnostics9030080 39

Eiren Sweetman, Alex Noble, Christina Edgar, Angus Mackay, Amber Helliwell, Rosamund Vallings, Margaret Ryan and Warren Tate
Current Research Provides Insight into the Biological Basis and Diagnostic Potential for Myalgic Encephalomyelitis/Chronic Fatigue Syndrome (ME/CFS)
Reprinted from: *Diagnostics* **2019**, *9*, 73, doi:10.3390/diagnostics9030073 59

Frank Twisk
Myalgic Encephalomyelitis or What? The International Consensus Criteria
Reprinted from: *Diagnostics* **2019**, *9*, 1, doi:10.3390/diagnostics9010001 73

Mark Vink and Friso Vink-Niese
Work Rehabilitation and Medical Retirement for Myalgic Encephalomyelitis/Chronic Fatigue Syndrome Patients. A Review and Appraisal of Diagnostic Strategies
Reprinted from: *Diagnostics* **2019**, *9*, 124, doi:10.3390/diagnostics9040124 81

Carly S. Holtzman, Shaun Bhatia, Joseph Cotler and Leonard A. Jason
Assessment of Post-Exertional Malaise (PEM) in Patients with Myalgic Encephalomyelitis (ME) and Chronic Fatigue Syndrome (CFS): A Patient-Driven Survey
Reprinted from: *Diagnostics* **2019**, *9*, 26, doi:10.3390/diagnostics9010026 115

Luis Nacul, Barbara de Barros, Caroline C. Kingdon, Jacqueline M. Cliff, Taane G. Clark, Kathleen Mudie, Hazel M. Dockrell and Eliana M. Lacerda
Evidence of Clinical Pathology Abnormalities in People with Myalgic Esncephalomyelitis/Chronic Fatigue Syndrome (ME/CFS) from an Analytic Cross-Sectional Study
Reprinted from: *Diagnostics* **2019**, *9*, 41, doi:10.3390/diagnostics9020041 129

Brett A. Lidbury, Badia Kita, Alice M. Richardson, Donald P. Lewis, Edwina Privitera, Susan Hayward, David de Kretser and Mark Hedger
Rethinking ME/CFS Diagnostic Reference Intervals via Machine Learning, and the Utility of Activin B for Defining Symptom Severity
Reprinted from: *Diagnostics* **2019**, *9*, 79, doi:10.3390/diagnostics9030079 145

Neil R. McGregor, Christopher W. Armstrong, Donald P. Lewis and Paul R. Gooley
Post-Exertional Malaise Is Associated with Hypermetabolism, Hypoacetylation and Purine Metabolism Deregulation in ME/CFS Cases
Reprinted from: *Diagnostics* **2019**, *9*, 70, doi:10.3390/diagnostics9030070 167

Alex A. Kashi, Ronald W. Davis and Robert D. Phair
The IDO Metabolic Trap Hypothesis for the Etiology of ME/CFS
Reprinted from: *Diagnostics* **2019**, *9*, 82, doi:10.3390/diagnostics9030082 . . . . **179**

About the Special Issue Editors

Brett A. Lidbury, Associate Professor, B.S. (Hons), Ph.D., FFSc (RCPA) Brett Lidbury is an Associate Professor with the National Centre for Epidemiology and Population Health (NCEPH), Research School of Population Health, The Australian National University (ANU) Canberra, Australia. He brings a laboratory background to his current role, with previous research programmes in infectious disease focused on virus–host interaction and viral pathogenesis. Discoveries in these fields included the elucidation of mechanisms for inflammatory regulation by Ross River virus (RRV, a mosquito-transmitted alphavirus), macrophage persistence by RRV, and muscle-joint pathology. RRV is associated with post-viral fatigue in Australia, and results from RRV research led to the current investigations into ME/CFS aetiology, which has taken a translational route with machine learning on patient data, as well as volunteer recruitment that requires clinical collaboration. Contributions to ME/CFS research include the identification of activin B as a potential serum biomarker, both alone and in combination with pathology test markers. The application of machine learning to pathology results and clinical observations is an ongoing research interest, with the aim of redefining diagnostic reference intervals that support an ME/CFS laboratory diagnosis and therefore assist clinicians.Lidbury is a member of the ME/CFS Discovery Research Network (MDRN) and is an investigator on the J.J. Mason Foundation-funded ME/CFS Biobank-Database programme in Australia.

Paul R. Fisher, Professor, BSc(Hons)(Qld), MSc(Qld), PhD(ANU) Professor Fisher has been the Professor and Head of Microbiology at La Trobe University, Melbourne, Australia since 2004. He has studied neurodegenerative and neurological disease, mitochondrial biology, and the roles of mitochondria in disease using two model systems to understand the cytopathologic pathways involved: 1. The eukaryotic microbe *Dictyostelium*, which is one of 10 model organisms recognized by the NIH for their value in biomedical research. *Dictyostelium* provides a tractable molecular genetic model for mitochondrial disease and neurodegenerative diseases; he is a world leader in this research. Using the *Dictyostelium* model, he specifically manipulates (separately and together) known disease genes and genes encoding proteins hypothesized to be involved in the associated cytopathological pathways. He then uses biochemical, molecular, and cell biological assays to determine the cellular consequences of disturbances in these pathways. The results support pathological roles for cellular stress signalling pathways in mitochondrial and neurodegenerative diseases. 2. Cultured cell lines from human disease patients and healthy control individuals. His laboratory's growing collection of cell lines currently includes a total of *ca.* 300 different lymphoblast (immortalized B cells) and fibroblast cell lines from healthy individuals and patients with Parkinson's disease, fragile-X-associated tremor and ataxia syndrome (FXTAS), and myalgic encephalomyelitis/chronic fatigue syndrome (ME/CFS). The aim is to study the roles of mitochondria and cellular stress signalling pathways in these diseases. This research requires advanced expertise in mitochondrial and molecular biology, biochemistry, and cell physiology, including the complete array of modern molecular techniques, as well as in the diverse statistical methods in the data analysis.

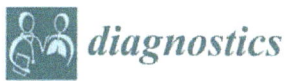

Editorial

Biomedical Insights that Inform the Diagnosis of ME/CFS

Brett A. Lidbury [1,*] and Paul R. Fisher [2]

[1] National Centre for Epidemiology and Population Health, Research School of Population Health, Australian National University, Canberra, ACT 2601, Australia
[2] Department of Physiology, Anatomy, and Microbiology, La Trobe University, Melbourne, VIC 3086, Australia; P.Fisher@latrobe.edu.au
* Correspondence: brett.lidbury@anu.edu.au

Received: 6 February 2020; Accepted: 6 February 2020; Published: 8 February 2020

It is well known that myalgic encephalomyelitis (ME) and chronic fatigue syndrome (CFS), whether considered as separate diseases or as the one chronic syndrome, continue to generate debate. Discussions on language, definitions and theoretical parameters continue, but whatever your position, one can now agree that ME and/or CFS (referred to hereafter as ME/CFS) is a disease with a physiological basis, rooted in biochemical and molecular dysfunction in the cells of sick individuals, and not attitudes that can be alleviated by psychological therapies. As a result, biomedical imperatives must now become the focus of research enquiry in order to find clinically translatable answers as soon as possible.

This book is intended as a landmark volume to mark this shift in thinking and to consolidate recent fundamental discoveries and biomedical insights as pathways towards tangible diagnostics, and eventual ME/CFS treatments. Australian researchers, with their collaborators locally and abroad, have been at the forefront of discovery in the biomedical realm, and this book draws together fundamental and applied insights that have emerged from scientific and clinical enquiry. The consolidation of up-to-date insights into ME/CFS was catalysed by a conference (https://www.emerge.org.au/symposium#.XbIv2iVS-3c) in March 2019 (Geelong, Australia), hosted by Emerge Australia, and several chapters in this volume are based on presentations from this meeting.

Section I—Reviews, Commentaries and Opinions

The book is arranged into two sections, with the first presenting the up-to-date commentaries and reviews of the broader ME/CFS literature.

Cortes Rivera et al. [1] provide a "comprehensive review" of the field that takes us from some of the early recorded outbreaks, attempts to recognise the aetiology of disease, a summary of ME/CFS clinical and population features, and impacts on contemporary biomedical thinking. The expertise of some authors was reflected also by valuable commentary on the genetic basis of ME/CFS, including epigenetic studies, with interesting lessons for complex disease in general. Central to the book's theme on "Biomedical Insights ...." are discoveries concerning ME/CFS patho-mechanism. Missailidis et al. [2] provides the required update on ME/CFS pathology as explained at the cellular level via biochemical and molecular alterations to function. Considering the array of triggers/causes of ME/CFS, but a similar range of symptoms, they suggest that patient stratification along these definitions is essential to understanding the molecular links to the whole person's clinical picture.

The commentary by Sweetman et al. [3] nicely follows the general reviews, and squarely addresses the question of whether biomedical science has assisted the clinic, with their views on the biomedical potential of fundamental discoveries augmented by the presentation of data from their own research laboratory. The answer, not surprisingly, is yes and no. However, they venture opinions on the frustrations experienced by both patients and clinicians due to "... a long period of debate among the health profession about the true nature of the illness. It has hindered funding for much needed research and has created inertia for researchers to join the research effort", while acknowledging the valuable discoveries of recent years, and the potential for progress in the near future. Such views are important to express, as they give impetus to a focused research effort, in spite of ongoing debate. Capturing an element of the debate, Twisk helpfully highlights a range of issues when considering ME as compared to the ME-ICC definitions (2011 International Consensus Criteria) [4]. In Twisk's view, the ICC has helpfully abandoned the "CFS" nomenclature, but continuing confusion exists since ME and ME-ICC definitions have not been harmonised.

To complete the review and commentary section of the book, Vink and Vink-Niese [5] review the situation pertaining to ME/CFS impairment and disability in relation to work, with a focus on diagnostic strategies and prognosis, as measured by the style and intensity of work possible post diagnosis. Of particular value is that the article draws upon the experience of one author (Vink), who is an occupational physician expert in the evaluation of patient disability, and discusses how to best facilitate a return to the workplace. To our knowledge, this is the first occasion that a specific examination of ME/CFS and its occupational impact has been published. Not only is the evidence reviewed, but advice is provided on how best to prepare ME/CFS patients for a return to work, if at all possible.

Section II—Research Results—Biomedical Insights and Diagnostics

The following section will highlight results obtained from primary biomedical research inquiry, and as such, represents contemporary thinking on the mechanisms of disease. For complex diseases like ME/CFS, research from diverse perspectives is essential. Section II starts with a qualitative study based on surveys and clinical observations, moving to new ways of using pathology laboratory data to provide marker patterns to assist diagnosis (as well as understand aetiology), with the final chapters highlighting exciting developments at the metabolomic and cellular levels of function.

Holtzman et al. [6] developed a survey, with community collaboration, to specifically assess PEM (post-exertional malaise). The surveys took the form of self-report questionnaires that were subsequently completed by over 1500 members of the patient community (35 countries, 41.1% from the USA). In the opinions of consulted community members, the most valuable PEM domains included onset triggers, timing and duration, the contribution of "personal characteristics", among other factors not previously investigated. The authors also proposed their study as a model of community collaboration, with valuable outcomes for patients, while declaring that they lacked knowledge of what case definitions were applied to individuals in the study cohort, and did not seek independent evaluation. As alluded to earlier, the variety of case definitions/criteria continues to bedevil progress on ME/CFS.

For patients who fulfil the diagnostic clinical criteria for ME/CFS, a feature of laboratory (pathology) tests is that all results across blood and biochemical markers report within the analyte reference intervals, suggesting no physiological dysfunction (but remain useful for excluding other health conditions). Nacul et al. [7] have confirmed this observation in the records of UK ME/CFS Biobank (UKMEB) participants, but found that for a normally non-requested blood test marker, creatine kinase (CK), severe cases had a significantly ($p < 0.001$) reduced serum concentration compared to healthy controls, with fluctuations in CK concentrations associated with symptom severity. Serum CK concentration variation persisted despite correction for disease duration, age, sex, and so on, encouraging further investigation of CK as a diagnostic marker.

The absence of pathology test results outside of the reference intervals was reported also by Lidbury et al. [8] for an Australian cohort recruited from the Melbourne region. For this investigation, the machine learning (ML) algorithm random forest (RF) was applied to identify predictor patterns from the pathology results, both for the direct comparison of ME/CFS to healthy control participants, as well as via the weighted standing time (WST) proxy for symptom severity. Serum urea and 24-hour urinary creatinine, markers of nitrogen metabolism, were found as the leading markers to differentiate ME/CFS from health, as well as degree of symptom severity. The role of the cytokine activin B as a serum marker was further examined along with the range of pathology tests, and was found to be significantly reduced in the serum of ME/CFS patients, in addition to being useful in differentiating moderate to severe symptom severity when added to RF models.

The identification of nitrogen markers within pathology test results link to deeper metabolomic analyses in samples from ME/CFS patients, as demonstrated by previous results from Gooley, Armstrong, and McGregor, who reported abnormalities in urea cycle metabolites. Further work by McGregor et al. [9] is presented here, which focused on biochemical alterations during self-reported PEM episodes. Glycolytic anomalies were indicated by glucose:lactate ratios, which correlated with a fall in the purine metabolite hypoxanthine. A "hypermetabolic event" was suggested by increases in the urinary excretion of methyl-histidine, mannitol, and acetate. In addition to these observations, data indicated a role for hypoacetylation, showing that multiple biochemical events from histone function to physical gut and muscle symptoms coincide with PEM.

The metabolomic biochemistry theme is further explored by Kashi et al. [10], who propose the indolamine-2,3-dioxygenase (IDO) metabolic trap hypothesis. The hypothesis explores the link of IDO biochemistry in the context of kynurenine pathways, and the amino acid transporter LAT1, through mathematical models of tryptophan metabolism. The formulation of the IDO hypothesis eventuated from understanding the history of outbreaks world-wide, database searches for common "damaging" mutations in human enzymes, and the synthesis of the hypothetical implications for ME/CFS through mathematical models. For example, the balance of tryptophan "steady-state" as physiological or pathological outcomes is presented, with the authors extending into experimental designs to test their hypothesis. As a disease with a "trigger", the disruption of steady-states, and thereafter perturbations in metabolism, these characteristics fit our understanding of ME/CFS aetiology.

Concluding Remarks

To reiterate, this book, as a Special Issue of the MDPI journal *Diagnostics*, stands as a landmark to consolidate the extent and value of biomedical research into ME/CFS, and associated clinical observations. Another metaphor may be a "rallying point", especially for those who have accepted the physiological basis of ME/CFS, but have been discouraged by ongoing disagreement among the research community and health professionals. In spite of debate, the evidence presented here and elsewhere provides sufficient impetus to explore ME/CFS as a biomedical challenge that can be solved.

Guided by the journal title, all contributors were encouraged to focus on elements within their research or practice that emphasised diagnostic utility and innovation. Having succeeded in presenting a collection of manuscripts spanning patient experience to pathology, physiology to molecular and cellular biology, we hope that this publication invites further insights from biomedical science, and finally acceptance that ME/CFS is a true disease with physiological foundations.

Conflicts of Interest: The authors declare no conflict of interest.

References

1. Cortes Rivera, M.; Mastronardi, C.; Silva-Aldana, C.T.; Arcos-Burgos, M.; Lidbury, B.A. Myalgic Encephalomyelitis/Chronic Fatigue Syndrome: A Comprehensive Review. Diagnostics 2019, 9, 91.
2. Missailidis, D.; Annesley, S.J.; Fisher, P.R. Pathological Mechanisms Underlying Myalgic Encephalomyelitis/Chronic Fatigue Syndrome. *Diagnostics* **2019**, *9*, 80.
3. Sweetman, E.; Noble, A.; Edgar, C.; Mackay, A.; Helliwell, A.; Vallings, R.; Ryan, M.; Tate, W. Current Research Provides Insight into the Biological Basis and Diagnostic Potential for Myalgic Encephalomyelitis/Chronic Fatigue Syndrome (ME/CFS). *Diagnostics* **2019**, *9*, 73.
4. Twisk, F. Myalgic Encephalomyelitis or What? The International Consensus Criteria. *Diagnostics* **2019**, *9*, 1
5. Vink, M.; Vink-Niese, F. Work Rehabilitation and Medical Retirement for Myalgic Encephalomyelitis/Chronic Fatigue Syndrome Patients. A Review and Appraisal of Diagnostic Strategies. *Diagnostics* **2019**, *9*, 124.

6. Holtzman, C.S.; Bhatia, S.; Cotler, J.; Jason, L.A. Assessment of Post-Exertional Malaise (PEM) in Patients with Myalgic Encephalomyelitis (ME) and Chronic Fatigue Syndrome (CFS): A Patient-Driven Survey. *Diagnostics* **2019**, *9*, 26.
7. Nacul, L.; de Barros, B.; Kingdon, C.C.; Cliff, J.M.; Clark, T.G.; Mudie, K.; Dockrell, H.M.; Lacerda, E.M. Evidence of Clinical Pathology Abnormalities in People with Myalgic Encephalomyelitis/Chronic Fatigue Syndrome (ME/CFS) from an Analytic Cross-Sectional Study. *Diagnostics* **2019**, *9*, 41.
8. Lidbury, B.A.; Kita, B.; Richardson, A.M.; Lewis, D.P.; Privitera, E.; Hayward, S.; de Kretser, D.; Hedger, M. Rethinking ME/CFS Diagnostic Reference Intervals via Machine Learning, and the Utility of Activin B for Defining Symptom Severity. *Diagnostics* **2019**, *9*, 79.
9. McGregor, N.R.; Armstrong, C.W.; Lewis, D.P.; Gooley, P.R. Post-Exertional Malaise Is Associated with Hypermetabolism, Hypoacetylation and Purine Metabolism Deregulation in ME/CFS Cases. *Diagnostics* **2019**, *9*, 70.
10. Kashi, A.A.; Davis, R.W.; Phair, R.D. The IDO Metabolic Trap Hypothesis for the Etiology of ME/CFS. *Diagnostics* **2019**, *9*, 82.

© 2020 by the authors. Licensee MDPI, Basel, Switzerland. This article is an open access article distributed under the terms and conditions of the Creative Commons Attribution (CC BY) license (http://creativecommons.org/licenses/by/4.0/).

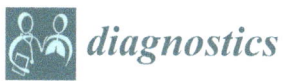

Review

Myalgic Encephalomyelitis/Chronic Fatigue Syndrome: A Comprehensive Review

Mateo Cortes Rivera [1,*], Claudio Mastronardi [2], Claudia T. Silva-Aldana [3], Mauricio Arcos-Burgos [4] and Brett A. Lidbury [5,*]

1. Facultad de Medicina, Grupo de Investigación Neuros, Universidad del Rosario, Bogotá 110211, Colombia
2. INPAC Research Group, Fundación Universitaria Sanitas, Bogotá 110211, Colombia
3. Center for Research in Genetics and Genomics-CIGGUR, GENIUROS Research Group, School of Medicine and Health Sciences, Universidad del Rosario, Bogotá 110211, Colombia
4. Group de Investigación en Psiquiatría (GIPSI), Instituto de Investigaciones Médicas, Facultad de Medicina, Universidad de Antioquia, Medellín 050002, Colombia
5. The National Centre for Epidemiology and Population Health, RSPH, College of Health and Medicine, The Australian National University, Canberra ACT 2601, Australia
* Correspondence: mateo.cortes@urosario.edu.co (M.C.R); brett.lidbury@anu.edu.au (B.A.L.)

Received: 22 May 2019; Accepted: 15 July 2019; Published: 7 August 2019

Abstract: Myalgic encephalomyelitis/chronic fatigue syndrome (ME/CFS) is a debilitating chronic disease of unknown aetiology that is recognized by the World Health Organization (WHO) and the United States Center for Disease Control and Prevention (US CDC) as a disorder of the brain. The disease predominantly affects adults, with a peak age of onset of between 20 and 45 years with a female to male ratio of 3:1. Although the clinical features of the disease have been well established within diagnostic criteria, the diagnosis of ME/CFS is still of exclusion, meaning that other medical conditions must be ruled out. The pathophysiological mechanisms are unclear but the neuro-immuno-endocrinological pattern of CFS patients gleaned from various studies indicates that these three pillars may be the key point to understand the complexity of the disease. At the moment, there are no specific pharmacological therapies to treat the disease, but several studies' aims and therapeutic approaches have been described in order to benefit patients' prognosis, symptomatology relief, and the recovery of pre-existing function. This review presents a pathophysiological approach to understanding the essential concepts of ME/CFS, with an emphasis on the population, clinical, and genetic concepts associated with ME/CFS.

Keywords: immunological; chronic fatigue syndrome; myalgic encephalomyelitis; biomarker; neuroimmune; Epstein Barr virus; hypothalamic–pituitary–adrenal axis

1. Introduction

Myalgic encephalomyelitis/chronic fatigue syndrome (ME/CFS) is a disabling clinical condition characterized by unexplained and persistent post exertional fatigue accompanied by a variety of symptoms related to cognitive, immunological, endocrinological, and autonomous dysfunction [1,2]. The estimated prevalence is estimated at 0.1–0.5% [3,4]. As a result of this debilitating condition, the burden for patients and caregivers is tremendous. In a recent review of the ME/CFS literature reported by The Institute of Medicine (IOM) of the United States (US), it was estimated that between 836,000 and 2.5 million Americans suffer from ME/CFS, causing an annual financial cost that ranges between 17–24 billion (USD) dollars per year [5]. The individual income losses are approximately $20,000 annually per household, and the unemployment rates among those who suffer this pathological condition are between 35–69% [5]. ME/CFS constitutes a particular enigmatic, debilitating and costly significant public health problem [6]. It is characterized by a substantial reduction in previous levels of occupational, educational, social and personal activities in a patient's lifetime. The disease affects all ages, races and socioeconomic groups and some studies showed that approximately three to four times as many women as men present the symptoms [3,7,8]. Table 1 shows the role of the main tissues involved in the pathogenesis of the disease following the hypothesis of the 3 pillars, explained later in the text.

Table 1. Features and function of main tissues representing the three pillars of myalgic encephalomyelitis/chronic fatigue syndrome (ME/CFS). HPA: hypothalamic–pituitary–adrenal.

System	Tissue/Cell	Feature	Ref.
Central Neurological System	Neuron	The symptomatology is related to a variety of sources of chronic neurological disturbance and associated distortions and chronicity in noxious sensory signaling and neuroimmune activation	[9]
	Glial cells	There is a significant blood–brain barrier permeability, microglia activation through toll-like receptors (TLR) signaling, secretion of IL-1B, upregulation of 5-HTT in astrocytes, reduced extracellular 5-HT levels, and hence a reduced activation of 5-HT receptors	[10]
Immune System	Lymphocytes Th1/Th2	Significant bias toward Th2 immune responses in CFS patients leading to an effector memory cell bias toward type 2 responsiveness	[11]
	NK cells	Reduction of cytotoxic activity in CFS, leading to a higher susceptibility of infection	[12]
	B cells	Persistence of autoreactive cells that can generate autoantibodies during common infections	[13]
Endocrine System	Hypothalamus–pituitary–adrenal (HPA) axis	Enhanced corticosteroid-induced negative feedback, basal hypocortisolism, attenuated diurnal variation, and a reduced responsivity to challenge	[14]

2. History

In the World Health Organization (WHO) International Classification of Diseases version 2016, both ME and CFS were coded identically and classified as other disorders of the nervous system; nevertheless, "fatigue syndrome", which non-expert clinicians may view as synonymous with CFS, is classified under mental and behavioral disorders [15]. This leads to confusion in the classification of the aetiology of the disease, mainly for primary care physicians.

Of the two current definitions, myalgic encephalomyelitis (ME) was the first to be defined. In 1934, multiple cases of an unknown illness were recorded around the world. The cases were confused with poliomyelitis or other medullary diseases, but it was eventually differentiated and first known as "neuromyasthenia" [5], with symptom attribution to psychological causes. The details changed from each patient, but in general, patients experienced a variety of symptoms including malaise, tender lymph nodes, sore throat, pain, and signs of encephalomyelitis [16]. As it occurs presently, the aetiology could not be clearly determined, and it was highly suspected to be infectious because of the flu-like prodrome in most of the affected patients. In 1959, the term "benign myalgic encephalomyelitis" eventually was chosen to reflect an inflammatory disease characterized by severe muscular pains and the evidence of parenchymal damage to the nervous system in the absence of mortality [5].

The landmark case from this era occurred in 1955, and became known as "Royal Free disease" through its association with an English hospital of the same name. Fifty-five nurses, doctors, assistants, and other health personnel were hospitalized on presenting a series of symptoms, which was unusual for the time. Interestingly, most of this hospitalized group contracted upper airway infection prior to the onset of the disease, as well as gastrointestinal alterations, acute vertigo and sore throat, which were followed thereafter by severe headache accentuated by movement and change of position, nuchal pain, pain in the limbs, extreme lassitude, and paranesthesia. Some cases reported more critical symptoms, including muscular cramps and twitching, objective sensory impairments, muscle tenderness, cranial nerve palsies, and ocular movement disorders, suggesting "epidemic neuromyasthenia" [17]. From that point, the efforts to look for the aetiology and the treatment of "myasthenia" began to grow.

In the 1970s, the European psychiatric society proposed that myalgic encephalomyelitis (ME) was a psychosocial phenomenon caused by either mass hysteria or the altered medical perception of the community, renaming the disease to "myalgia nervosa". With this redefinition and no organic explanations of the disease, the medical community began to consider the psychiatric component to understand the condition. This perception among medical professionals vastly limited the research efforts to study ME in fields different from psychiatry and psychology [5,18]. Later on, some researchers demonstrated the severe long-term disability of the disease and abolished the term "benign." [15].

In 1986, Ramsay [17] published the first diagnostic criteria for myalgic encephalomyelitis, which is a condition characterized by a unique and chronic form of muscle fatigability even after a minor degree of physical effort, spending three or more days to restore full muscle power. At the end of the 1980s, two cases of an illness resembling mononucleosis attracted the attention of some medical communities [19]. The disease was then defined as "chronic or recurrent debilitating fatigue and various combinations of other symptoms, including a sore throat, lymph node pain and tenderness, headache, myalgia, and arthralgia" [5]. Since this time, the illness was largely linked with Epstein-Barr virus (EBV) infection onset and was known as "chronic Epstein-Barr virus syndrome".

In 1987, the US Center for Disease Control and Prevention (CDC) convened a working group to reach a consensus on the clinical criteria of the disease. After much debate about the disease nomenclature, the CDC reached the consensus of "chronic fatigue syndrome", but noticed that the term "myalgic encephalomyelitis" was the name that was most accepted in other parts of the world. That was the origin of ME/CFS, the term for this condition, that is currently accepted worldwide [15,20]. In 1994 Fukuda proposed a clinical and investigative protocol in order to recreate a comprehensive and integrated approach to study ME/CFS.

The definition that was proposed by Fukuda considers chronic fatigue as "self-reported persistent or relapsing fatigue lasting six or more consecutive months" and requires a clinical evaluation to identify or rule out other medical or psychological conditions that may explain the symptomatology [21]. A diagnosis of ME/CFS involves the absence of other fatigue-associated conditions, unexplained fatigue for at least six months, and at least four of eight minor symptoms. Although this definition had been widely criticized for being overly inclusive, it is still used in the clinical evaluation and diagnosis of the disease. As well as the 1994 criteria, up to 20 other clinical criteria have emerged [1], with the other notable clinical consensus criteria being the 2003 Canadian Criteria, which was an update in 2011–12 to the International Consensus Criteria [2,22].

ME was recognized by the World Health Organization (WHO) in 1969 as a defined organic neurological disorder. However, in the daily medical practice globally, the concept of ME was not well recognized. The disease formerly described as 'epidemic neuromyasthenia' in the US is now more likely to be diagnosed as Chronic Fatigue Syndrome (CFS). Unfortunately, it was not until the ICD-10 that CFS was included in the medical classification of diseases in the US, with inclusions such as benign myalgic encephalomyelitis and post-viral fatigue syndrome [23]. Also, as a prolonged atypical illness associated with serological evidence of a persistent Epstein-Barr infection, it was associated with infectious mononucleosis syndrome [24]. However, six years later, Holmes described the first combination of nonspecific symptoms of the syndrome, introducing major and minor criteria for the ME/CFS in the clinical practice [25].

Since the definition of this syndrome, the main issue to diagnose the condition has been the absence of objective parameters to facilitate an accurate clinical assessment of the patient. Patients with ME/CFS were frequently maligned and told they did not have a real physical illness, but rather a psychological condition [26]. Through years of molecular research and clinical investigation, several clinical definitions have been established in the literature. However, the most widely used in clinical trials have been the Fukuda criteria and the international criteria, both with an inability to separate the ME from the CFS [26,27]. Therefore, a case of ME/CFS is defined by the presence of an unexplained, persistent, and relapsing chronic fatigue of new onset that is not alleviated by rest, which results in a significant reduction in the quality of life, and a concurrent occurrence of four or more of the following eight symptoms that must have persisted during six or more consecutive months:

1. "Brain fog" described as impairment in short-term memory or concentration severe enough to cause a reduction in previous levels of personal activities; 2. A sore throat; 3. Tender cervical or axillary nodes; 4. Muscle pain; 5. Multipoint pain without joint swelling; 6. Headaches; 7. Unrefreshing sleep; 8. Post-exertional malaise lasting more than 24 h [21].

Even though over the last few decades clinicians have reached a consensus to diagnose ME/CFS, the underlying aetiology is not well understood [1]. It is noteworthy that prior to a ME/CFS diagnosis, patients are mostly healthy, fully functional and have a good quality of life. Approximately 50–80% of patients with ME/CFS start suddenly with a flu-like illness, from which patients do not recover. ME/CFS is commonly found after infection by a virus, bacteria, or parasite, suggesting an immunological dysfunction as the possible beginning of the multi-systemic impairment, which is accompanied by a strong genetic predisposition, as shown in a twin analysis [26,28].

There has been an increasing effort to investigate the aetiology and maintenance of symptoms, including for patients with no infectious prodrome. Life stressors are shown to cause a negative impact on the neuroendocrine circuits of stress, leading to other complications besides immunological impairment [26]. Stress can be triggered by inflammatory components. Interestingly, one of the hypotheses that attempts to explain the aetiological component of the condition suggests the involvement of inflammatory cascades impairing either the functionality of the blood–brain barrier or the gut barrier [6] with other studies indicating that infections and immunological dysfunction contribute to the development and maintenance of symptoms, probably interacting with genetic and psychosocial factors [1].

Viral involvement is a well-supported pathophysiological theory due to the high index of an infectious onset in at least half of the patients, and confirmed findings of biochemical dysregulation of the 2-5A synthetase/ribonuclease L antiviral defense pathway in monocytes [2]. The alteration of this pathway and the reduced cytotoxic activity of the NK cells in ME/CFS patients are recognized as the main findings of the immunological impairment on ME/CFS patients [29]. In addition to immune and viral aetiology, the attenuation of the hypothalamus–pituitary–adrenal (HPA) axis is documented in adult and adolescent ME/CFS patients, with marked evidence of systemic hypocortisolism, which is an aspect that can influence the immunological and neuronal homeostasis of the individual [30]. Also, previous studies have reported enhanced sympathetic nervous activity, as well as increased levels of catecholamines in ME/CFS, evidencing a neuroactive pattern in the pathophysiology of the syndrome [31]. The alterations of these three biological systems will be further discussed.

The purpose of this review is to propose a coherent connection between the three pillars of the pathophysiology of the ME/CFS described in the literature: the immunological system, the neuroendocrine system, and the central nervous system, leading to a clear explanation of the symptomatology of the disease in the absence of a reference standard.

3. Epidemiology

The prevalence of ME/CFS varies among different studies depending on how this pathological condition is defined, the population surveyed, and the employed methodology. Terminological variations and inconsistencies in how definition and labels are used in different studies of ME/CFS pose a challenge to compare different global cohorts [32]. Therefore, there is a need to unify the diagnostic terminology, and this constitutes a goal in the investigation process.

Fatigue is commonly experienced by patients presenting different pathological conditions. Thus, it is necessary that any clinical measurement of fatigue differentiate between ordinary fatigue and a symptom of a pathological disease [33]. It is essential to be aware that the boundaries between normal and abnormal fatigue are arbitrary. For instance, some authors argued that fatigue should be considered unusual when the fatigued person views himdelf or herself to be ill [34,35]. A number of surveys conducted around the world proposed that the prevalence of fatigue among the adult population is considerable. The Office of the Privacy Commissioner of Canada (OPC) survey of psychiatric morbidity in the United Kingdom (UK) found that 27% of all adults reported significant fatigue in an ordinary week, and pointed out that the prevalence of chronic fatigue was 13.4% in that population [36]. A comparable study from the United States reported a prevalence of 6% of unexplained fatigue lasting more than two weeks [37,38]. One study involving the population of 143,000 people between 18–64 years of age from England reported an incidence of 4.7% of the included cases in the population and an overall prevalence rate of 0.20% [33]. Lawrie et al. estimated the annual incidence of CFS as 370 per 100,000 and the prevalence as 740 per 100,000 individuals in a study executed in Edinburgh, Scotland [39].

ME/CFS is an endemic disorder that affects all racial/ethnic groups and is seen across all socioeconomic strata. Most studies of gender differences report higher rates in women [8]. However, it has been suggested that gender differences may occur as an artefact of recruiting samples in a gender-biased manner from different specialist centers. For example, in a prospective cross-sectional cohort study performed in a rheumatology center in Spain, statistical tests were omitted to determine the significance of the gender, suggesting a possible bias [40]. Nonetheless, many community-based studies indicate that there may be a real gender difference [41,42].

The median duration of the illness is approximately seven years, a quarter of those with the disease are unemployed or disabled, and the average affected family forgoes approximately $20,000 in annual earnings and wages [43]. Kroenke et al. found a comparison with the disability experience in some medical conditions such as untreated hyperthyroidism and myocardial infarction [44].

The prognosis of patients with ME/CFS is variable. For some patients, an improvement in symptoms is a more commonly reported outcome than full recovery, and the prognosis in this case is less disappointing, especially among patients in primary care [45]. Some of the most prominent risk factors that predict progression are the severity of the symptoms at the time of onset, the standard of early management of the disease, having a mother with the syndrome, and comorbid diagnosis of fibromyalgia. The attribution of CFS to a physical cause and poor control over the symptoms have been associated with worse outcomes in those patients [46]. Death in patients with ME/CFS is usually caused by another co-existing illness, in which cancer and cardiovascular abnormalities are the most common causes of death among this population [47,48].

4. Clinical Manifestations

Myalgic encephalomyelitis/chronic fatigue syndrome (ME/CFS) is a complex condition with multiple systemic dysfunction. The primary symptom is the post-exertional fatigue accompanied by various neurological, cardiovascular, respiratory, and gastrointestinal manifestations [49]. Although an attempt was made to systematize the clinical signs of the disease through some major and minor criteria, clinical heterogeneity is far from being covered. However, most of the clinical trials accept and use the Fukuda and/or the CDC criteria for patient selection. Research efforts continue seeking biomarkers to aid aetiological understanding, clinical selection, and treatment options for this debilitating condition [26].

In order to make the diagnosis of ME/CFS, the patients must have the following criteria shown in Table 2 for at least six months in adults, and three months in children.

Table 2. Common symptom range and key features of myalgic encephalomyelitis/chronic fatigue syndrome patients (ME/CFS).

Symptom	Description	Reference
Fatigue	Fatigue is not the result of ongoing exertion, is not relieved by rest, and is medically unexplained. Fatigue can worsen with prolonged upright posture or even low-energy consumption tasks.	[50]
Sleep Dysfunction	Sleep is unrefreshing with disturbed quantity or rhythm that can include daytime hypersomnia, night time insomnia, and day/night reversal.	[3]
Muscle Pain	Muscle pain is more common in the pediatric population and can be explained by a comorbid fibromyalgia.	[51]
Joint Pain	Joint pain is not a common condition and can be related to autoimmune comorbidities.	
Cognitive Dysfunction	Slow mental processing speed, impaired working memory, poor learning of new information, difficulty with word retrieval, increased distractibility, decreased concentration and attention span, and inability to multitask; all of which are collectively described by patients as "brain fog".	[52]
Headaches	Frequently, patients suffer chronic, daily, new onset headaches, which can fluctuate in severity from week to week. If they are episodic, a diagnosis of migraine should be considered.	[3]
Post-Exertional Malaise	Normal activity or moderate exertion is followed by worsening of malaise, intense fatigue, and other symptoms. Recovery is difficult for the patient and usually takes more than 24 h.	
One of the following: (a) Autonomic Manifestations (b) Neuroendocrine Manifestations (c) Immune Dysfunction	Autonomic manifestations: orthostatic hypotension, exercise intolerance, sweating abnormalities digestive, urinary and sexual alterations. Neuroendocrine manifestations: Tolerance for stress, anxiety, or panic attacks, anorexia, recurrent feeling of feverishness Immune manifestations: Tender lymphadenopathy, sore throat, new sensitivities to food or medications.	[26]

Other unspecific symptoms also reported by patients include dizziness, nausea, anorexia, headaches, and night sweats [49]. The onset of the disease may vary depending on demographic factors. For instance, most patients that attend tertiary care health medical doctors frequently report an acute onset of symptoms after an infectious illness; nevertheless, in the general population attending primary care, the onset of fatigue is gradual [53,54].

The fatigue in patients suffering ME/CFS is more intense and different from usual tiredness related to physical exercise. It may combine cognitive and physical exhaustion, weakness, heaviness, general malaise, light headedness, and sleepiness. These characteristics are the main tool that the primary care physician has to be able to differentiate ME/CFS from other common causes of fatigue, including fatigue associated with cancer.

Post-exertional malaise (PEM) is considered one of the distinguishing symptoms of ME/CFS. It can be used by the clinicians to differentiate it from other conditions with similar symptomatology such as depression. PEM refers to severe fatigue after minimal physical or mental/cognitive exertion. The mental fatigue is described by the patients as "brain fog" and includes poor concentration, forgetting words in speech and poor short-term memory [54].

The autonomic dysfunction may elicit a central alteration of the autonomic nervous system, which provides unconscious control of basic systemic functions [49]. The symptoms of the autonomic dysfunction include dizziness and fainting upon standing up, inability to alter heart rate with exercise, sweating abnormalities, digestion difficulties due to slow digestion, and urinary, sexual and visual problems [54]. This autonomic dysfunction is related to one of the most common comorbidities found in the syndrome, the Postural Orthostatic Tachycardia Syndrome (POTS), which is defined by Reynolds et al. as the presence of orthostatic intolerance and an increased heart rate of more than 30 beats per minute from baseline [53].

All of these signs are suggestive of ME/CFS, but are not specific. Patients feel tired; they may have drooped and crooked postures with rounded shoulders when sitting in a chair. Some patients need to lie down on the examination table while they wait to be seen by the physician; others go to the hospital in a wheelchair [26]. Some patients may present periorbital hyperpigmentation indicating allergies, and puffy eyes, meaning fatigue or oedema. Patients with a sore throat are more likely to report a viral reactivation accompanied by tender lymphadenopathy in the cervical, axillary and inguinal areas [54]. Examination of the pupils may show oscillation of the pupils or diminished pupillary accommodation due to the imbalance of the central sympathetic and parasympathetic nervous system [55].

5. Pathophysiology

5.1. Immune System

The pathophysiological mechanism of ME/CFS is unclear [56]. In the context of the immune system, hypotheses include altered central nervous system functioning resulting from abnormal responses to common antigens; the activation of inflammatory, cell-mediated immune (CMI) response, and enhancement of oxidative and nitrosative pathways; a neuroendocrine disturbance, and autoimmune responses against neuronal and other cells and proteins [29].

Numerous studies have sought evidence for a disturbance in the immunity system. A decreased function of natural killer (NK) cells, an alteration in cytokine profile, and the reduced responses of T cell to mitogens, and other specific antigens, have been reported in several studies [56]. The immunological findings encompass a low-grade inflammation, as indicated by an increased production of nuclear factor kB (NF-κB), cyclooxygenase-2 (COX-2), and inducible nitric oxide synthase (iNOS); immune activation, with increased expression of activation markers; increased levels of proinflammatory cytokines, including IL-1, IL-4, IL-5, IL-6, and IL-12 and lowered levels of IL-8, IL-13, and IL-15; immunosuppression, as indicated in decreased NK cell cytotoxicity; autoimmune reactions; oxidative and nitrosative stress (O&NS) damage to membrane fatty acids, proteins and DNA; lowered antioxidant levels; mitochondrial dysfunction; bacterial translocation, and the alteration of antiviral response elements, such as the 2-5 oligoadenylate synthetase/RNase L pathway [29,56,57].

5.2. Inflammation and Oxidative Stress

Studies have reported that ME/CFS is accompanied by systemic inflammation, while others define ME/CFS as a low-grade inflammatory disease characterized by: (a) increased levels of pro-inflammatory cytokines and high concentrations of acute phase reactants; (b) diminished levels of antioxidants, including zinc and coenzyme Q10 and antioxidant enzymes; (c) O&NS damage to fatty acids, proteins and DNA; (d) dysfunctional mitochondria; (e) a lowered w3/w9 polyunsaturated fatty acid ratio; (f) increased translocation of Gram-negative bacteria; and (g) aberrations in intracellular signal transduction and apoptosis pathways [58].

The high level of pro-inflammatory cytokines is an important feature of the pathophysiology and may explain some of the clinical manifestations of the disease, such as chronic fatigue and flu-like symptoms [56]. The most supported origin of this inflammatory state is the association with an infectious pathogen, especially a viral infection. A viral infection could rapidly activate antiviral pathways, e.g., IFN-γ-indicated pathways, which would quickly allow the establishment of a systemic inflammatory state [59].

The evidence that immunoinflammatory pathways are activated are:

(a) chronic low-grade inflammation, as indicated by elevated production or levels of tumor necrosis factor-alpha (TNF-α) and other pro-inflammatory cytokines such as IL-1β and IL-6;
(b) Cellular-mediated immune (CMI) response activation, as indicated by increased neopterin levels, a well-known biomarker of the immunological stimulation;
(c) immunological phenotypic change including Th1 to Th2 shift, increased CD26 expression on T cells, defective T regulatory cell functions, and T cell exhaustion [11,60,61]; and
(d) increased bacterial translocation sustained by the leaky gut theory of increased IgA levels against lipopolysaccharides (LPS) of Gram-negative bacteria [29,58].

Oxidative stress is defined as a disturbance to the equilibrium status of pro-oxidant and antioxidant systems in favor of pro-oxidation. The term is used to describe chemical reactions involved in the production of free radicals and other reactive molecules that potentially induce cellular injury [62].

ME/CFS patients have a significant activation of the oxidative and nitrosative stress, which appears to be a critical feature in the pathophysiology of the disease; for example, studies have reported the elevation of oxidative stress biomarkers in blood (notably isoprostane, oxidized LDL, and iso-prostaglandin F2), and the reduced antioxidant capacity as represented by glutathione levels [62,63]. These findings suggest that oxidative stress could be implicated in the pathophysiology of ME/CFS by an excessive free radical formation, but not by the depletion of antioxidant reserves [58,62]. The damaging effects of the O&NS to fatty acids or proteins transform them into immunogenic targets for the immune system as it loses immunogenic tolerance [59,64]. This mechanism might explain the high incidence of IgM-mediated autoimmune responses directed against O&NS-modified epitopes in ME/CFS.

An important aspect that allows the integration of the immunological phenomena is the relationship between mitochondrial damage and the increase of oxidative stress [64]. Increased ROS leads to damage of the electron transport chain leading to depleted adenosine-5′-triphosphate (ATP) production which in turn causes a deficiency in oxidative phosphorylation and impaired mitochondrial function [62,65]. Mitochondrial aetiology for ME/CFS is a prominent feature of current thinking, and whether immune dysregulation explains all aspects is yet to be determined [66–68].

Viral infections, including ROS/RNS-induced damage and inflammatory cytokines can activate a key transcription factor NF-κB, which could play a triggering role and propel an inflammatory cascade in patients. Once activated, NF-κB is translocated from the cytoplasm to the nucleus to bind the DNA promoter sequences of several inflammatory mediators such as IL-1β, IL-6, TNFα; and O&NS mediators, such as cyclooxygenase-2 (COX-2) and inducible NO synthase (iNOS) [64,69]. This upregulation could link the interaction between the increase in oxidative stress and the immunological overreaction in these patients. However, the directionality of this interaction is not clear yet. It is believed that the immune response to an external pathogen could be the cause of the activation of unbridled oxidative stress, which in turn perpetuates a steady inflammatory cascade [59,70].

5.3. NK Alteration

The NK cells are granular lymphocytes that play an important role at the interface between innate and adaptive immunity [29,71]. NK cells are important effectors of the innate immune system, as they responsible for the lysis of tumor and virally infected cells without affecting healthy host cells. [72]. The surface markers in NK cells indicate different subtypes with different functions. For example, two subsets of NK population known as $CD56^{bright}$ $CD16^{dim/-}$ and $CD56^{dim}$ CD16+ have different functions [73]. The former subset plays a predominately immunosurveillance role with potent cytokine production, whereas the latter subset is primarily cytotoxic and can kill infected and tumor cells [29,74]. CD16, or FcγRIIIA, is a low-affinity receptor for the Fc portion of immunoglobulin G, and CD56 is an adhesion molecule that mediates the homotypic adhesion in immunological cells [75]. For the proper interaction with the cells, NK cells are recruited mainly by interferon and chemoattractive chemokines, including CCL22, CX3CL1, and CXCL8, with an alteration of intracellular Ca^{+2} concentration impacting lytic potential [76]. Decreased NK cell function and associations of NK impairment with viral infection/reactivation have been observed in ME/CFS patients.

A study examining 41 ME/CFS patients reported a decreased frequency of peripheral blood CD3-CD57+ lymphocytes; primarily representing NK cells, whereas frequencies of CD3+CD57+ cells, representing cytotoxic T lymphocytes, were unperturbed, suggesting an immunological selectivity in the disease [74,77,78]. However, another study found a significantly lower frequency of CD3+ lymphocytes and a higher CD4 T-cell representation in ME/CFS patients [79], whereas several studies found no significant changes in the immunological profile between ME/CFS patients and controls [80].

Transient receptor potential (TRP) ion channels are involved in diverse physiological processes, such as the sensation of a wide range of stimuli and modulation of ion entry to the cytoplasm [81].

Recently, the TRPM3 ion channel was shown to display a significantly lower expression on the cell surface of NK, and B cells form ME/CFS patients when compared with healthy controls. This finding suggests an impaired Ca^{+2} mobilization in the NK cells of ME/CFS patients, which prevents the mobilization of secretory vesicles leading to a reduction in NK cell cytotoxic activity [56,66]. Interestingly, one study recently demonstrated an alteration in the signaling of the MAPK pathway that was associated with a decrease of the intracellular concentrations of Ca^{+2} in NK isolated cells of patients with ME/CFS, suggesting a fundamental alteration in the lytic function of these immune cells [29]. Additional studies reported findings for a number of SNPs in genes for acetylcholine receptors (AChR) and TRP ion channels from the isolated NK cells from ME/CFS patients. These investigations reported a significant reduction in NK lysis in these patients compared with unfatigued controls [82].

Interestingly, other studies established that mitochondria play a key role in the function of innate immunity cells, including NK cells. A recent discovery that mitochondria express a range of AChR subtypes, including nicotinic α3 subunit receptor, suggests that nAChR may impact the mitochondrial function directly to regulate oxidative stress [29,75]. In the face of dysregulation in several neurotransmitters, including acetylcholine, the mitochondrial stress associated with the activation of these nicotinic receptors would lead to an alteration in intracellular dynamics in several immune cells, including NK cells.

5.4. Immunoglobulins

Levels of total serum immunoglobulin G (IgG) and the IgG subclass are reduced in CFS patients. Some studies report decreased IgG1 and IgG3 levels; others observed deficiencies in all IgG subclasses or only in the IgG3 levels in some patients. These deficiencies may be correlated with antiviral activity in these patients and contribute to the pathogenesis of the disease [83]. ME/CFS is accompanied by increased serum levels of IgA and, to a lesser extent, IgM against the LPS of commensal Gram-negative enterobacteria [84]. It is well known that persistent inflammation in the syndrome can cause the mucosal barrier to become more permeable, whereby wider spaces between the cells of the gut wall cause a loss of the protective barrier. This may induce increased bacterial translocation, and thus an increase of serum endotoxin concentrations, which might trigger an immune response [85]. The increased serum IgA and IgM levels against the LPS of the Gram-negative enterobacteria in ME/CFS indicate the presence of increased gut permeability and an immune response mounted against the LPS of the enterobacteria [83]. Although there are no exact figures to pathologize the levels of IgA in CFS, an elevation of this immunoglobulin can help the primary care physician establish the progress of systemic inflammation in the natural history of the disease.

5.5. Autoimmunity

Maes et al. reported in a study analyzing the IgM levels from the serum of ME/CFS patients, that the syndrome is characterized by an IgM-related immune response directed against disrupted lipid membrane components, by-products of lipid peroxidation, S-farnesyl-L-cysteine, and NO-modified amino acids, which are not usually detected by the immune system and, due to oxidative and nitrosative damage, have become immunogenic [58]. These findings suggest that an underlying infection may be present in these individuals, and that the immune system is chronically activated in response to a pathogen [56]. The onset of autoimmune responses in ME/CFS may be explained by different mechanisms, including the creation of new epitopes due to the effects of O&NS; inflammatory processes that produce a state of immunologic overreaction; and increased bacterial translocation, with new immunogenic molecules coming into contact with the immune system [86].

Recently, a subset of patients with ME/CFS was shown to display an array of autoantibodies directed against neurotransmitters and neuronal components including serotonin, anti-neural antibodies, gangliosides, and mu-opioid, dopamine D2, muscarinic, and 5-HT1A receptors [87]. Thus, the neurotransmitter alteration could explain many of the disease symptoms such as the neurocognitive dysfunction, sleep alterations, or even a central fatigue theory.

Anti-conjugated oleic, palmitic, and myristic acid, malondialdehyde, azelaic acid, and S-farnesyl-L-cysteine autoantibodies levels are significantly higher in ME/CFS patients than in normal control [58,59,88]. This increased autoantibody production presumably reflects cellular damage or breakdown, which represent increased autoantibody production to self-epitopes that became immunogenic due to oxidative stress [56]. ME/CFS is also accompanied by increased anti-conjugated NO• adducts, e.g., NO-tyrosine, NO-phenylalanine, NO-arginine, NO-tryptophan [83]. The IgM responses to these conjugated NO-derivatives represent an autoimmune response to nitrosylated self-epitopes that became immunogenic due to nitrosative damage.

Several studies described autoantibodies in ME/CFS, mostly against nuclear and membrane structures and neurotransmitter receptors, as pointed out earlier. Antinuclear antibodies (ANA) were found between 13–68% of the ME/CFS patients, dsDNA antibodies were found in 12% of patients, further autoantibodies against endothelial and neuronal cells were described in 30% and 16% of patients, respectively [89].

Antibodies against the muscarinic M1 acetylcholine receptor (AChR) were reported in 15% of ME/CFS patients and were highly associated with muscle weakness and muscle pain [87,90]. Antibodies against B1 and B2 adrenergic receptors were found in 29% of patients with ME/CFS compared to healthy controls [91]. The association of B2 receptors autoantibodies with immune markers suggest an activation of B and T cells expressing B2 adrenoreceptors [92]. Disturbance of these receptors and M1 AChR function may explain the symptoms related to autonomic dysregulation, and some of the most common comorbidities of the syndrome, for example, postural orthostatic tachycardia syndrome (POTS) [53].

There is compelling evidence that all of the immunological alterations seen in the pathophysiology of ME/CFS are associated with autoimmunity, suggesting a possible hallmark for the understanding of the disease. Nowadays, the search for autoantibodies is of great importance allowing the development of potential biomarkers for the diagnosis of the disease and thus providing further advances for therapeutic interventions [93].

5.5.1. B Cell Impairment

The profile of B cell subpopulations could be different in ME/CFS compared with controls. However, this variation is still not fully elucidated within the pathophysiology of the disease [94]. The constant interaction of B cells with an infectious pathogen leads to the dysfunction of the immunological tolerance, losing mechanisms that generally prevent the development of autoreactivity. New memory B cells with autoreactivity, which normally would be eliminated by the thymus, arise and persist in these individuals [13]. When the patient is exposed to a new infection, these B cells could produce antibodies that react both to microbe and autoantigens. This is the basis of the mimicry theory behind autoimmune disease [95]. Abundant studies have proved this theory with immunological biomarkers; ME/CFS is associated with a significant increase in the amount of B cell with a $CD20^+$ $CD5^+$ phenotype, which is correlated with autoantibody production and with overexpression of CD21 markers, which acts as a receptor for some viruses, including EBV [56,96].

5.5.2. 5′-Oligoadenylate Synthetase/RNase L Pathway

The association between the onset of ME/CFS with a viral infection has always been a fundamental pillar in the understanding of the pathophysiology of the disease, as the viral exposition has been one of the most supported triggers of the disease. As a result, interest in the antiviral pathways in these individuals has increased widely, and its disturbance may explain the onset of the immunological dysfunction partially. One of the principal interferon-activated antiviral pathways involves the activation of the 2′-5′-oligoadenylate (2-5A) synthetase/RNase L system, which is an innate immunity pathway that responds to a pathogen-associated molecular pattern to induce the degradation of viral and cellular RNAs to block viral infections and propagation [97,98]. It is composed of three types of enzymatic activity: 2-5A synthetase, 2-5A degrading enzymes, and RNase L, which drive the antiviral and antiproliferative effects of type I interferons [98–100].

On a theoretical basis, some intracellular antigens are capable of deregulating the 2-5A synthetase/RNase L pathway in patients with ME/CFS [97]. Severe deregulation of the 2-5A synthetase/RNase L pathway is accompanied by the down-regulation of apoptotic activity in the peripheral blood mononuclear cells (PBMC) of patients due to the accumulation of proteolytic cleavage products. The initial up-regulation of apoptosis in these cells due to the alteration of the antiviral pathways is followed by a subsequent down-regulation [95]. Therefore, down-regulated apoptotic activity implicates a suppressed ability to eliminate intracellular antigens, similar to EBV or Mycoplasma spp. [99,101].

As well as triggering the 2-5A synthetase/RNase L activation, type I IFN induces the expression of protein kinase R (PKR) [97]. The activation of this enzyme, as typically seen during viral infection or cellular stress, results in a blockade of protein synthesis and consequent cell death through the activation of some transcription factors [102]. Recently, the role of PKR related to metabolism, inflammatory processes, cancer, and neurodegenerative diseases has gained interest because of its relevance; it does not act just as an antiviral agent, but also as a cell growth regulator [103]. However, there is conflicting data regarding the activity of PKR in ME/CFS patients, so the further investigation of PKR activity in CFS patients is warranted [101].

5.5.3. Central Nervous System Alteration

Neuroinflammation

One of the reasons why ME/CFS is profoundly disabling is due to the neuropsychologic symptoms that patients experience, including cognitive impairment, decreased alertness, impaired memory and concentration, and depressive symptoms. In addition, they also experience widespread chronic pain, including headaches, muscle, and joint pain [104]. These findings suggest that the central nervous system (CNS) is deeply involved in the pathophysiology of the disease [105,106].

Previous studies with functional imaging showed hypoperfusion and a reduction of the biosynthesis of neurotransmitters such as glutamate, aspartate, and gamma aminobutyric acid (GABA) in the frontal, temporal, cingulate and occipital cortices and basal ganglia. Using single photon emission computed tomography (SPECT), some studies found ME/CFS-related perfusion defects in the frontal and temporal lobes and impaired cerebral blood flow [107,108]. A voxel-based morphometry study demonstrated volume reduction of the bilateral prefrontal cortices in ME/CFS patients, and the volume reduction level in the right prefrontal cortex was associated with the severity of fatigue and the reduced functional status [109]. The reaction time was slower and the amplitude of electroencephalography-derived premovement-related cortical potential was also reduced in CFS in comparison with healthy individuals [108]. In this section, we will explain the neurological dysfunction and the possible interactions with other systems in ME/CFS patients.

With pro-inflammatory activity recognized for ME/CFS, it has been suggested that neuroinflammation is involved in its pathogenesis and progression [104]. Neuroinflammation is evidenced in ME/CFS patients by the activation of glial cells, specifically microglia and astrocytes. The activated glia exhibits an increase in the expression of the 18-kDa translator protein (TSPO). This protein can be assessed by PET to ascertain the inflammatory activation within the CNS [105]. Conversely, this constant interaction between the CNS and the proinflammatory cytokines results in "sickness behavior", which is a state that is characterized by malaise, lassitude, fatigue, numbness, reduced appetite, reduced social interactions, fatigue, and weight loss, which is similar in many aspects to major depression [110,111]. Additionally, Hornig et al. demonstrated a significant increase in the levels of proinflammatory cytokines in the cerebrospinal fluid of patients with CFS/ME. They made a network analysis that revealed a markedly disturbed immune signature in the cerebrospinal fluid of the patients that is consistent with immune activation in the central nervous system, and a shift toward an allergic or

T helper type-2 pattern associated with autoimmunity [112]. Later, the same author re-analyzed the cerebrospinal fluid from a patient cohort with CFS/ME and found suggestive patterns of disturbances in interleukin 1 signaling and autoimmunity-type patterns of immune activation in patients with atypical clinical characteristics [113].

Although the mechanisms underlying neuroinflammation in ME/CFS are unclear [104], it appears that positive feedback between the inflammatory state and the neuronal overactivation takes place [114]. On one hand, patients have to exert a significant effort to perform daily activities, which results in enhanced neural activation that leads to an increased production of pro-inflammatory cytokines, reactive oxygen species, and nitrogen species [65,66,106]. The central inflammatory component can also be triggered by the immunologic response to an initial infectious process [6]. Thus, the overwhelmingly increased inflammatory state cannot be countered by anti-inflammatory mechanisms, thereby encouraging the development of ME/CFS [115].

Neuronal Sensitization

Central sensitization is a characteristic of neuropathic pain that underlies chemical, functional and structural changes in the CNS [116]. It is manifested as an exaggerated response to noxious stimuli, a reduced threshold for pain, and spread sensitivity around the innervation territory of the injured nerve. It may be produced by the constant stimulation of inflammatory molecules, affecting peripheral sensitivity to further non-noxious stimuli [117]. Furthermore, sensitized neurons may continue to fire after the initial stimulation has ceased: a phenomenon that is referred as "kindling" [6]. Thus, an insidious peripheral-central neurogenic sensitization loop takes place, which would conceivably have the power to modulate the impact of symptoms in ME/CFS [118].

Peripheral pain can contribute to this sensitization by a process that manifest in hyperalgesia and contributes to ME/CFS symptomatology. This phenomenon takes place under long-term potentiation (LTP), in the context of temporal summation effected by repetitive nociception stimulation [119]. Thus, most of the pain symptoms displayed during ME/CFS may be produced by changes in synapse transmission in some of the primary structures involved in pain modulation such as serotonin and glutamate attenuation in encephalic pain modulation structures [117,120].

Glial Activation

The inflammatory response within the CNS favors a proper environment to cause peripheral sensitization. These nociceptive afferents not only interact with post-synaptic neurons, but they also trigger glial responses [104,121]. Calcium ion influx into glial cells, especially astrocytes, causes central terminals of the nociceptive pathway to release neuroactive-signalling molecules that activate the surrounding microglia [122]. These include the primary neuroexcitatory neurotransmitters such as glutamate, nitric oxide (NO), and potent pro-inflammatory cytokines such as tumor necrosis factor alpha (TNF-α) and IL-1B [6,107]. Activated microglia responds similarly to systemic inflammation by inducing superoxide and NO production. Superoxide and NO are free radical substrates of the peroxynitrite (ONOO-) radical, and hence sources of oxidative and nitrosative (O&NS) stress damage [123]. The enhanced glial activation results in neuroexcitation, neuroinflammation, and neurodegeneration through molecular alteration by oxidative stress, which is supported by neuroimaging studies that evidence a significant reduction in white and grey matter volumes in ME/CFS patients [124].

This glial activation due to systemic inflammation may be one of the causes of chronic pain in patients with ME/CFS, involving pathological processes of allodynia and hyperalgesia, via the impact of bidirectional neuroglial signaling [6]. Glia can be activated by neuronal stimulation and the inflammatory cytokines that they release may in turn link to neuronal glutamate receptors enhancing neuroexcitation [117,121]. Collectively, the overactivation of glia by neural and immunological signals can favor sickness behavior and peripheral symptoms that are observed in patients with ME/CFS.

Recently, overall research into glial activation due to systemic inflammation has been deepened. Some toxins have been described that are specifically capable of activating the glial cells called "gliotoxins", which are produced by certain species of bacteria, fungi and viruses [125]. This activation could generate a gliopathy in the CNS. However, gliopathies have also been shown to be initiated by other molecules and neurotransmitters directly related to a systemic inflammatory state such as the pro-inflammatory cytokines TNF-α and IL-6, and high concentrations of glutamate and other pain-related neurotransmitters such as substance P [6,126].

5.5.4. Alterations of Serotonin Transmission

Serotonin (5-HT) is a monoamine that is involved in the pathophysiology of many neuropsychiatric conditions that share some symptoms with ME/CFS, especially the extreme fatigue that does not improve with rest [127]. Central fatigue represents the contribution of the CNS to muscle fatigue; in other words, it is the progressive decline in the capacity to produce voluntary muscle force as exercise continues [128,129]. It is characterized by a decreased ability to contract muscle fibers adequately during motor activity, and is observed separately from muscle fatigue [129,130]. The cellular mechanism remains unknown, but the evidence suggests that central fatigue correlates with increased levels of 5-HT and its metabolites in the CNS [131,132].

It is known that the 5-HT1A receptor negatively regulates the activity of 5-HT neurons via the Gi protein, and is expressed as both a presynaptic autoreceptor on raphe neurons and as a significant postsynaptic receptor in the hippocampus, cortical, hypothalamic and spinal regions involved in mood, emotion, stress responses, and motor activity [127,128]. Unlike motoneurons excitation via the 5-HT 2B/C receptors, 5HT1A-mediated inhibition only occurred during prolonged stimulation of the dorsolateral funiculus and appeared to depend on the spillover of 5-HT to the initial axon segment, which does not receive serotoninergic innervation [133]. During high levels of release, 5-HT spills over to reach extra-synaptic receptor sites in the initial axon segment, and inhibits the generation of action potentials [130]. This prevents the hyperactivity of motoneurons, promotes motor unit rotations, and reduces detrimental muscle activity. All these findings have identified the 5-HT1A receptor as a critical contributor of central fatigue [129]. Thus, it is widely proposed that the obvious disability due to extreme fatigue may be because of punctual alterations in the serotoninergic transmission [134].

Several hypotheses aimed at defining the aetiology of these alterations have been proposed in the literature, but the ones that have more significant support at present are the consequences for the systemic inflammatory state and changes in the genotype of the proteins involved in the serotonergic pathway [135]. Inflammatory cytokines are known to act centrally to alter the metabolism and release of neurotransmitters including serotonin. For instance, inflammatory cytokines such as TNF-α and IL-1β acutely activate the serotoninergic transporter (SERT) through the stimulation of the p38 MAPK pathway and increase the concentration of other catecholamines in specific brain regions such as the anterior hypothalamus [110,136]. SERT transport serotonin from the synaptic cleft into the presynaptic neuron and together with 5-hydroxytryptamine transporter (5-HTT) is involved in the termination of the serotoninergic signaling [137]. Genetic studies reported specific polymorphisms in different components of the serotoninergic neurotransmission such as the 5-HT1A receptor and the serotoninergic transporter 5-HTT in patients suffering from ME/CFS [110,131].

It appears that the neuroimmune dysregulation occurring in patients with ME/CFS is capable of explaining the neuropsychiatric symptoms reported in this pathological condition. Thus, treatments toward the reduction of this inflammatory state and consequently neuroinflammation may in turn reduce the severity of the symptoms of this disease.

5.5.5. Neuroendocrine

HPA Axis in ME/CFS

The interest in the role of the hypothalamic-pituitary-adrenal (HPA) axis in CFS developed from the careful observations that clinical conditions in which there is low circulating cortisol are characterized by debilitating fatigue [138]. Thus, Addison's disease, glucocorticoid withdrawal, and bilateral adrenalectomy are all associated with fatigue and with other symptoms that are also seen in CFS, such as arthralgia, myalgia, sleep disturbance, and mood disorder [84,139]. These observations gave rise to the hypothesis that one of the features of the fatigue in ME/CFS is low circulating levels of cortisol [138].

Reviewing the literature, there is a wealth of studies that have conflicting conclusions about the dysfunction in the HPA axis in patients with ME/CFS. It seems that some of the reasons for the inconsistencies in the data include the heterogeneous nature of ME/CFS itself [30]. The hypofunction of the HPA axis as manifested by a low salivary cortisol-awakening response is the most replicated biological finding in ME/CFS adult patients [140,141]. Moreover, low baseline levels of HPA axis hormones; aberrant diurnal hormone variation; reduced HPA axis response to physical and psychological stressors; and enhanced sensitivity to glucocorticoids have been also reported in patients suffering from this disease [30]. Approximately half of the studies that have measured unstimulated cortisol and ACTH levels in blood or saliva, and others that determined the diurnal variation of urinary cortisol, reported some evidence for lowered cortisol levels at some point in the day in patients with ME/CFS [140]. However, there is no convincing evidence that any HPA axis disturbance is specific to ME/CFS, or that it is a primary cause of the disorder rather than being related to the many possible consequences or comorbidities of the illness [138].

One of the hypotheses that could explain the low cortisol levels reported in patients with ME/CFS is related to the nature of the dysregulation of the stress response. It is noteworthy to remark that since 1998, Scott et al. [142] have suggested the ME/CFS is a stress-related disorder. They hypothesized that initial stress might cause an elevation in corticotropin release hormone (CRH) with a consequent down-regulation of CRH receptors (CRHR) on the pituitary corticotrophs neurons. This down-regulation fails to normalize after the alleviation of stress or the subsequent reduction of CRH levels because of the abnormal plasticity in the CRH receptor. Thus, the hypofunctioning of the HPA axis is the consequence of a "stressed crash" or "exhaustion" phenomenon whereby the stress-induced HPA axis hyperfunction switches into HPA axis hypofunction following prolonged stress. Long-standing stress can result in an exhaustion of the stress response whereby the HPA axis is proposed to lose its ability to cope with environmental stress, coupled with decreased cortisol output [138,139]. Since plasma cortisol is mainly controlled by ACTH, there is a linear relationship between these two hormones in patients with ME/CFS [31,143].

Different interrelationships among hormones of the HPA axis, the sympathetic/adrenal medulla (SAM) system, and the thyroid system between ME/CFS patients and healthy controls have been reported in a number of studies [14,31,144]. This neuroendocrine imbalance affects the homeostasis of another major system that is involved in the pathophysiology of the disease: the immune system. It is well-known that the interaction between glucocorticoids and immune cells is crucial for the optimal development of the host immunological response [145]. There is bidirectional communication between immune-inflammatory pathways and the HPA axis. For example, HPA axis hormones exhibit negative feedback on the immune system, downregulating inflammatory responses, whereas pro-inflammatory cytokines stimulate the HPA axis to produce more HPA axis hormones [84,139].

Therefore, the findings in ME/CFS could be explained by at least two different mechanisms:

(a) Activation of immune-inflammatory pathways is secondary to HPA axis hypofunction by the attenuation of negative feedback of the HPA axis hormones on the immune system, and
(b) chronic activation of immune-inflammatory pathways play a causative role in HPA axis hypofunction [143].

In conclusion, the repeated activation of immune-inflammatory pathways in ME/CFS, including increased levels of pro-inflammatory cytokines, may be influenced by the HPA axis hypofunction [138]. Glucocorticoids have anti-inflammatory and adverse immune-regulatory effects by attenuating Th1 cell-mediated immune responses and promoting Th2-mediated and Treg functions [140,143].

Consequently, there are syntheses of cytokines and the activity of transcription factors, such as NF-κB, which modulates the viability of immune cells (e.g., monocytes and lymphocytes), impedes NO production, blocks promoter sites of pro-inflammatory genes (e.g., IL-1, IL-2, and IL-6), and activates anti-inflammatory genes such as IL-10. These glucocorticoid effects are mediated by binding to their glucocorticoid receptors (GCRs) in the immune cells [139].

Regardless of whether disruption of the HPA axis is primary or secondary, a more significant comprehension of the complexities of the pathophysiology of the ME/CFS has been gained by understanding the changes in the HPA axis. This knowledge could profoundly improve the symptomatic treatment of ME/CFS by adequately controlling the hormone dysfunction.

Hypocortisolism

Patients with ME/CFS show dysfunction of the HPA axis resulting in hypocortisolism, and an attenuated cortisol awakening response. Cortisol is the principal end product of the HPA axis and is involved in the regulation of several bodily systems. Two recent meta-analyses found that the cortisol awakening response (CAR) is the most common finding in the experience of fatigue, and may be relevant in the pathophysiology of the post-exertional malaise, which is a crucial feature of ME/CFS [146]. The CAR describes a surge in cortisol levels upon awakening and has two components: (1) the total cortisol output within this period, and (2) the dynamic response, usually referring to the change in cortisol output from waking to peak levels [147].

Urinary sampling for cortisol is sometimes utilized in research designs, but offers only a summary index of cortisol production over a period [146,148]. Evidence from eight control studies indicated decreased within-person CAR and circadian cortisol variation within ME/CFS. However, a lack of validating studies prevents overly robust conclusions about the importance of these biomarkers in the pathophysiology of the CFS.

The cause of hypocortisolism in patients with ME/CFS remains unclear [145]. Some authors suggest that it may be caused by impaired central nervous system signaling of the adrenal glands, such as limited adrenocorticotrophic hormone (ACTH) output; decreased adrenal gland body size; a compensatory shift toward hypocortisolism after a period of HPA hyperactivity following chronic stress; and enhanced negative feedback of the HPA axis and reduced response of ACTH [148,149].

There is evidence suggesting that stressors, including emotional distress, may exacerbate ME/CFS symptoms, with fatigue being the most prevalent [138]. Emotional distress reactions, such as environmental challenges, may trigger physical symptoms in ME/CFS [150]. This finding has led to the proposal of a standard endocrinological pathway that may underlie the development of "stress-related" disorders, and which would potentially help explain common symptoms of enhanced stress sensitivity [141]. It can be concluded that using stress reduction interventions, such as perceived stress management skills in patients suffering from ME/CFS, could be useful to mitigate the symptomatology [143,148]. ME/CFS patients reveal a flatter cortisol awakening response, as well as a flatter diurnal slope of salivary cortisol output compared to healthy individuals [31], particularly in patients with early adverse life stressors [146]. It is plausible that persons with better stress management skills have less anxiety and negative mood, which in turn relates to lower evening cortisol levels and better HPA control over pro-inflammatory cytokine production [148].

6. Cortisol Treatments for Patients With CFS

Since the identification of endocrinological alterations in patients with ME/CFS, treatments with corticosteroids were assessed, most of them with positive effects in the symptomatology of the patients. Some studies that managed patients with ME/CFS with low doses of hydrocortisone showed favorable results in the reduction of symptoms, especially regarding a reduction in the fatigue levels in the short term [151,152].

7. Genetic Predisposition

As described previously, ME/CFS is a complex condition with a multifactorial aetiology involving multiple mechanisms [153]. As a focus of this review is to exhibit the impact of dysregulation of the neuro-immuno-endocrine relationships, we aimed at summarizing several findings reporting genetic polymorphisms in key neuroimmunoendocrine-related genes that might be involved in the ME/CFS condition. There are plenty of studies that have analyzed the gene expression in the peripheral blood of patients with ME/CFS, and have proposed candidates genes related to the risk of developing the disease [154–160]. Unfortunately, many of these studies did not confirm their finding with PCR, making some of the proposed results unreliable [161,162]. There are a few studies that have analyzed twins with the condition; however, a study conducted in 2001 using 146 female-female twin pairs with ME/CFS provided evidence that supported a familial aggregation of this syndrome [163]. More recent studies have proposed similar conclusions using principle components and latent class analyses to select genes that can have a heritable component, which is mostly involved in the HPA axis and cytokines [164,165].

A common approach to address the symptom heterogeneity of the disease in many studies is to subtype the patient population, allowing the research to focus on the analysis of the biological differences that underlie more specific manifestations of the disease [166]. Some authors attempted to subtype ME/CFS patients based on differences in gene expression profiles in order to approach particular etiological factors [162,167,168]. A symptom-based approximation of the disease has had success in identifying musculoskeletal, inflammatory, and neurological subtypes [169]. One of those studies enrolled patients with a defined ME/CFS phenotype and compared them to healthy blood donors using a microarray that represents the entire human genome and with quantitative PCR (qPCR) confirmation. They clustered the mean relative quantity of mRNA transcripts in patients with ME/CFS and identified seven subtypes of genes with similar profiles of expression. Relative quantification of the mRNA is an approach to determine the quantity of target mRNA in samples with a relation between them [170]. Analysis of mean age and sex ratios for each subtype revealed differences between males and females in the severity of the disease; differences in social functioning and emotional roles; and differences in the severity of individual symptoms between subtypes [162]. However, it is difficult to directly compare and interpret subtypes in various studies because of the differences in the study design, the subject selection, and the inherent variability of the data, among other differences.

The attempt to determine the genetic aetiology of ME/CFS is further obfuscated by diagnostic errors, phenotypic heterogeneity, and environmental effects [171].

7.1. Epigenetic Modification

Molecular studies using DNA methylation microarrays indicate that methylation plays an essential role in the regulation of several genes involved in the relationship with the pathophysiology of the disease [172]. The interaction between the environment and the development of the disease is highly supported, and may be explained by the epigenetic modification of some candidate genes [173]. This idea has been amply supported by an increasing number of studies that have carefully examined the epigenetic changes associated with the neuro-immuno-endocrinology axis of the disease pathophysiology [174–176]. The methylation of DNA is one of the most studied epigenetic modifications. It mainly occurs on the cytosines of the CpG dinucleotide sites across the genome, and regulates the gene expression without disrupting the nucleotide sequence, and may arise through genetic, stochastic, and environmental factors [176]. To date, there are plenty of studies relating the ME/CFS with epigenomic changes. De Vega et al. found significant differences in DNA methylation between CFS patients and healthy controls at 1192 CpG sites in 826 genes, with differential DNA methylation occurring in promoters, gene regulatory elements and within coding regions [175]. Most of these genes are involved in the adaptive immune response and the preservation of an inflammatory state [171]. It is known that epigenetic modifications are mechanisms that modify the long-term gene expression in response to an environmental stimulus [114,115,176,177]. Clearly, the infectious prodrome observed in a vast majority of cases of ME/CFS is indicative of the importance of this infectious exposure in genetic regulation. However, it is still not clear if the relationship between the epigenetic modifications of genes related to the adaptive immune response is the reason why individuals with ME/CFS are predisposed to contract viral infections, or if the infection is the necessary environmental stimulus for the epigenetic modification. Future research is required in order to correctly solve doubts about the epigenetic impact on ME/CFS.

7.2. Mechanisms

In the following section, an attempt will be made to demonstrate the genetic importance in the physiopathological mechanisms most supported in the literature. These mechanisms primarily include the neurotransmitter dysregulation, the alteration in the HPA axis, and the immune-inflammatory responses [178–180].

7.3. Neurotransmitter Dysregulation

The most common neurotransmitter alteration related to the ME/CFS in the literature is the serotoninergic system [153]. Some polymorphisms in the serotonin transporter, receptors, and synthetic enzymes are highly linked with ME/CFS. In a case-control study, Narita et al. identified a polymorphism in the serotonin transporter gene 5′ upstream region (5-HTTLPR) in ME/CFS patients, but not in controls [97,155]. Besides, in another case-control study, three were located in the 5-HT receptor subtype HTR2A (rs1923884, rs6311, and rs6313) and identified as associated with ME/CFS [180]. Also, two polymorphisms in the adrenergic signaling pathway were found to be more abundant in ME/CFS patients than in controls: the β2-adrenergic receptor and the catechol-O-methyl transferase (COMT) [87,181].

The enzymatic activity of COMT has been shown to be inversely related to the levels of catecholamines [182]. Considering previous studies that observed ME/CFS patients with elevated levels of norepinephrine and epinephrine, the COMT low-activity met/met genotype appears to be more prevalent amongst adolescents with ME/CFS [159].

Another neurotransmitter involved in disease pathophysiology is acetylcholine, although from a limited number of studies. A small sample study identified a cholinergic receptor SNP (mAChM3R) that featured prominently in ME/CFS patients, which is consistent with the alteration of NK cells in these patients [183]. Another study found antibodies against mAChM3R (a muscarinic receptor) in a population with ME/CFS, and in which a modest positive response occurred with reduced symptom presentation following the anti-CD20 intervention [87,184].

All of these studies have identified a genetic predisposition in the dysfunction of some central and peripheral neurotransmitters in patients with CFS/ME, which may explain much of the symptomatology of the disease, mainly related to the nervous system such as pain or muscle weakness.

7.4. Alteration in HPA Axis

In light of genetic analysis, a study identified that a genetic variation in POMC and NR3C1 might contribute to the pathophysiology of subgroups of patients with ME/CFS [184]. This finding is consistent with other reports of the association between the disease, and polymorphisms in NR3C1 [185]. NR3C1 is a glucocorticoid receptor gene that is influential in regulating the HPA axis function and blood glucocorticoid levels that have been highly related to the neuroendocrine pathophysiology of the disease [157].

7.5. Immune-Inflammatory RESPONSES

As previously described, immune dysregulation and the inflammatory reactions contribute to the pathophysiology of ME/CFS, and a genetic predisposition may contribute to the spread and persistence of a mild systemic inflammatory state. A study that investigated the human leucocyte antigen (HLA) class II alleles, and the receptor for advanced glycation end product (RAGE), found a significant association between HLA-DRB1 and multiple RAGE polymorphisms with the pathogenesis of ME/CFS [186]. Also, a previous study identified a clear association between the HLA-DQA1 alleles and the ME/CFS [187]. Although multiple studies have taken into account the existing relationship within the polymorphisms of cytokine receptors, none of them reported reliable and reproducible data with the disease [183,188].

8. Management

In the pharmacological approach to the management of ME/CFS, trials have had a poor external validity, and have proven to be inconsistent and inconclusive. The only systematic review of the pharmacological management of ME/CFS identified 20 drug therapies from 26 studies, and 18 applied the Fukuda criteria as the primary tool for inclusion criteria [189]. Eleven medications were shown to be either slightly, mildly, or moderately effective in their respective study groups. Outcomes were measured with clinician-administered and self-administered surveys or scales. From those 11 drugs, six of them had significant results in the fatigue outcome. This group included medications that were individually studied in clinical trials such as dextroamphetamine [190] and nefazodone [191], both with inconclusive results. Other drugs involved in the systematic review included rintatolimod, acetyl-L-carnitine, and intravenous immunoglobulin. Each one of these drugs has individual studies reporting some improvements in severe symptoms, especially in fatigue and cognitive impairment [192–195]. However, as stated earlier, none of them had the epidemiological significance to be the gold standard in the pharmacological treatment of ME/CFS.

There are multiple mechanisms of action in the pharmacological therapies that are used for the management of ME/CFS. Dextroamphetamine is a well-known CNS stimulant and a sympathomimetic that induces the release of dopamine in the mesocorticolimbic circuits. Nefazodone is a serotoninergic modulating antidepressant, and acetyl-L-carnitine is an acid ester of carnitine that facilitates the movement of acetyl-CoA inside the mitochondria during the oxidation of fatty acids, with proven neuroprotective action [196]. There are medications whose mechanisms target a proposed pathophysiology of ME/CFS; one example is rintatolimod, which is an inducer of the interferon activity without helicase activation [192]. Rintatolimod has been studied due to its selectivity in its mechanism of action, its safety for the patient, and the initial success in open-label trials [197].

In the symptomatic management, the studies show results with meaningful outcomes. In the cognitive disability and functional status, Bonnet and Young respectively discussed the effects of moclobemide and lisdexamfetamine dimesylate [198,199]. However, the results given by Bonnet and Young were limited due to the questionnaires that were used to assess the cognitive and functional status and the sample used for the study. For fatigue and post-exertional malaise, some studies have evaluated low-dose hydrocortisone (5–10 mg daily), and found a short-term improvement in fatigue, but with a relapse of the symptoms once the drug is discontinued [152].

The fact that the pathophysiology of the ME/CFS is still not understood entirely opens the possibility of studying a number of non-pharmacological options, some of them with good results in the symptomatological relief [200]. One area of those non-pharmacological approaches is dietary interventions, including the mitoprotective diet, consisting of caloric restriction, fasting diets, and ketogenic diets [201]. The mitoprotective diet has a crucial role in the regulation of the mitochondrial dysfunction due to oxidative stress, which is a well-known pathophysiological feature [202,203]. The impairment of the energetic balance due to reduced mitochondrial capacity in the skeletal muscles of ME/CFS patients has mainly been studied and, as previously seen, is one of the hallmarks of the disease. This dysfunction can be attributed to many triggers, including chronic viral infections; these infections have the potential to create a cycle that disrupts the mitobioenergetics of affected cells, increasing the oxidative stress damage by alteration of the anti-oxidants components of the cell [204]. The improvement of this mitochondrial dysfunction, and the subsequent O&NS damage, is shown to have an inverse relationship with fatigue severity scores in patients with ME/CFS [205]. With this background, the caloric restriction of the diet can lead to adaptive responses that affect the inflammatory pathway, the energy metabolism, the DNA repair and the modulation of the O&NS [206]. However, the exact mechanism of this diet is not well understood. Along with mitoprotective diets, natural antifatigue supplements have also had promising results in animal models enhancing exercise tolerance [207].

One of the constituents of mitoprotective diets is the ketogenic diet, which is defined as a high-fat, deficient carbohydrate diet that mimics the effects of caloric restriction or the fasting diets. The ketone bodies acetoacetate and β-hydroxybutyrate are produced during lipolysis through the generation of acetyl-CoA, as occurs in a fasting state or with a minimal intake of carbohydrates. The mitochondrial effects of the ketogenic diet are similar to those observed during the caloric restriction by a similar mechanism as described earlier. In experimental studies with animals, it has been found that the β-hydroxybutyrate is an endogenous and specific inhibitor of class I histone deacetylases, resulting in global changes of genes transcription, including the ones involved in the oxidative stress resistance factors [208,209]. However, the effects of the ketogenic diet are not all beneficial for the patient, and may not contribute to the complete recovery of the disease, as ME/CFS has other pathophysiological pathways, as described herein.

There is also literature that demonstrates mitoprotective roles in specific medications, such as sodium dichloroacetate, which enhances the activity of the mitochondrial enzyme pyruvate dehydrogenase [210]. However, it has been seen that this medication does not work in all patients [211], thus generating more doubts about the hypothesis of whether mitochondria is the only etiology of the disease.

Table 3. Current therapeutic strategies for ME/CFS.

Medication	Examples	Intervention	Adverse Reactions
NSAIDs	Ibuprofen, Naproxen	Relieve frequent or severe joint and muscle pain, headaches, reduce fevers and inflammation [212].	Gastrointestinal distress and bleeding
Tricyclic antidepressants	Amitriptyline, Doxepin, Nortriptyline, Desipramine	Symptom relieve, improve sleep, and relieve pain in much lower doses than those used to treat depression. Has anti-anxiety effect and improve locomotor activity [213].	Sedation, urinary retention, sexual dysfunction, weight-gain comorbidities.
Selective serotonin-reuptake inhibitors	Fluoxetine, Sertraline, Paroxetine	Helpful for anxiety/depression and other mood disorders in patients with ME/CFS, as well as patients with chronic neuropathic pain [214].	No specific adverse reactions have been described in the RCT
Antiviral Drugs	Rintatolimod, Valganciclovir	Enhance the NK-function and influence the 2-5A-synthetase pathway, producing an objective improvement in exercise tolerance and a reduction in ME/CFS-related concomitant medication usage [193,215].	Is a well-tolerated medication in the right dosage
Monoclonal Antibodies	Rituximab	Decrease the activity and number B-cell by inhibiting CD20, thus reducing inflammation. Studies demonstrate symptoms alleviation and improvement in quality of life within a 12-month follow-up [216,217].	Neutropenia, and increase of severe infections
Complementary and alternative medicine	Nutritional supplements, Acetyl-L-carnitine, Essential fatty acids, Magnesium, Vitamins, Coenzyme Q10 plus	Nutritional supplements may improve ME/CFS-related physical and mental fatigue in patients with specific nutritional deficiencies [215]. There are discrepant results in most of the RCT, and further research is needed in order to conclude a specific therapeutic role.	No specific adverse reactions have been described in the RCT of nutritional supplements
Corticosteroids	Hydrocortisone, Frudocortisone	Associated with statistical improvement in ME/CFS symptoms, especially in physical fatigue [218].	Adrenal suppression, mood disorders, weight-gain comorbidities.

See Reference [219] for additional details.

There are other trials and reviews of pharmacological and non-pharmacological therapeutic option for ME/CFS; most of these are directed toward the reduction of the inflammation and the oxidative stress with the objective of symptomatologic relief [219]. Table 3 briefly summarizes the current therapeutic approaches that are being studied. That is the case of the probiotic interventions showing good outcomes in the management of gastrointestinal symptoms observed in the ME/CFS, reducing the cytokine levels entering the systemic circulation by the leaky gut phenomena [220]. However, as for most of the therapeutic options, the studies have inconclusive results due to limited data and validation.

9. Discussion

In this comprehensive review, a holistic approach to a new disease has been presented. It is evident that diagnostic tests for clinical practice are not specific to the condition, which is reflected in the high rates of underdiagnoses (85–90%). When reviewing the historical perspective of ME/CFS, the relevance of infectious prodrome in the understanding of pathophysiology was identified. The first clinicians to describe the syndrome, as reviewed earlier, immediately associated the disease with an ongoing infection. Nowadays, with a significant core of research, it is known that the disease has its pathophysiological sustenance in "three pillars" that continuously interact with each other: the immune system, the nervous system, and the neuroendocrine network. Table 1 offers a brief summary of the main features of the tissues involved in the "three pillars" hypothesis. As can be seen in Table 3, current therapeutic strategies target several elements of the proposed neuro-immunoendocrine network, which also supports the "three pillars" hypothesis that we are discussing in this review.

The immune system is involved in modulating neural plasticity, learning, and memory, although the precise link between these two seemingly distinct systems was, until recently, unclear [54]. The connection may be explained by the coevolution of the nervous and immune systems, as the two systems share mechanisms of stimulation, cell communication and signaling, gene regulation, and supracellular organization. The immune system supports the central nervous system (CNS) and aids functional recovery by facilitating the renewal, migration and cell lineage specification of neural progenitor cells [221].

The immune system is involved in the stress response, since stress activates the immune system, leading to peripheral inflammation that may ultimately contribute to the onset of a part of the symptomatology of the disease [222]. Indeed, stress has been shown to be an essential predisposing factor in the development of several neurodegenerative and psychiatric disorders [223]. The hypothalamic–pituitary–adrenal (HPA) axis and the systemic sympatho-adrenomedullary (SAM) system are essential modulators of stress response systems [224]. The HPA axis is an endocrine pathway that regulates standard stress response and merges with the immune system to maintain homeostasis [138,139]. Therefore, stress stimulates the release of glucocorticoids, particularly cortisol, which is able to cross the BBB and alter the transcription of proteins in the brain [225]. Glucocorticoids bind to the glucocorticoid receptor (GR), resulting in disassociation from the heat-shock protein, and promoting a structural change of the receptor that enables the glucocorticoid-GR complex to enter the nucleus. The glucocorticoid-GR complex binds to the glucocorticoid response element on the DNA, resulting in the activation of transcription of immune-mediator genes, among others [223,226]. Therefore, stress hormones, such as cortisol, have the ability to regulate the immune system. However, HPA is not the only neuroendocrinological network that can interact with the immune system. The SAM is also activated by stress, leading to the release of catecholamines (e.g., epinephrine and norepinephrine) in the adrenal medulla in response to stress [134,227]. Catecholamines have been found to regulate the synthesis of immune system mediators through β-adrenergic receptor stimulation [226], suggesting an alternative pathway that links the neuroendocrine and immunological systems.

ME/CFS patients show heightened negative feedback inhibition of the HPA axis, which is associated with hypocortisolism and heightened GR sensitivity [224]. As a result, patients with ME/CFS often show heightened immune responses owing to the combined effects of chronic stress with activated microglia [130,223] and increased HPA-axis sensitivity [224]. The HPA axis has been of great importance for the understanding of the pathophysiology of the disease, since the consequences of its alteration, such as hypocortisolism, have allowed us to understand the persistence of an altered immune status, the high risk of infections and the generation of humoral autoreactivity.

Although the metabolic sphere is not part of the aetiopathological pillars of the disease, it is clear that it is a physiological aspect compromised in patients with ME/CSF. The dysregulation of the energetic metabolism can be understood as the tip of the iceberg, which will trigger the symptomatology experienced by the patient. However, the etiology of this metabolic imbalance in ME/CSF has not yet been understood, which is most likely because it is a pathological process that is the product of complex multisystemic interactions. Studies on metabolism and CFS suggest irregularities in energy metabolism, amino acid metabolism, nucleotide metabolism, nitrogen metabolism, hormone metabolism, and oxidative stress metabolism [228,229]. The overwhelming body of evidence suggests an oxidative environment with the minimal utilization of mitochondria for efficient energy production, leading to thoughts of some type of etiology in this organelle, but as we have seen previously, apparently the mitochondria are affected with the course of the disease [230]. As well as throughout the review, more studies are needed to understand which is the metabolic pathway that is first affected or which is the most altered in order to understand where to direct the etiological search in this complicated disease.

ME/CFS remains a challenge for the biomedical community. Pathophysiological research should follow two strategies. The first consists of distinguishing ME/CFS from other disorders. The characteristic pathophysiology of chronic fatigue in neurological disorders, or during cancer, or in inflammatory diseases such as rheumatoid arthritis, should be compared with the fatigue in ME/CFS. The second strategy consists of investigating the similarities and dissimilarities in functional somatic syndromes. Modern neurosciences offer some explanatory models, which might bridge the gap between somatic and psychological models for ME/CFS and other functional somatic syndromes [225].

Due to the unclear aetiology, diagnostic uncertainty, and the resultant heterogeneity of the ME/CFS, there are no established treatment recommendations in the clinical practice [32]. Systematic reviews have investigated the effectiveness of several ME/CFS treatments [231,232]. Cognitive behavior therapy (CBT) and graded exercise therapy (GET) are some of the few interventions that are proposed as beneficial in improving quality of life [233], but these remain controversial and have been recently criticized by others [234].

In practice, pharmacological or non-pharmacological treatments have been directed toward relieving symptoms and improving quality of life [32]. Table 3 shows some of the treatments that are being studied for the relief of symptomatology in patients with CFS/ME. Several randomized control trials have shown improvement in the most disabling symptoms with the use of certain drugs [189,213,218,231,235]. Additionally, there are studies that have proven significant improvement of the symptomatology using a drug together with an adjuvant; this is the case of the use of the selective inhibitors of the reuptake of serotonin, which were studied alongside Dengzhanshengmai capsules, which are a traditional Chinese medicine, resulting in a significant improvement in general fatigue, as well as in mental and physical health [214]. However, it should be clarified that more studies are required to reproduce these conclusions and results in order to provide more scientific sustenance so that a pharmaceutical indication can exist. There has also been insufficient evidence of the effectiveness of pharmacological, supplementary, complementary, and other interventions [32,54]; treatment with anticholinergics, hormones, nicotinamide adenine dinucleotide, and antidepressants have been studied without conclusive results [236,237]. Similar to many patients with other chronic diseases for which conventional medicine has been unable to provide relief, those with ME/CFS use alternative treatments with unknown outcomes. These treatments include megavitamins, energy healing, herbal therapies, and special diets [219]. However, controlled studies to clarify the real effectiveness of these therapies do not exist.

Longitudinal studies of varying duration have shown that although 17–64% of the patients with ME/CFS improve, less than 10% fully recover, and another 10–20% worsen during follow-up [238]. Older age, longer illness duration, fatigue severity, comorbid psychiatric illness, and a physical attribution are some risk factors that worsen the prognosis of the patient [46]. As expected, children and adolescents appear to recover more rapidly and tend not to have recurrences of the disease in the future.

During this review we have seen that various biomarkers have been chosen to explain many of the pathophysiological processes involved in the aetiology of the disease; nonetheless the results of the different studies on these biomarkers are inconclusive, and do not define a clear pathological process. This review proposes a physiopathological hypothesis, using many of the results that have emerged from the molecular studies of ME/CFS. Although the scientific community has come to propose reproducible molecular bases, only the molecular explanation of some of the symptomatology of the disease has been achieved. For example, the biomolecular reason for fatigue and lack of energy has clearly been explained by many authors, such as Rasa et. al., proposing both a mitochondrial dysfunction and an alteration in the use of energy by myocytes [239]. However, in this example, the mitochondrial alteration does not necessarily explain the totality of the symptomatology and the aetiology of this alteration is still not clear. Other studies have proposed an infectious aetiology; however, as with other attempts, not all patients that have ME/CFS have an infection in the onset of the disease [42,240]. Taking this into account, we can conclude that the studies on the biomarkers involved in the disease present frustrating results for the research groups that aim to understand the biomolecular bases of the disease in order to generate strategies for effective treatments.

More knowledge about the psychoneurobiology of ME/CFS and the natural history of the disease is needed to improve our understanding of this illness, and thereafter to allow the development of more effective treatments that can significantly improve the quality of life for patients, and lead them to recover their functionality in the shortest possible time.

Author Contributions: C.M., B.A.L., M.A.-B., C.T.S.-A. and M.C.R. conceived the general idea of the project, researched the scientific literature and wrote the review. All of the authors read and commented on the final version of the present manuscript and endorse its submission.

Funding: This work was funded by Institutional Funds of Universidad del Rosario. B.A.L. was supported by the J.J. Mason and H.S. Williams Memorial Foundation (The Mason Foundation), grant number CT23141–23142.

Conflicts of Interest: The authors declare no conflict of interests.

References

1. Brurberg, K.G.; Fønhus, M.S.; Larun, L.; Flottorp, S.; Malterud, K. Case definitions for chronic fatigue syndrome/myalgic encephalomyelitis (CFS/ME): A systematic review. *BMJ Open* **2014**, *4*, e003973. [CrossRef] [PubMed]
2. Carruthers, B.M.; Jain, A.K.; DeMeirleir, K.L.; Peterson, D.; Klimas, N.G.; Lerner, A.M.; Bested, A.C.; Flor-Henry, P.; Joshi, P.; Powles, A.C.P.; et al. Myalgic Encephalomyelitis/Chronic Fatigue Syndrome: Clinical Working Case Definition, Diagnostic and Treatment Protocols. *J. Chronic Fatigue Syndr.* **2003**, *11*, 7–36. [CrossRef]
3. Rowe, P.C.; Underhill, R.A.; Friedman, K.J.; Gurwitt, A.; Medow, M.S.; Schwartz, M.S.; Speight, N.; Stewart, J.M.; Vallings, R.; Rowe, K.S. Myalgic Encephalomyelitis/Chronic Fatigue Syndrome Diagnosis and Management in Young People: A Primer. *Front. Pediatr.* **2017**, *5*, 121. [CrossRef] [PubMed]
4. Reeves, W.C.; Jones, J.F.; Maloney, E.; Heim, C.; Hoaglin, D.C.; Boneva, R.S.; Morrissey, M.; Devlin, R. Prevalence of chronic fatigue syndrome in metropolitan, urban, and rural Georgia. *Popul. Health Metr.* **2007**, *5*, 1–10. [CrossRef] [PubMed]
5. Clayton, E.W.; Biaggionni, I.; Cockshell, S.; Vermeculen, R.; Snell, C.; Rove, K. *Beyond Myalgic Encephalomyelitis/Chronic Fatigue Syndrome: Redefining an Illness*; The National Academies Press: Washington, DC, USA, 2015.
6. Glassford, J.A.G. The neuroinflammatory etiopathology of myalgic encephalomyelitis/chronic fatigue syndrome (ME/CFS). *Front. Physiol.* **2017**, *8*, 1–9. [CrossRef]
7. Słomko, J.; Newton, J.L.; Kujawski, S.; Tafil-Klawe, M.; Klawe, J.; Staines, D.; Marshall-Gradisnik, S.; Zalewski, P. Prevalence and characteristics of chronic fatigue syndrome/myalgic encephalomyelitis (CFS/ME) in Poland: A cross-sectional study. *BMJ Open* **2019**, *9*, e023955. [CrossRef] [PubMed]
8. Castro-Marrero, J.; Faro, M.; Aliste, L.; Sáez-Francàs, N.; Calvo, N.; Martínez-Martínez, A.; de Sevilla, T.F.; Alegre, J. Comorbidity in Chronic Fatigue Syndrome/Myalgic Encephalomyelitis: A Nationwide Population-Based Cohort Study. *Psychosomatics* **2017**, *58*, 533–543. [CrossRef]

9. Komaroff, A.L. Advances in Understanding the Pathophysiology of Chronic Fatigue Syndrome. *JAMA* **2019**. [CrossRef]
10. Noda, M.; Ifuku, M.; Hossain, M.S.; Katafuchi, T. Glial Activation and Expression of the Serotonin Transporter in Chronic Fatigue Syndrome. *Front. Psychiatry* **2018**, *9*, 589. [CrossRef]
11. Skowera, A.; Cleare, A.; Blair, D. High levels of type 2 cytokine-producing cells in chronic fatigue syndrome. *Clin. Exp. Immunol.* **2004**, *135*, 294–302. [CrossRef]
12. Rivas, J.L.; Palencia, T.; Fernández, G.; García, M. Association of T and NK Cell Phenotype with the Diagnosis of Myalgic Encephalomyelitis/Chronic Fatigue Syndrome (ME/CFS). *Front. Immunol.* **2018**, *9*, 1028. [CrossRef] [PubMed]
13. Bradley, A.S.; Ford, B.; Bansal, A.S. Altered functional B cell subset populations in patients with chronic fatigue syndrome compared to healthy controls. *Clin. Exp. Immunol.* **2013**, *172*, 73–80. [CrossRef] [PubMed]
14. Tomas, C.; Newton, J.; Watson, S. A review of hypothalamic-pituitary-adrenal axis function in chronic fatigue syndrome. *ISRN Neurosci.* **2013**, *2013*, 784520. [CrossRef] [PubMed]
15. Lloyd, A.R.; Wakefield, D.; Boughton, C.; Dwyer, J. What Is Myalgic Encephalomyelitis? *Lancet* **1988**, *331*, 1286–1287. [CrossRef]
16. Anderson, V.R.; Jason, L.A.; Hlavaty, L.E. A Qualitative Natural History Study of ME/CFS in the Community. *Health Care Women Int.* **2016**, *35*, 1–21. [CrossRef] [PubMed]
17. Ramsay, A.M. 'Epidemic neuromyasthenia' 1955–1978. *Postgrad. Med. J.* **1978**, *54*, 718–721. [CrossRef] [PubMed]
18. Hashimoto, N. History of chronic fatigue syndrome. *Nihon Rinsho* **2007**, *65*, 975–982.
19. Holmes, G.P.; Kaplan, J.E.; Gantz, N.M.; Komaroff, A.L.; Schonberger, L.B.; Straus, S.E.; Jones, J.F.; Dubois, R.E.; Cunningham-Rundles, C.; Pahwa, S.; et al. Chronic Fatigue Syndrome: A Working Case Definition. *Ann. Int. Med.* **1988**, *108*, 387. [CrossRef]
20. Twisk, F.N.M. A critical analysis of the proposal of the Institute of Medicine to replace myalgic encephalomyelitis and chronic fatigue syndrome by a new diagnostic entity called systemic exertion intolerance disease. *Curr. Med. Res. Opin.* **2015**, *31*, 1333–1347. [CrossRef]
21. Fukuda, K.; Straus, S.E.; Hickie, I.; Sharpe, M.C.; Dobbins, J.G.; Komaroff, A. The chronic fatigue syndrome: A comprehensive approach to its definition and study. International Chronic Fatigue Syndrome Study Group. *Ann. Int. Med.* **1994**, *121*, 953–959. [CrossRef]
22. Carruthers, B.M.; van de Sande, M.I.; De Meirleir, K.L.; Klimas, N.G.; Broderick, G.; Mitchell, T.; Staines, D.; Powles, A.C.; Speight, N.; Vallings, R.; et al. Myalgic encephalomyelitis: International Consensus Criteria. *J. Intern. Med.* **2011**, *270*, 327–338. [CrossRef]
23. Wojcik, W.; Armstrong, D.; Kanaan, R. Chronic fatigue syndrome: Labels, meanings and consequences. *J. Psychosom. Res.* **2011**, *70*, 500–504. [CrossRef]
24. Tobi, M.; Ravid, Z. Prolonged Atypical Illness Associated woth serological evidence of persistent Epstein-barr virus infection. *Lancet* **1982**, *319*, 61–64. [CrossRef]
25. Sharpe, M.C.; Archard, L.C.; Banatvala, J.E. A report chronic fatigue syndrome: Guidelines for research. *J. R. Soc. Med.* **1991**, *84*, 118–121. [CrossRef]
26. Bested, A.C.; Marshall, L.M. Review of Myalgic Encephalomyelitis/Chronic Fatigue Syndrome: An evidence-based approach to diagnosis and management by clinicians. *Rev. Environ. Health* **2015**, *30*, 223–249. [CrossRef]
27. Nacul, L.; Kingdon, C.C.; Bowman, E.W.; Curran, H.; Lacerda, E.M.; Diseases, T.; Street, K. Differing case definitions point to the need for an accurate diagnosis of myalgic encephalomyelitis/chronic fatigue syndrome. *Fatigue* **2017**, *5*, 1–4. [CrossRef]
28. Sullivan, P.; Evengard, B.; Jacks, A. Twin analyses of chronic fatigue in a Swedish national sample. *Psychol. Med.* **2005**, *35*, 1327–1336. [CrossRef]
29. Marshall-Gradisnik, S.; Huth, T.; Chacko, A.; Johnston, S.; Smith, P.; Staines, D. Natural killer cells and single nucleotide polymorphisms of specific ion channels and receptor genes in myalgic encephalomyelitis/chronic fatigue syndrome. *Appl. Clin. Genet.* **2016**, *9*, 39–47. [CrossRef]
30. Nijhof, S.L.; Rutten, J.M.T.M.; Kimpen, J.L.L.; Putte, E.M.V.D. The role of hypocortisolism in chronic fatigue syndrome. *Psychoneuroendocrinology* **2014**, *42*, 199–206. [CrossRef]

31. Wyller, V.B.; Vitelli, V.; Sulheim, D.; Fagermoen, E.; Winger, A.; Godang, K.; Bollerslev, J. Altered neuroendocrine control and association to clinical symptoms in adolescent chronic fatigue syndrome: A cross-sectional study. *J. Transl. Med.* **2016**, *14*, 1–12. [CrossRef]
32. Afari, N.; Buchwald, D. Chronic fatigue syndrome: A review. *Am. J. Psychiatry* **2003**, *160*, 221–236. [CrossRef]
33. Nacul, L.C.; Lacerda, E.M.; Pheby, D.; Campion, P.; Molokhia, M.; Fayyaz, S.; Leite, J.C.D.C.; Poland, F.; Howe, A.; Drachler, M.L. Prevalence of myalgic encephalomyelitis/chronic fatigue syndrome (ME/CFS) in three regions of England: A repeated cross-sectional study in primary care. *BMC Med.* **2011**, *9*, 91. [CrossRef]
34. Ranjith, G. Epidemiology of chronic fatigue syndrome. *Occup. Med.* **2005**, *55*, 13–19. [CrossRef]
35. Pawlikowska, T.; Chalder, T.; Hirsch, S.R.; Wallace, P.; Wright, D.J.M.; Wessely, S.C. Population based study of fatigue and psychological distress. *Br. Med. J.* **1994**, *308*, 763–766. [CrossRef]
36. Skapinakis, P.; Lewis, G.; Meltzer, H. Clarifying the relationship between unexplained chronic fatigue and psychiatric morbidity: Results from a community survey in Great Britain. *Int. Rev. Psychiatry* **2003**, *15*, 57–64. [CrossRef]
37. Nijrolder, I.; Van Der Windt, D.A.W.M.; Twisk, J.W.; Van Der Horst, H.E. Fatigue in primary care: Longitudinal associations with pain. *Pain* **2010**, *150*, 351–357. [CrossRef]
38. Cathébras, P.J.; Robbins, J.M.; Kirmayer, L.J.; Hayton, B.C. Fatigue in primary care: Prevalence, psychiatric comorbidity, illness behavior, and outcome. *J. Gen. Int. Med.* **1992**, *7*, 276–286. [CrossRef]
39. Lawrie, S.M.; Manders, D.N.; Geddes, J.R.; Pelosi, A.J. A population-based incidence study of chronic fatigue. *Psychol. Med.* **1997**, *27*, 343–353. [CrossRef]
40. Faro, M.; Sàez-Francás, N.; Castro-Marrero, J.; Aliste, L.; Fernández de Sevilla, T.; Alegre, J. Gender differences in chronic fatigue syndrome. *Reumatol. Clin.* **2016**, *12*, 72–77. [CrossRef]
41. Capellil, E.; Zola, R.; Loruss, L.; Sardi, L.V.F.; Ricevutp, G.; Immunologia, L.; Animale, B.; Pavia, U.; Ospedaliera, A.; Mellini, M.; et al. Chronic Fatigue Syndrome/Myalgic Encepahlomyelitis: An Update. *Int. J. Immunopathol. Pharmacol.* **2010**, *23*, 981–989. [CrossRef]
42. Underhill, R.A. Myalgic encephalomyelitis, chronic fatigue syndrome: An infectious disease. *Med. Hypotheses* **2015**, *85*, 765–773. [CrossRef]
43. Reynolds, K.J.; Vernon, S.D.; Bouchery, E.; Reeves, W.C. The economic impact of chronic fatigue syndrome. *Cost Eff. Resour. Allocat.* **2004**, *2*, 1–9.
44. Kroenke, K.; Wood, D.R.; Mangelsdorff, D.; Meier, N.J.; Powell, J.B. Chronic Fatigue in Primary Care. *JAMA* **1988**, *260*, 929–934. [CrossRef]
45. Griffith, J.P.; Zarrouf, F.A. A systematic review of chronic fatigue syndrome: Don't assume it's depression. *Prim. Care Companion J. Clin. Psychiatry* **2008**, *10*, 120–128. [CrossRef]
46. Cairns, R.; Hotopf, M. A systematic review describing the prognosis of chronic fatigue syndrome. *Occup. Med.* **2005**, *55*, 20–31. [CrossRef]
47. Jason, L.A.; Corradi, K.; Gress, S.; Williams, S.; Torres-Harding, S. Causes of Death Among Patients with Chronic Fatigue Syndrome. *Health Care Women Int.* **2006**, *27*, 615–626. [CrossRef]
48. McManimen, S.; Devendorf, A.; Brown, A. Mortality in Patients with CFS/ME. *Fatigue* **2016**, *4*, 195–207.
49. Wallis, A.; Ball, M.; McKechnie, S.; Butt, H.; Lewis, D.P.; Bruck, D. Examining clinical similarities between myalgic encephalomyelitis/chronic fatigue syndrome and d-lactic acidosis: A systematic review. *J. Transl. Med.* **2017**, *15*, 1–22. [CrossRef]
50. Vermeulen, R.C.; Kurk, R.M.; Visser, F.C.; Sluiter, W.; Scholte, H.R. Patients with chronic fatigue syndrome performed worse than controls in a controlled repeated exercise study despite a normal oxidative phosphorylation capacity. *J. Transl. Med.* **2010**, *8*, 93. [CrossRef]
51. Clauw, D.J. Perspectives on fatigue from the study of chronic fatigue syndrome and related conditions. *PM R* **2010**, *2*, 414–430. [CrossRef]
52. Cockshell, S.J.; Mathias, J.L. Cognitive functioning in chronic fatigue syndrome: A meta-analysis. *Psychol. Med.* **2010**, *40*, 1253–1267. [CrossRef]
53. Reynolds, G.K.; Lewis, D.P.; Richardson, A.M.; Lidbury, B.A. Comorbidity of postural orthostatic tachycardia syndrome and chronic fatigue syndrome in an Australian cohort. *J. Intern. Med.* **2014**, *275*, 409–417. [CrossRef]
54. Prins, J.B.; van der Meer, J.W.M.; Bleijenberg, G.; Meer, J.W.M.V.D. Review Chronic fatigue syndrome. *Rev. Lit. Arts Am.* **2006**, *367*, 346–355.

55. Lowenstein, O.; Feinberg, R.; Loewenfeld, I.I.E. Pupillary Movements During Acute and Chronic Fatigue A New Test for the Objective Evaluation of Tiredness. *Investig. Ophthalmol.* **1963**, *2*, 138–158.
56. Lorusso, L.; Mikhaylova, S.V.; Capelli, E.; Ferrari, D.; Ngonga, G.K.; Ricevuti, G. Immunological aspects of chronic fatigue syndrome. *Autoimmun. Rev.* **2009**, *8*, 287–291. [CrossRef]
57. Nguyen, T.; Johnston, S. Impaired calcium mobilization in natural killer cells from chronic fatigue syndrome/myalgic encephalomyelitis patients is associated with transient receptor potential melastatin 3 ion channels. *J. Transl. Immunol.* **2016**, *187*, 284–293. [CrossRef]
58. Maes, M.; Mihaylova, I.; Kubera, M.; Leunis, J.C.; Twisk, F.N.M.; Geffard, M. IgM-mediated autoimmune responses directed against anchorage epitopes are greater in Myalgic Encephalomyelitis/Chronic Fatigue Syndrome (ME/CFS) than in major depression. *Metab. Brain Dis.* **2012**, *27*, 415–423. [CrossRef]
59. Maes, M.; Twisk, F.N.M.; Kubera, M.; Ringel, K. Evidence for inflammation and activation of cell-mediated immunity in Myalgic Encephalomyelitis/Chronic Fatigue Syndrome (ME/CFS): Increased interleukin-1, tumor necrosis factor-α, PMN-elastase, lysozyme and neopterin. *J. Affect. Disord.* **2012**, *136*, 933–939. [CrossRef]
60. Torres-Harding, S.; Sorenson, M.; Jason, L.A.; Maher, K.; Fletcher, M.A. Evidence for T-helper 2 shift and association with illness parameters in chronic fatigue syndrome (CFS). *Bull. IACFS/ME* **2008**, *16*, 19–33.
61. Jafari-Shakib, R.; Ajdary, S.; Amiri, Z.M.; Mohammadi, A.M.; Nourijelyani, K.; Mortazavi, H.; Shokrgozar, M.A.; Nikbin, B.; Khamesipour, A. CD26 expression on CD4+T cells in patients with cutaneous leishmaniasis. *Clin. Exp. Immunol.* **2008**, *153*, 31–36. [CrossRef]
62. Kennedy, G.; Spence, V.A.; McLaren, M.; Hill, A.; Underwood, C.; Belch, J.J.F. Oxidative stress levels are raised in chronic fatigue syndrome and are associated with clinical symptoms. *Free Radic. Biol. Med.* **2005**, *39*, 584–589. [CrossRef]
63. Kennedy, G.; Khan, F.; Hill, A.; Underwood, C.; Belch, J.J.F. Biochemical and vascular aspects of pediatric chronic fatigue syndrome. *Arch. Pediatr. Adolesc. Med.* **2010**, *164*, 817–823. [CrossRef]
64. Maes, M. Inflammatory and oxidative and nitrosative stress pathways underpinning chronic fatigue, somatization and psychosomatic symptoms. *Curr. Opin. Psychiatry* **2009**, *22*, 75–83. [CrossRef]
65. Morris, G.; Maes, M. Mitochondrial dysfunctions in Myalgic Encephalomyelitis/chronic fatigue syndrome explained by activated immuno-inflammatory, oxidative and nitrosative stress pathways. *Metab. Brain Dis.* **2014**, *29*, 19–36. [CrossRef]
66. Schoeman, E.M.; Van Der Westhuizen, F.H.; Erasmus, E.; van Dyk, E.; Knowles, C.V.Y.; Al-Ali, S.; Ng, W.F.; Taylor, R.W.; Newton, J.L.; Elson, J.L. Clinically proven mtDNA mutations are not common in those with chronic fatigue syndrome. *BMC Med. Genet.* **2017**, *18*, 1–4. [CrossRef]
67. Ross, P.B.; Germain, A.; Ye, K.; Keinan, A.; Gu, Z.; Hanson, M.R. Mitochondrial DNA variants correlate with symptoms in myalgic encephalomyelitis/chronic fatigue syndrome. *J. Transl. Med.* **2016**, *14*, 1–12.
68. Finsterer, J.; Mahjoub, S.Z. Is chronic fatigue syndrome truly associated with haplogroups or mtDNA single nucleotide polymorphisms? *J. Transl. Med.* **2016**, *14*, 1–2. [CrossRef]
69. Tomas, C.; Brown, A.; Strassheim, V.; Elson, J.; Newton, J.; Manning, P. Cellular bioenergetics is impaired in patients with chronic fatigue syndrome. *PLoS ONE* **2017**, *12*, 1–15. [CrossRef]
70. Rutherford, G.; Manning, P.; Newton, J.L. Understanding Muscle Dysfunction in Chronic Fatigue Syndrome. *J. Aging Res.* **2016**, *2016*. [CrossRef]
71. Klimas, N.G.; Salvato, F.R.; Morgan, R.; Fletcher, M.A. Immunologic abnormalities in chronic fatigue syndrome. *J. Clin. Microbiol.* **1990**, *28*, 1403–1410.
72. Mavilio, D.; Lombardo, G.; Benjamin, J.; Kim, D.; Follman, D.; Marcenaro, E.; O'Shea, M.A.; Kinter, A.; Kovacs, C.; Moretta, A.; et al. Characterization of CD56-/CD16+ natural killer (NK) cells: A highly dysfunctional NK subset expanded in HIV-infected viremic individuals. *Proc. Natl. Acad. Sci. USA* **2005**, *102*, 2886–2891. [CrossRef]
73. Rebuli, M.E.; Pawlak, E.A.; Walsh, D.; Martin, E.M.; Jaspers, I. Distinguishing Human Peripheral Blood NK Cells from CD56dimCD16dimCD69+CD103+ Resident Nasal Mucosal Lavage Fluid Cells. *Sci. Rep.* **2018**, *8*, 3394. [CrossRef]
74. Michel, T.; Poli, A.; Cuapio, A.; Briquemont, B.; Iserentant, G.; Ollert, M.; Zimmer, J. Human CD56^{bright} NK Cells: An Update. *J. Immunol.* **2016**, *196*, 2923–2931. [CrossRef]
75. Poli, A.; Michel, T.; Thérésine, M.; Andrès, E.; Hentges, F.; Zimmer, J. CD56bright natural killer (NK) cells: An important NK cell subset. *Immunology* **2009**, *126*, 458–465. [CrossRef]

76. Brenu, E.W.; Huth, T.K.; Hardcastle, S.L.; Fuller, K.; Kaur, M.; Johnston, S.; Ramos, S.B.; Staines, D.R.; Marshall-Gradisnik, S.M. Role of adaptive and innate immune cells in chronic fatigue syndrome/myalgic encephalomyelitis. *Int. Immunol.* **2014**, *26*, 233–242. [CrossRef]
77. Brenu, E.W.; van Driel, M.L.; Staines, D.R.; Ashton, K.J.; Hardcastle, S.L.; Keane, J.; Tajouri, L.; Peterson, D.; Ramos, S.B.; Marshall-Gradisnik, S.M. Longitudinal investigation of natural killer cells and cytokines in chronic fatigue syndrome/myalgic encephalomyelitis. *J. Transl. Med.* **2012**, *10*, 1. [CrossRef]
78. Lugli, E.; Marcenaro, E.; Mavilio, D. NK cell subset redistribution during the course of viral infections. *Front. Immunol.* **2014**, *5*, 1–7. [CrossRef]
79. Curriu, M.; Carrillo, J.; Massanella, M.; Rigau, J.; Alegre, J.; Puig, J.; Garcia-Quintana, A.M.; Castro-Marrero, J.; Negredo, E.; Clotet, B.; et al. Screening NK-, B- and T-cell phenotype and function in patients suffering from Chronic Fatigue Syndrome. *J. Transl. Med.* **2013**, *11*, 1–13. [CrossRef]
80. Theorell, J.; Indre, B.-L.; Tesi, B.; Schlums, H.; Johnsgaard, M.S.; Babak, A.-A.; Strand, E.B.; Bryceson, Y.T. Unperturbed cytotoxic lymphocyte phenotype and function in myalgic encephalomyelitis/chronic fatigue syndrome patients. *Front. Immunol.* **2017**, *8*, 1–15. [CrossRef]
81. Nilius, B.; Owsianik, G. The transient receptor potential family of ion channels. *Genom. Biol.* **2011**, *12*, 218. [CrossRef]
82. Marshall-gradisnik, S.M.; Smith, P.; Brenu, E.W.; Nilius, B.; Ramos, S.B.; Staines, D.R. Examination of Single Nucleotide Polymorphisms (SNPs) in Transient Receptor Potential (TRP) Ion Channels in Chronic Fatigue Syndrome Patients. *Immunol. Immunogenet. Insights* **2015**, *7*, 1–6. [CrossRef]
83. Maes, M.; Mihaylova, I.; Leunis, J.C. Increased serum IgA and IgM against LPS of enterobacteria in chronic fatigue syndrome (CFS): Indication for the involvement of gram-negative enterobacteria in the etiology of CFS and for the presence of an increased gut-intestinal permeability. *J. Affect. Disord.* **2007**, *99*, 237–240. [CrossRef]
84. Maes, M.; Twisk, F.N.M.; Kubera, M.; Ringel, K.; Leunis, J.C.; Geffard, M. Increased IgA responses to the LPS of commensal bacteria is associated with inflammation and activation of cell-mediated immunity in chronic fatigue syndrome. *J. Affect. Disord.* **2012**, *136*, 909–917. [CrossRef]
85. Maes, M.; Leunis, J.C. Normalization of leaky gut in chronic fatigue syndrome (CFS) is accompanied by a clinical improvement: Effects of age, duration of illness and the translocation of LPS from gram-negative bacteria. *Neuroendocrinol. Lett.* **2008**, *29*, 902.
86. Sotzny, F.; Blanco, J.; Capelli, E.; Castro-Marrero, J.; Steiner, S.; Murovska, M.; Scheibenbogen, C. Myalgic Encephalomyelitis/Chronic Fatigue Syndrome—Evidence for an autoimmune disease. *Autoimmun. Rev.* **2018**, *17*, 601–609. [CrossRef]
87. Loebel, M.; Grabowski, P.; Heidecke, H.; Bauer, S.; Hanitsch, L.G.; Wittke, K.; Meisel, C.; Reinke, P.; Volk, H.D.; Fluge, O.; et al. Antibodies to β adrenergic and muscarinic cholinergic receptors in patients with Chronic Fatigue Syndrome. *Brain Behav. Immun.* **2016**, *52*, 32–39. [CrossRef]
88. Maes, M.; Kubera, M.; Uytterhoeven, M.; Vrydags, N.; Bosmans, E. Increased plasma peroxides as a marker of oxidative stress in myalgic encephalomyelitis/chronic fatigue syndrome (ME/CFS). *Med. Sci. Monit.* **2011**, *17*, SC11. [CrossRef]
89. Ortega-Hernandez, O.-D.; Cuccia, M.; Bozzini, S.; Bassi, N.; Moscavitch, S.; Diaz-Gallo, L.-M.; Blank, M.; Agmon-Levin, N.; Shoenfeld, Y. Autoantibodies, Polymorphisms in the Serotonin Pathway, and Human Leukocyte Antigen Class II Alleles in Chronic Fatigue Syndrome. *Ann. N. Y. Acad. Sci.* **2009**, *1173*, 589–599. [CrossRef]
90. Tanaka, S.; Kuratsune, H.; Hidaka, Y.; Hakariya, Y.; Tatsumi, K.I.; Takano, T.; Kanakura, Y.; Amino, N. Autoantibodies against muscarinic cholinergic receptor in chronic fatigue syndrome. *Int. J. Mol. Med.* **2003**, *12*, 225–230. [CrossRef]
91. Scheibenbogen, C.; Loebel, M.; Freitag, H.; Krueger, A.; Bauer, S.; Antelmann, M.; Doehner, W.; Scherbakov, N.; Heidecke, H.; Reinke, P.; et al. Immunoadsorption to remove β2 adrenergic receptor antibodies in Chronic Fatigue Syndrome CFS/ME. *PLoS ONE* **2018**, *13*, 1–15. [CrossRef]
92. Ortega-Hernandez, O.D.; Shoenfeld, Y. Infection, vaccination, and autoantibodies in chronic fatigue syndrome, cause or coincidence. *Ann. N. Y. Acad. Sci.* **2009**, *1173*, 600–609. [CrossRef]
93. Klimas, N.; Broderick, G.; Fletcher, M.A. Biomarkers for CFS. *Brain Behav. Immun.* **2012**, *26*, 1202–1210. [CrossRef]

94. Mensah, F.; Bansal, A.; Berkovitz, S.; Sharma, A.; Reddy, V.; Leandro, M.J.; Cambridge, G. Extended B cell phenotype in patients with myalgic encephalomyelitis/chronic fatigue syndrome: A cross-sectional study. *Clin. Exp. Immunol.* **2016**, *184*, 237–247. [CrossRef]
95. Blomberg, J.; Gottfries, C.G.; Elfaitouri, A.; Rizwan, M.; Rosén, A. Infection elicited autoimmunity and Myalgic encephalomyelitis/chronic fatigue syndrome: An explanatory model. *Front. Immunol.* **2018**, *9*, 229. [CrossRef]
96. Cherukuri, A.; Cheng, P.C.; Pierce, S.K. The Role of the CD19/CD21 Complex in B Cell Processing and Presentation of Complement-Tagged Antigens. *J. Immunol.* **2001**, *167*, 163–172. [CrossRef]
97. Nijs, J.; de Meirleir, K. Impairments of the 2-5A synthetase/RNase L pathway on chronic fatigue syndrome. *In Vivo* **2005**, *19*, 1013–1022.
98. Silverman, R.H. Viral Encounters with 2′,5′-Oligoadenylate Synthetase and RNase L during the Interferon Antiviral Response. *J. Virol.* **2007**, *81*, 12720–12729. [CrossRef]
99. Bisbal, C.; Silhol, M.; Laubenthal, H.; Kaluza, T.; Carnac, G.; Milligan, L.; Roy, F.L.E.; Salehzada, T. The 2 J -5 J Oligoadenylate/RNase L/RNase L Inhibitor Pathway Regulates Both MyoD mRNA Stability and Muscle Cell Differentiation. *Mol. Cell. Biol.* **2000**, *20*, 4959–4969. [CrossRef]
100. Banerjee, S.; Li, G.; Li, Y.; Gaughan, C.; Baskar, D.; Parker, Y.; Lindner, D.J.; Weiss, S.R.; Silverman, R.H. RNase L is a negative regulator of cell migration. *Oncotarget* **2015**, *6*, 44360. [CrossRef]
101. Su Suhadolnik, R.J.; Lombardi, V.; Peterson, D.L.; Welsch, S.; Cheney, P.R.; Furr, E.G.; Horvath, S.E.; Charubala, R.; Reichenbach, N.L.; Pfleiderer, W.; et al. Biochemical Dysregulation of the 2-5A Synthetase/RNase L Antiviral Defense Pathway in Chronic Fatigue Syndrome Biochemical Dysregulation of the 2-5A Synthetase/RNase L Antiviral Defense Pathway in Chronic Fatigue Syndrome. *J. Chronic Fatigue Syndr.* **1999**, *5*, 223–242. [CrossRef]
102. Garcia, M.A.; Gil, J.; Ventoso, I.; Guerra, S.; Domingo, E.; Rivas, C.; Esteban, M. Impact of Protein Kinase PKR in Cell Biology: From Antiviral to Antiproliferative Action. *Microbiol. Mol. Biol. Rev.* **2006**, *70*, 1032–1060. [CrossRef]
103. Garcia-Ortega, M.B.; Lopez, G.J.; Jimenez, G.; Garcia-Garcia, J.A.; Conde, V.; Boulaiz, H.; Carrillo, E.; Perán, M.; Marchal, J.A.; Garcia, M.A. Clinical and therapeutic potential of protein kinase PKR in cancer and metabolism. *Expert Rev. Mol. Med.* **2017**, *19*, 1–13. [CrossRef]
104. Nakatomi, Y.; Mizuno, K.; Ishii, A.; Wada, Y.; Tanaka, M.; Tazawa, S.; Onoe, K.; Fukuda, S.; Kawabe, J.; Takahashi, K.; et al. Neuroinflammation in Patients with Chronic Fatigue Syndrome/Myalgic Encephalomyelitis: An 11C-(R)-PK11195 PET Study. *J. Nucl. Med.* **2014**, *55*, 945–950. [CrossRef]
105. Chen, M.-K.; Guilarte, T.R. Translocator Protein 18kDA (TSPO): Molecular Sensor of Brain Injury & Repair. *Pharmacol. Ther.* **2009**, *118*, 1–17.
106. De Lange, F.P.; Kalkman, J.S.; Bleijenberg, G.; Hagoort, P.; Werf, S.P.V.; Van Der Meer, J.W.M.; Toni, I. Neural correlates of the chronic fatigue syndrome—An fMRI study. *Brain* **2004**, *127*, 1948–1957. [CrossRef]
107. Ji, R.-R.; Berta, T.; Nedergaard, M. Glia and Pain: Is chronic pain a gliopathy? *Pain* **2013**, *154*, 10–28. [CrossRef]
108. Siemionow, V.; Fang, Y.; Calabrese, L.; Sahgal, V.; Yue, G.H. Altered central nervous system signal during motor performance in chronic fatigue syndrome. *Clin. Neurophysiol.* **2004**, *115*, 2372–2381. [CrossRef]
109. Finkelmeyer, A.; He, J.; Maclachlan, L.; Watson, S.; Gallagher, P.; Newton, J.L.; Blamire, A.M. Grey and white matter differences in Chronic Fatigue Syndrome—A voxel-based morphometry study. *NeuroImage Clin.* **2018**, *17*, 24–30. [CrossRef]
110. Zhu, C.B.; Blakely, R.D.; Hewlett, W.A. The proinflammatory cytokines interleukin-1beta and tumor necrosis factor-alpha activate serotonin transporters. *Neuropsychopharmacology* **2006**, *31*, 2121–2131. [CrossRef]
111. Dantzer, R. Cytokine, Sickness Behaviour, and Depression. *Immunol. Allergy Clin. N. Am.* **2009**, *29*, 247–264. [CrossRef]
112. Hornig, M.; Gottschalk, G.; Peterson, D.L.; Knox, K.K.; Schultz, A.F.; Eddy, M.L.; Che, X.; Lipkin, W.I. Cytokine network analysis of cerebrospinal fluid in myalgic encephalomyelitis/chronic fatigue syndrome. *Mol. Psychiatry* **2016**, *21*, 261–269. [CrossRef]
113. Hornig, M.; Gottschalk, C.G.; Eddy, M.L.; Che, X.; Ukaigwe, J.E.; Peterson, D.L.; Lipkin, W.I. Immune network analysis of cerebrospinal fluid in myalgic encephalomyelitis/chronic fatigue syndrome with atypical and classical presentations. *Transl. Psychiatry* **2017**, *7*, e1080. [CrossRef]

114. Morris, G.; Berk, M.; Galecki, P.; Walder, K.; Maes, M. The Neuro-Immune Pathophysiology of Central and Peripheral Fatigue in Systemic Immune-Inflammatory and Neuro-Immune Diseases. *Mol. Neurobiol.* **2016**, *53*, 1195–1219. [CrossRef]
115. Komaroff, A.L. Inflammation correlates with symptoms in chronic fatigue syndrome. *Proc. Natl. Acad. Sci. USA* **2017**, *114*, 8914–8916. [CrossRef]
116. Campbell, J.N.; Meyer, R.A. Mechanisms of neuropathic pain. *Neuron* **2006**, *52*, 77–92. [CrossRef]
117. Meeus, M.; Nijs, J. Central sensitization: A biopsychosocial explanation for chronic widespread pain in patients with fibromyalgia and chronic fatigue syndrome. *Clin. Rheumatol.* **2007**, *26*, 465–473. [CrossRef]
118. Pereira, M.P.; Agelopoulos, K.; Köllner, J.; Neufang, G.; Schmelz, M.; Ständer, S. Selective Nerve Fibre Activation in Patients with Chronic Generalized Pruritus May Indicate a Central Sensitization Mechanism. *Acta Derm. Venereol.* **2019**. [CrossRef]
119. Herring, B.E.; Nicoll, R.A. Long-Term Potentiation: From CaMKII to AMPA Receptor Trafficking. *Annu. Rev. Physiol.* **2016**, *78*, 351–365. [CrossRef]
120. Miwa, S.; Takikawa, O. Chronic fatigue syndrome and neurotransmitters. *Nihon Rinsho* **2007**, *65*, 1005–1010.
121. Ren, K.; Dubner, R. Neuron-glia crosstalk gets serious: Rolein pain hypersensitivity. *Curr. Opin. Anaesthesiol.* **2008**, *21*, 570–579. [CrossRef]
122. Zhao, H.; Alam, A.; Chen, Q.; A Eusman, M.; Pal, A.; Eguchi, S.; Wu, L.; Ma, D. The role of microglia in the pathobiology of neuropathic pain development: What do we know? *Br. J. Anaesth.* **2017**, *118*, 504–516. [CrossRef]
123. Ricci, G.; Volpi, L.; Pasquali, L.; Petrozzi, L.; Siciliano, G. Astrocyte-neuron interactions in neurological disorders. *J. Biol. Phys.* **2009**, *35*, 317–336. [CrossRef]
124. Puri, B.K.; Jakeman, P.M.; Agour, M.; Gunatilake, K.D.R.; Fernando, K.A.C.; Gurusinghe, A.I.; Treasaden, I.H.; Waldman, A.D.; Gishen, P. Regional grey and white matter volumetric changes in myalgic encephalomyelitis (chronic fatigue syndrome): A voxel-based morphometry 3 T MRI study. *Br. J. Radiol.* **2012**, *85*, e270–e273. [CrossRef]
125. Svahn, K.S.; Göransson, U.; Chryssanthou, E.; Olsen, B.; Sjölin, J.; Strömstedt, A.A. Induction of gliotoxin secretion in Aspergillus fumigatus by bacteria-associated molecules. *PLoS ONE* **2014**, *9*, e93685. [CrossRef]
126. Hulsebosch, C.E. Gliopathy ensures persistent inflammation and chronic pain after spinal cord injury. *Exp. Neurol.* **2008**, *214*, 6–9. [CrossRef]
127. Cao, Y.; Li, Q. The variation of the 5-hydroxytryptamine system between chronic unpredictable mild stress rats and chronic fatigue syndrome rats induced by forced treadmill running. *NeuroReport* **2017**, *28*, 630–637. [CrossRef]
128. Drevets, W.C.; Thase, M.; Moses, E.; Price, J.; Ph, D.; Kupfer, D.J.; Mathis, C. Serotonin-1A receptor imaging in recurrent depression: Replication and Literature Review. *Nucl. Med. Biol.* **2009**, *34*, 865–877. [CrossRef]
129. Liu, J.Z.; Yao, B.; Siemionow, V.; Sahgal, V.; Wang, X.; Sun, J.; Yue, G.H. Fatigue induces greater brain signal reduction during sustained than preparation phase of maximal voluntary contraction. *Brain Res.* **2005**, *1057*, 113–126. [CrossRef]
130. Cotel, F.; Exley, R.; Cragg, S.J.; Perrier, J.F. Serotonin spillover onto the axon initial segment of motoneurons induces central fatigue by inhibiting action potential initiation. *Proc. Natl. Acad. Sci. USA* **2013**, *110*, 4774–4779. [CrossRef]
131. Meyer, B.; Nguyen, C.B.T.; Moen, A.; Fagermoen, E.; Sulheim, D.; Nilsen, H.; Wyller, V.B.; Gjerstad, J. Maintenance of chronic fatigue syndrome (CFS) in Young CFS patients is associated with the 5-HTTLPR and SNP rs25531 A> G Genotype. *PLoS ONE* **2015**, *10*, 1–11. [CrossRef]
132. Yamashita, M.; Yamamoto, T. Tryptophan circuit in fatigue: From blood to brain and cognition. *Brain Res.* **2017**, *1675*, 116–126. [CrossRef]
133. Maratta, R.; Fenrich, K.K.; Zhao, E.; Neuber-Hess, M.S.; Rose, P.K. Distribution and density of contacts from noradrenergic and serotoninergic boutons on the denditres of neck flexor motoneurons in the adult cat. *J. Comp. Neurol.* **2015**, *1*, 1–40.
134. Zuo, L.J.; Yu, S.Y.; Hu, Y.; Wang, F.; Piao, Y.S.; Lian, T.H.; Yu, Q.J.; Wang, R.D.; Li, L.X.; Guo, P.; et al. Serotonergic dysfunctions and abnormal iron metabolism: Relevant to mental fatigue of Parkinson disease. *Sci. Rep.* **2016**, *6*, 1–9. [CrossRef]

135. Maes, M.; Ringel, K.; Kubera, M.; Anderson, G.; Morris, G.; Galecki, P.; Geffard, M. In myalgic encephalomyelitis/chronic fatigue syndrome, increased autoimmune activity against 5-HT is associated with immuno-inflammatory pathways and bacterial translocation. *J. Affect. Disord.* **2013**, *150*, 223–230. [CrossRef]
136. Farooq, R.K.; Asghar, K.; Kanwal, S.; Zulqernain, A. Role of inflammatory cytokines in depression: Focus on interleukin-1β. *Biomed. Rep.* **2017**, *6*, 15–20. [CrossRef]
137. Hensler, J.G. *Serotonin in Mood and Emotion*; Elsevier: Amsterdam, The Netherlands, 2010; Volume 21, pp. 367–378.
138. Morris, G.; Anderson, G.; Maes, M. Hypothalamic-Pituitary-Adrenal Hypofunction in Myalgic Encephalomyelitis (ME)/Chronic Fatigue Syndrome (CFS) as a Consequence of Activated Immune-Inflammatory and Oxidative and Nitrosative Pathways. *Mol. Neurobiol.* **2017**, *54*, 6806–6819. [CrossRef]
139. Hochberg, Z.E.; Pacak, K.; Chrousos, G.P. The Neuroendocrinology of Chronic Fatigue Syndrome. *Endocr. Rev.* **2003**, *24*, 236–252.
140. Tak, L.M.; Cleare, A.J.; Ormel, J.; Manoharan, A.; Kok, I.C.; Wessely, S.; Rosmalen, J.G. Meta-analysis and meta-regression of hypothalamic-pituitary-adrenal axis activity in functional somatic disorders. *Biol. Psychol.* **2011**, *87*, 183–194. [CrossRef]
141. Torres-Harding, S.; Sorenson, M.; Jason, L.; Reynolds, N.; Brown, M.; Maher, K.; Fletcher, M.A. The associations between basal salivary cortisol and illness symptomatology in CFS. *J. Appl. Biobehav. Res.* **2008**, *13*, 157–180. [CrossRef]
142. Scott, L.V.; Burnett, F.; Medbak, S.; Dinan, T.G. Naloxone-mediated activation of the hypothalamic-pituitary-adrenal axis in chronic fatigue syndrome. *Psychol. Med.* **1998**, *28*, 285–293. [CrossRef]
143. Papadopoulos, A.S.; Cleare, A.J. Hypothalamic-pituitary-adrenal axis dysfunction in chronic fatigue syndrome. *Nat. Rev. Endocrinol.* **2012**, *8*, 22–32. [CrossRef]
144. Ruiz-Núñez, B.; Tarasse, R.; Vogelaar, E.F.; Janneke Dijck-Brouwer, D.A.; Muskiet, F.A. Higher Prevalence of "Low T3 Syndrome" in Patients with Chronic Fatigue Syndrome: A Case-Control Study. *Front. Endocrinol.* **2018**, *9*, 97. [CrossRef]
145. Tanriverdi, F.; Karaca, Z.; Unluhizarci, K.; Kelestimur, F. The hypothalamo-pituitary-adrenal axis in chronic fatigue syndrome and fibromyalgia syndrome. *Stress* **2007**, *10*, 13–25. [CrossRef]
146. Hall, D.; Lattie, E.G.; Antoni, M.H.; Fletcher, M.A.; Czaja, S.; Perdomo, D.; Klimas, N.G. Stress Manegement Skills, Cortisol Awakening Response and Post-Exertional Malaise in CFS. *Psychoneuroendocrinology* **2014**, *49*, 26–31. [CrossRef]
147. Powell, D.J.H.; Liossi, C.; Moss-Morris, R.; Schlotz, W. Unstimulated cortisol secretory activity in everyday life and its relationship with fatigue and chronic fatigue syndrome: A systematic review and subset meta-analysis. *Psychoneuroendocrinology* **2013**, *38*, 2405–2422. [CrossRef]
148. Lattie, E.G.; Antoni, M.H.; Fletcher, M.A.; Penedo, F.; Czaja, S.; Lopez, C.; Perdomo, D.; Sala, A.; Nair, S.; Fu, S.H.; et al. Stress management skills, neuroimmune processes and fatigue levels in persons with chronic fatigue syndrome. *Brain Behav. Immun.* **2012**, *26*, 849–858. [CrossRef]
149. Ehlert, U.; Gaab, J.; Heinrichs, M. Psychoneuroendocrinological contributions to the etiology of depression, posttraumatic stress disorder, and stress-related bodily disorders: The role of the hypothalamus-pituitary-adrenal axis. *Biol. Psychol.* **2001**, *57*, 141–152. [CrossRef]
150. Lopez, C.; Antoni, M.; Penedo, F.; Weiss, D.; Cruess, S.; Segotas, M.C.; Helder, L.; Siegel, S.; Klimas, N.; Fletcher, M.A. A pilot study of cognitive behavioral stress management effects on stress, quality of life, and symptoms in persons with chronic fatigue syndrome. *J. Psychosom. Res.* **2011**, *70*, 328–334. [CrossRef]
151. McKenzie, R.; O'Fallon, A.; Dale, J.; Demitrack, M.; Sharma, G.; Deloria, M.; Garcia-Borreguero, D.; Blackwelder, W.; Straus, S.E. Low-dose hydrocortisone for treatment of chronic fatigue syndrome: A randomized controlled trial. *JAMA* **1998**, *280*, 1061–1066. [CrossRef]
152. Cleare, A.J.; Heap, E.; Malhi, G.S.; Wessely, S.; O'Keane, V.; Miell, J. Low-dose hydrocortisone in chronic fatigue syndrome: A randomised crossover trial. *Lancet* **1999**, *353*, 455–458. [CrossRef]
153. Wang, T.; Yin, J.; Miller, A.H.; Xiao, C. A systematic review of the association between fatigue and genetic polymorphisms. *Brain Behav. Immun.* **2017**, *62*, 230–244. [CrossRef]
154. Johnston, S.; Staines, D.; Klein, A.; Marshall-Gradisnik, S. A targeted genome association study examining transient receptor potential ion channels, acetylcholine receptors, and adrenergic receptors in Chronic Fatigue Syndrome/Myalgic Encephalomyelitis. *BMC Med. Genet.* **2016**, *17*, 1–7. [CrossRef]

155. Narita, M.; Nishigami, N.; Narita, N.; Yamaguti, K.; Okado, N.; Watanabe, Y.; Kuratsune, H. Association between serotonin transporter gene polymorphism and chronic fatigue syndrome. *Biochem. Biophys. Res. Commun.* **2003**, *311*, 264–266. [CrossRef]
156. Hanson, M.R.; Gu, Z.; Keinan, A.; Ye, K.; Germain, A.; Ross, P.B. Association of mitochondrial DNA variants with myalgic encephalomyelitis/chronic fatigue syndrome (ME/CFS) symptoms. *J. Transl. Med.* **2016**, *14*, 1–2. [CrossRef]
157. oertzel, B.N.; Pennachin, C.; de Souza Coelho, L.; Gurbaxani, B.; Maloney, E.M.; Jones, J.F. Combinations of single nucleotide polymorphisms in neuroendocrine effector and receptor genes predict chronic fatigue syndrome. *Pharmacogenomics* **2006**, *7*, 475–483. [CrossRef]
158. De Vega, W.C.; Herrera, S.; Vernon, S.D.; McGowan, P.O. Epigenetic modifications and glucocorticoid sensitivity in Myalgic Encephalomyelitis/Chronic Fatigue Syndrome (ME/CFS). *BMC Med. Genom.* **2017**, *10*, 1–14. [CrossRef]
159. Hall, K.T.; Kossowsky, J.; Oberlander, T.F.; Ted, J.; Saul, J.P.; Wyller, V.B.; Fagermoen, E.; Sulheim, D.; Gjerstad, J.; Winger, A.; et al. Genetic Variation in catechol-O-methyltransferase modifies effects of clonidine treatment in CFS. *Pharmacogenomics* **2016**, *16*, 454–460. [CrossRef]
160. Löbel, M.; Mooslechner, A.A.; Bauer, S.; Günther, S.; Letsch, A.; Hanitsch, L.G.; Grabowski, P.; Meisel, C.; Volk, H.D.; Scheibenbogen, C. Polymorphism in COMT is associated with IgG$_3$ subclass level and susceptibility to infection in patients with chronic fatigue syndrome. *J. Transl. Med.* **2015**, *13*, 1–8. [CrossRef]
161. Vernon, S.D.; Unger, E.R.; Dimulescu, I.M.; Ravjeevan, M.; Reeves, W.C. Utility of the blood for gene expression profiling and biomarker discovery in chronic fatigue syndrome. *Dis. Mark.* **2002**, *18*, 193–199. [CrossRef]
162. Kerr, J.R.; Petty, R.; Burke, B.; Gough, J.; Fear, D.; Sinclair, L.I.; Mattey, D.L.; Richards, S.C.; Montgomery, J.; Baldwin, D.A.; et al. Gene expression subtypes in patients with chronic fatigue syndrome/myalgic encephalomyelitis. *J. Infect. Dis.* **2008**, *197*, 1171–1184. [CrossRef]
163. Buchwald, D.; Herrell, R.; Ashton, S.; Belcourt, M.; Schmaling, K.; Sullivan, P.; Neale, M.; Goldberg, J. A twin study of chronic fatigue. *Psychosom. Med.* **2001**, *63*, 936–943. [CrossRef]
164. Crawley, E.; Smith, G.D. Is chronic fatigue syndrome (CFS/ME) heritable in children, and if so, why does it matter? *Arch. Dis. Child.* **2007**, *92*, 1058–1061. [CrossRef]
165. Ciregia, F.; Giusti, L.; Da Valle, Y.; Donadio, E.; Consensi, A.; Giacomelli, C.; Sernissi, F.; Scarpellini, P.; Maggi, F.; Lucacchini, A.; et al. A multidisciplinary approach to study a couple of monozygotic twins discordant for the chronic fatigue syndrome: A focus on potential salivary biomarkers. *J. Transl. Med.* **2013**, *11*, 1. [CrossRef]
166. Whistler, T.; Unger, E.R.; Nisenbaum, R.; Vernon, S.D. Integration of gene expression, clinical, and epidemiologic data to characterize Chronic Fatigue Syndrome. *J. Transl. Med.* **2003**, *1*, 1–8. [CrossRef]
167. Jonsjö, M.A.; Wicksell, R.K.; Holmström, L.; Andreasson, A.; Bileviciute-Ljungar, I.; Olsson, G.L. Identifying symptom subgroups in patients with ME/CFS – relationships to functioning and quality of life. *Fatigue Biomed. Health Behav.* **2017**, *5*, 33–42. [CrossRef]
168. Jason, L.A.; Corradi, K.; Torres-Harding, S.; Taylor, R.R.; King, C. Chronic fatigue syndrome: The need for subtypes. *Neuropsychol. Rev.* **2005**, *15*, 29–58. [CrossRef]
169. Zaturenskaya, M.; Jason, L.A.; Torres-Harding, S.; Tryon, W.W. Subgrouping in Chronic Fatigue Syndrome Based on Actigraphy and Illness Severity. *Open Biol. J.* **2009**, *2*, 20–26. [CrossRef]
170. Čikoš, Š.; Bukovská, A.; Koppel, J. Relative quantification of mRNA: Comparison of methods currently used for real-time PCR data analysis. *BMC Mol. Biol.* **2007**, *8*, 1–14. [CrossRef]
171. Presson, A.P.; Sobel, E.M.; Papp, J.C.; Suarez, C.J.; Whistler, T.; Rajeevan, M.S.; Vernon, S.D.; Horvath, S. Integrated weighted gene co-expression network analysis with an application to chronic fatigue syndrome. *BMC Syst. Biol.* **2008**, *2*, 1–21. [CrossRef]
172. Trivedi, M.S.; Oltra, E.; Sarria, L.; Rose, N.; Beljanski, V.; Fletcher, M.A.; Klimas, N.G.; Nathanson, L. Identification of Myalgic Encephalomyelitis/Chronic Fatigue Syndrome-associated DNA methylation patterns. *PLoS ONE* **2018**, *13*, e0201066. [CrossRef]
173. Falkenberg, V.R.; Whistler, T.; Murray, J.R.; Unger, E.R.; Rajeevan, M.S. Acute Psychosocial Stress-Mediated Changes in the Expression and Methylation of Perforin in Chronic Fatigue Syndrome. *Genet. Epigenet.* **2013**, *5*, 1–9. [CrossRef]

174. Suarez-alvarez, B.; Rodriguez, R.M.; Fraga, M.F.; López-Larrea, C. DNA methylation: A promising landscape for immune system-related diseases. *Trends Genet.* **2012**, *28*, 506–514. [CrossRef]
175. De Vega, W.C.; Vernon, S.D.; McGowan, P.O. DNA Methylation Modifications Associated with Chronic Fatigue Syndrome. *PLoS ONE* **2014**, *9*, 1–11. [CrossRef]
176. Petronis, A. Epigenetics as a unifying principle in the aetiology of complex traits and diseases. *Nature* **2010**, *465*, 721–727. [CrossRef]
177. Martino, D.; Loke, Y.J.; Gordon, L.; Ollikainen, M.; Cruickshank, M.N.; Saffery, R.; Craig, J.M. Longitudinal, genome-scale analysis of DNA methylation in twins from birth to 18 months of age reveals rapid epigenetic change in early life and pair-specific effects of discordance. *Genom. Biol.* **2013**, *14*, 1–14. [CrossRef]
178. Rajeevan, M.S.; Dimulescu, I.; Murray, J.; Falkenberg, V.R.; Unger, E.R. Pathway-focused genetic evaluation of immune and inflammation related genes with chronic fatigue syndrome. *Hum. Immunol.* **2015**, *76*, 553–560. [CrossRef]
179. Smith, A.K.; Fang, H.; Whistler, T.; Unger, E.R.; Rajeevan, M.S. Convergent genomic studies identify association of GRIK2 and NPAS2 with chronic fatigue syndrome. *Neuropsychobiology* **2011**, *64*, 183–194. [CrossRef]
180. Smith, A.K.; Dimulescu, I.; Falkenberg, V.R.; Narasimhan, S.; Heim, C.; Vernon, S.D.; Rajeevan, M.S. Genetic evaluation of the serotonergic system in chronic fatigue syndrome. *Psychoneuroendocrinology* **2008**, *33*, 188–197. [CrossRef]
181. Sommerfeldt, L.; Portilla, H.; Jacobsen, L.; Gjerstad, J.; Wyller, V.B. Polymorphisms of adrenergic cardiovascular control genes are associated with adolescent chronic fatigue syndrome. *Acta Paediatr.* **2011**, *100*, 293–298. [CrossRef]
182. Meyer-lindenberg, A.; Kohn, P.D.; Kolachana, B.; Kippenhan, S.; McInerney-Leo, A.; Nussbaum, R.; Weinberger, D.R.; Berman, K.F. Midbrain dopamine and prefrontal function in humans: Interaction and modulation by COMT genotype. *Nat. Neurosci.* **2005**, *8*, 594–596. [CrossRef]
183. Marshall-gradisnik, S.; Johnston, S.; Chacko, A.; Nguyen, T.; Smith, P.; Staines, D. Single nucleotide polymorphisms and genotypes of transient receptor potential ion channel and acetylcholine receptor genes from isolated B lymphocytes in myalgic encephalomyelitis/chronic fatigue syndrome patients. *J. Int. Med. Res.* **2016**, *44*, 1381–1394. [CrossRef]
184. Smith, A.K.; White, P.D.; Aslakson, E. Polymorphisms in genes regulating the HPA axis associated with empirically delineated classes of unexplained chronic fatigue. *Pharmacogenomics* **2006**, *7*, 387–394. [CrossRef]
185. Rajeevan, M.S.; Smith, A.K.; Dimulescu, I. Glucocorticoid receptor polymorphisms and haplotypes associated with chronic fatigue syndrome. *Genes Brain Behav.* **2007**, *6*, 167–176. [CrossRef]
186. Bozzinp, S.; Silvestrp, A.D.E.; Pizzocher, C.; Loruss, L.; Martinettp, M.; Cuccin, M. Molecular study of receptor for advanced glycation endproduct gene promoter and identification of specific hla haplotypes possibly involved in chronic fatigue syndrome' Genetics and Microbiology Department, University ofPavia; ' Biometric Unit, Founda. *Int. J. Immunopathol. Pharmacol.* **2009**, *22*, 745–754.
187. Smith, J.; Fritz, E.L.; Kerr, J.R.; Cleare, A.J.; Wessely, S. Association of chronic fatigue syndrome with human leucocyte antigen class II alleles. *J. Clin. Pathol.* **2005**, *58*, 860–863. [CrossRef]
188. Petty, R.D.; McCarthy, N.E.; Dieu, R.L.; Kerr, J.R. MicroRNAs hsa-miR-99b, hsa-miR-330, hsa-miR-126 and hsa-miR-30c: Potential Diagnostic Biomarkers in Natural Killer (NK) Cells of Patients with Chronic Fatigue Syndrome (CFS)/Myalgic Encephalomyelitis (ME). *PLoS ONE* **2016**, *11*, 1–19. [CrossRef]
189. Collatz, A.; Johnston, S.C.; Staines, D.R.; Marshall-Gradisnik, S.M. A Systematic Review of Drug Therapies for Chronic Fatigue Syndrome/Myalgic Encephalomyelitis. *Clin. Ther.* **2016**, *38*, 1263–1271. [CrossRef]
190. Olson, L.G.; Ambrogetti, A.; Sutherland, D.C. A Pilot Randomized Controlled Trial of Dexamphetamine in Patients with Chronic Fatigue Syndrome. *Psychosomatics* **2003**, *44*, 38–43. [CrossRef]
191. Hickie, I. Nefazodone for Patients with Chronic Fatigue Syndrome. *Aust. N. Z. J. Psychiatry* **1999**, *33*, 278–280. [CrossRef]
192. Mitchell, W.M. Efficacy of rintatolimod in the treatment of chronic fatigue syndrome/myalgic encephalomyelitis (CFS/ME). *Expert Rev. Clin. Pharmacol.* **2016**, *9*, 755–770. [CrossRef]
193. Strayer, D.R.; Carter, W.A.; Stouch, B.C.; Stevens, S.R.; Bateman, L.; Cimoch, P.J.; Lapp, C.W.; Peterson, D.L.; Mitchell, W.M. A double-blind, placebo-controlled, randomized, clinical trial of the TLR-3 agonist rintatolimod in severe cases of chronic fatigue syndrome. *PLoS ONE* **2012**, *7*, 1–9. [CrossRef]

194. Malaguarnera, M.; Gargante, M.P.; Cristaldi, E.; Colonna, V.; Messano, M.; Koverech, A.; Neri, S.; Vacante, M.; Cammalleri, L.; Motta, M. Acetyl l-carnitine (ALC) treatment in elderly patients with fatigue. *Arch. Gerontol. Geriatr.* **2008**, *46*, 181–190. [CrossRef]
195. Kerr, J.R.; Cunniffe, V.S.; Kelleher, P.; Bernstein, R.M.; Bruce, I.N. Successful intravenous immunoglobulin therapy in 3 cases of parvovirus B19-associated chronic fatigue syndrome. *Clin. Infect. Dis.* **2003**, *36*, 100–106. [CrossRef]
196. Zanelli, S.; Solenski, N.; Rosenthal, R.; Fiskum, G. Mechanisms of ischemic Neuroprotection by Acetyl-L-carnetine. *Ann. N. Y. Acad. Sci.* **2005**, *1053*, 153–161. [CrossRef]
197. Mitchell, W.M.; Nicodemus, C.F.; Carter, W.A.; Horvath, J.C.; Strayer, D.R. Discordant biological and toxicological species responses to TLR3 activation. *Am. J. Pathol.* **2014**, *184*, 1062–1072. [CrossRef]
198. Bonnet, U. Moclobemide: Therapeutic Use and Clinical Studies. *CNS Drug Rev.* **2003**, *9*, 97–140. [CrossRef]
199. Young, J.L. Use of lisdexamfetamine dimesylate in treatment of executive functioning deficits and chronic fatigue syndrome: A double blind, placebo-controlled study. *Psychiatry Res.* **2013**, *207*, 127–133. [CrossRef]
200. Blitshteyn, S.; Chopra, P. Chronic Fatigue Syndrome: From Chronic Fatigue to More Specific Syndromes. *Eur. Neurol.* **2018**, *80*, 73–77. [CrossRef]
201. Craig, C. Mitoprotective dietary approaches for Myalgic Encephalomyelitis/Chronic Fatigue Syndrome: Caloric restriction, fasting, and ketogenic diets. *Med. Hypotheses* **2015**, *85*, 690–693. [CrossRef]
202. Shungu, D.; Weiduschat, N.; Murrough, J.; Mao, X. Increased ventricular lactate in chronic fatigue syndrome. III. Relationships to cortical glutathione and clinical symptoms implicate oxidative stress in disorder pathophysiology. *NMR Biomed.* **2012**, *25*, 1073–1087. [CrossRef]
203. Maes, M.; Mihaylova, I.; Kubera, M.; Uyttterhoeven, M.; Vrydags, N.; Bosmans, E. Increased 8-hydroxy-deoxyguanosine, a marker of oxidative damage to DNA, in major depression and myalgic encephalomyelitis/chronic fatigue syndrome. *Neuroendocrinol. Lett.* **2009**, *30*, 675–682.
204. Anand, S.K.; Tikoo, S.K. Viruses as modulators of mitochondrial functions. *Adv. Virol.* **2013**, *2013*, 1–17. [CrossRef]
205. Maes, M.; Mihaylova, I.; Kubera, M.; Uyttterhoeven, M.; Vrydags, N.; Bosmans, E. Coenzyme Q10 deficiency in myalgic encephalomyelitis/chronic fatigue syndrome (ME/CFS) is related to fatigue, autonomic and neurocognitive symptoms and is another risk factor explaining the early mortality in ME/CFS due to cardiovascular disorder. *Neuro Endocrinol. Lett.* **2009**, *30*, 470–476.
206. Mattson, M.P. Challenging oneself intermittently to improve health. *Dose-Response* **2014**, *12*, 600–618. [CrossRef]
207. Wang, X.; Qu, Y.; Zhang, Y.; Li, S.; Sun, Y.; Chen, Z.; Teng, L.; Wang, D. Antifatigue Potential Activity of Sarcodon imbricatus in acute excise-treated and chronic fatigue syndrome in mice via regulation of Nrf2-mediated oxidative stress. *Oxid. Med. Cell. Longev.* **2018**, *2018*, 9140896. [CrossRef]
208. Shimazu, T.; Hirschey, M.D.; Newman, J.; He, W.; Moan, N.L.; Grueter, C.a.; Lim, H.; Laura, R.; Stevens, R.D.; Newgard, C.B.; et al. Suppression of Oxidative Stress by B-Hydroxybutyrate, an Endogenous Histone Deacetylase Inhibitor. *Science* **2013**, *339*, 211–214. [CrossRef]
209. Bjørklund, G.; Dadar, M.; Pen, J.J.; Chirumbolo, S.; Aaseth, J. Chronic fatigue syndrome (CFS): Suggestions for a nutritional treatment in the therapeutic approach. *Biomed. Pharmacother.* **2019**, *109*, 1000–1007. [CrossRef]
210. Comhaire, F. Treating patients suffering from myalgic encephalopathy/chronic fatigue syndrome (ME/CFS) with sodium dichloroacetate: An open-label, proof-of-principle pilot trial. *Med. Hypotheses* **2018**, *114*, 45–48. [CrossRef]
211. Comhaire, F. Why do some ME/CFS patients benefit from treatment with sodium dichloroacetate, but others do not? *Med. Hypotheses* **2018**, *120*, 65–67. [CrossRef]
212. Theoharides, T.C.; Asadi, S.; Weng, Z.; Zhang, B. Serotonin-selective reuptake inhibitors and nonsteroidal anti-inflammatory drugs–important considerations of adverse interactions especially for the treatment of myalgic encephalomyelitis/chronic fatigue syndrome. *J. Clin. Psychopharmacol.* **2011**, *31*, 403–405. [CrossRef]
213. Kumar, A.; Garg, R. Protective effects of antidepressants against chronic fatigue syndrome-induced behavioral changes and biochemical alterations. *Fundam. Clin. Pharmacol.* **2009**, *23*, 89–95. [CrossRef]
214. Li, D.Q.; Li, Z.C.; Dai, Z.Y. Selective serotonin reuptake inhibitor combined with dengzhanshengmai capsule improves the fatigue symptoms: A 12-week open-label pilot study. *Int. J. Clin. Exp. Med.* **2015**, *8*, 11811–11817.

215. Beth Smith, M.E.; Haney, E.; McDonagh, M.; Pappas, M.; Daeges, M.; Wasson, N.; Fu, R.; Nelson, H.D. Treatment of myalgic encephalomyelitis/chronic fatigue syndrome: A systematic review for a National Institutes of health pathways to prevention workshop. *Ann. Intern. Med.* **2015**, *162*, 841–850. [CrossRef]
216. Fluge, Ø.; Bruland, O.; Risa, K.; Storstein, A.; Kristoffersen, E.K.; Sapkota, D.; Næss, H.; Dahl, O.; Nyland, H.; Mella, O. Benefit from B-lymphocyte depletion using the anti-CD20 antibody rituximab in chronic fatigue syndrome. A double-blind and placebo-controlled study. *PLoS ONE* **2011**, *6*, e26358. [CrossRef]
217. Fluge, Ø.; Risa, K.; Lunde, S.; Alme, K.; Rekeland, I.G.; Sapkota, D.; Kristoffersen, E.K.; Sørland, K.; Bruland, O.; Dahl, O.; et al. B-Lymphocyte Depletion in Myalgic Encephalopathy/Chronic Fatigue Syndrome. An Open-Label Phase II Study with Rituximab Maintenance Treatment. *PLoS ONE* **2015**, *10*, e0129898. [CrossRef]
218. Chambers, D.; Bagnall, A.M.; Hempel, S.; Forbes, C. Interventions for the treatment, management and rehabilitation of patients with chronic fatigue syndrome/myalgic encephalomyelitis: An updated systematic review. *J. R. Soc. Med.* **2006**, *99*, 506–520.
219. Castro-Marrero, J.; Sáez-Francás, N.; Santillo, D.; Alegre, J. Treatment and management of chronic fatigue syndrome/myalgic encephalomyelitis: All roads lead to Rome. *Br. J. Pharmacol.* **2017**, *174*, 345–369. [CrossRef]
220. Corbitt, M.; Campagnolo, N.; Staines, D.; Marshall-Gradisnik, S. A Systematic Review of Probiotic Interventions for Gastrointestinal Symptoms and Irritable Bowel Syndrome in Chronic Fatigue Syndrome/Myalgic Encephalomyelitis (CFS/ME). *Probiotics Antimicrob. Proteins* **2018**, *1*, 1–12. [CrossRef]
221. Molina-Holgado, E.; Molina-Holgado, F. Mending the broken brain: Neuroimmune interactions in neurogenesis: REVIEW. *J. Neurochem.* **2010**, *114*, 1277–1290.
222. Yirmiya, R.; Goshen, I. Immune modulation of learning, memory, neural plasticity and neurogenesis. *Brain Behav. Immun.* **2011**, *25*, 181–213. [CrossRef]
223. De Pablos-Velasco, P.; Parhofer, K.G.; Bradley, C.; Eschwège, E.; Gönder-Frederick, L.; Maheux, P.; Wood, I.; Simon, D. Current level of glycaemic control and its associated factors in patients with type 2 diabetes across Europe: Data from the PANORAMA study. *Clin. Endocrinol.* **2014**, *80*, 47–56. [CrossRef]
224. Yehuda, R.; Bierer, L.; Sarapas, C.; Makotkine, I.; Andrew, R. Cortisol metabolic predictors of response to psychotherapy for symtpms of PTSD in survivors of the World Trade Center attacks on September 11, 2001. *Psychoneuroendocrinology* **2009**, *34*, 1304–1312. [CrossRef]
225. Wessely, S.; White, P.D. There is only one functional somatic syndrome. *Br. J. Psychiatry* **2004**, *185*, 95–96. [CrossRef]
226. Rhen, T.; Cidlowski, J.A. Antiinflammatory Action of Glucocorticoids—New Mechanisms for Old Drugs. *N. Engl. J. Med.* **2005**, *353*, 1711–1723. [CrossRef]
227. Liberzon, I.; King, A.P.; Britton, J.C.; Phan, K.L.; Abelson, J.L.; Taylor, S.F. Paralimbic and Medial Prefrontal Cortical Involvement in Neuroendocrine Responses to Traumatic Stimuli. *Am. J. Psychiatry* **2007**, *164*, 1250–1258. [CrossRef]
228. Armstrong, C.W.; McGregor, N.R.; Butt, H.L.; Gooley, P.R. Metabolism in chronic fatigue syndrome. *Adv. Clin. Chem.* **2014**, *66*, 121–172.
229. Germain, A.; Ruppert, D.; Levine, S.M.; Hanson, M.R. Metabolic profiling of a myalgic encephalomyelitis/chronic fatigue syndrome discovery cohort reveals disturbances in fatty acid and lipid metabolism. *Mol. Biosyst.* **2017**, *13*, 371–379. [CrossRef]
230. Gerwyn, M.; Maes, M. Mechanisms Explaining Muscle Fatigue and Muscle Pain in Patients with Myalgic Encephalomyelitis/Chronic Fatigue Syndrome (ME/CFS): A Review of Recent Findings. *Curr. Rheumatol. Rep.* **2017**, *19*, 1. [CrossRef]
231. Lloyd, A.; Hickie, I.; Wakefield, D.; Boughton, C.; Dwyer, J.; Australia, S. A Double-Blind, Placebo-Controlled Trial of Intravenous Immunoglobulin Therapy in Patients with Chronic Fatigue Syndrome. *Am. J. Med.* **1989**, *89*, 561. [CrossRef]
232. Price, J.R.; Mitchell, E.; Tidy, E.; Hunot, V. Cognitive behaviour therapy for chronic fatigue syndrome in adults. *Cochrane Database Syst. Rev.* **2008**. [CrossRef]
233. White, P.D.; Goldsmith, K.A.; Johnson, A.L.; Potts, L.; Walwyn, R.; DeCesare, J.C.; Baber, H.L.; Burgess, M.; Clark, L.V.; Cox, D.L.; et al. Comparison of adaptive pacing therapy, cognitive behaviour therapy, graded exercise therapy, and specialist medical care for chronic fatigue syndrome (PACE): A randomised trial. *Lancet* **2011**, *377*, 823–836. [CrossRef]

234. Wilshire, C.E.; Kindlon, T. Response: Sharpe, Goldsmith and Chalder fail to restore confidence in the PACE trial findings. *BMC Psychol.* **2019**, *7*, 19. [CrossRef]
235. Peterson, P.K.; Pheley, A.; Schroeppel, J.; Schenck, C.; Marshall, P.; Kind, A.; Haugland, J.M.; Lambrecht, L.J.; Swan, S.; Goldsmith, S. A Preliminary Placebo-Controlled Crossover Trial of Fludrocortisone for Chronic Fatigue Syndrome. *Arch. Intern. Med.* **1998**, *158*, 908. [CrossRef]
236. Rowe, P.C.; Calkins, H.; DeBusk, K.; McKenzie, R.; Anand, R.; Sharma, G.; Cuccherini, B.A.; Soto, N.; Hohman, P.; Snader, S.; et al. Fludrocortisone Acetate to Treat Neurally Mediated Hypotension in CFS. *JAMA* **2001**, *285*, 52–59. [CrossRef]
237. Vercoulen, J.H.; Swanink, C.M.; Fennis, J.F.; Galama, J.M.; van der Meer, J.W.; Bleijenberg, G. Randomised, double-blind, placebo-controlled study of fluoxetine in chronic fatigue syndrome. *Lancet* **1996**, *347*, 858–861. [CrossRef]
238. Vercoulen, J.H.; Swanink, C.M.; Fennis, J.F.; Galama, J.M.; van der Meer, J.W.; Bleijenberg, G. Prognosis in chronic fatigue syndrome: A prospective study on the natural course. *J. Neurol. Neurosurg. Psychiatry* **1996**, *60*, 489–494. [CrossRef]
239. Rasa, S.; Nora-Krukle, Z.; Henning, N.; Eliassen, E.; Shikova, E.; Harrer, T.; Scheibenbogen, C.; Murovska, M.; Prusty, B.K. Chronic viral infections in myalgic encephalomyelitis/chronic fatigue syndrome (ME/CFS). *J. Transl. Med.* **2018**, *16*, 268. [CrossRef]
240. Ahn, B.H.; Kim, H.S.; Song, S.; Lee, I.H.; Liu, J.; Vassilopoulos, A.; Deng, C.X.; Finkel, T. A role for the mitochondrial deacetylase Sirt3 in regulating energy homeostasis. *Proc. Natl. Acad. Sci. USA* **2008**, *105*, 14447–14452. [CrossRef]

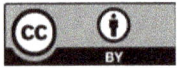

© 2019 by the authors. Licensee MDPI, Basel, Switzerland. This article is an open access article distributed under the terms and conditions of the Creative Commons Attribution (CC BY) license (http://creativecommons.org/licenses/by/4.0/).

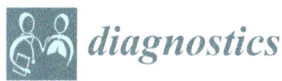

Review

Pathological Mechanisms Underlying Myalgic Encephalomyelitis/Chronic Fatigue Syndrome

Daniel Missailidis, Sarah J. Annesley and Paul R. Fisher *

Department of Physiology Anatomy and Microbiology, La Trobe University, VIC 3086, Australia
* Correspondence: P.Fisher@latrobe.edu.au; Tel.: +61-4-3756-8771

Received: 18 June 2019; Accepted: 19 July 2019; Published: 20 July 2019

Abstract: The underlying molecular basis of myalgic encephalomyelitis/chronic fatigue syndrome (ME/CFS) is not well understood. Characterized by chronic, unexplained fatigue, a disabling payback following exertion ("post-exertional malaise"), and variably presenting multi-system symptoms, ME/CFS is a complex disease, which demands a concerted biomedical investigation from disparate fields of expertise. ME/CFS research and patient treatment have been challenged by the lack of diagnostic biomarkers and finding these is a prominent direction of current work. Despite these challenges, modern research demonstrates a tangible biomedical basis for the disorder across many body systems. This evidence is mostly comprised of disturbances to immunological and inflammatory pathways, autonomic and neurological dysfunction, abnormalities in muscle and mitochondrial function, shifts in metabolism, and gut physiology or gut microbiota disturbances. It is possible that these threads are together entangled as parts of an underlying molecular pathology reflecting a far-reaching homeostatic shift. Due to the variability of non-overlapping symptom presentation or precipitating events, such as infection or other bodily stresses, the initiation of body-wide pathological cascades with similar outcomes stemming from different causes may be implicated in the condition. Patient stratification to account for this heterogeneity is therefore one important consideration during exploration of potential diagnostic developments.

Keywords: myalgic encephalomyelitis; chronic fatigue syndrome; ME/CFS; diagnosis; metabolism; mitochondria; inflammation; immune system; signaling; gut microbiota

---

1. Introduction

Myalgic encephalomyelitis/chronic fatigue syndrome (ME/CFS) encompasses diverse symptoms that manifest variably across a range of body systems, the characteristic symptoms being chronic unexplained fatigue (lasting more than 6 months) and post-exertional malaise (PEM)—a disabling and exacerbated disease state following bouts of physical or mental exertion that exceed a patient-specific threshold. ME/CFS also entails a varied kaleidoscope of other symptoms including muscle weakness, migraine, flu-like symptoms, cognitive impairment ("brain fog"), and sensitivities to a variety of external stimuli that may include light, sound, or specific odors. This can be accompanied by comorbidities, such as fibromyalgia, postural orthostatic tachycardia (POTS), and Ehlers–Danlos syndrome.

A major challenge for this field of study has been the varied usage of multiple diagnostic case criteria that may render comparison between studies difficult depending on the composition of the participant cohort. Furthermore, these criteria are slow processes of exclusion that leave patients without the support or acknowledgment that they need for extended periods and they may be subjected to a protracted, harsh, and insensitive diagnostic gauntlet. These problems are further compounded by medical guidelines in some developed countries that are out of date regarding ME/CFS clinical practice and require urgent overdue revision.

Case definitions, such as the commonly termed Oxford [1] or Fukuda [2] criteria, are most often utilized throughout the UK and USA, respectively, yet may fail to discriminate between generalized chronic fatigue and ME/CFS which specifically also involves PEM, which aids in characterizing this disorder as a discrete clinical entity. Also in usage are the Canadian Consensus Criteria [3] and International Consensus Criteria [4], which mandate PEM for a diagnosis of ME/CFS and therefore may be considered more specific definitions. While the presence of PEM is an optional component of the Fukuda criteria, PEM is, unfortunately, not required for research participation by all studies using this or other less strict definitions. Consequently, the discovery of a reliable diagnostic biomarker is perhaps the most common recurring theme in modern ME/CFS research. Despite myriad relevant study outcomes [5–16], no such discovery has yet been widely validated or implemented as a suitable diagnostic biomarker of ME/CFS.

Not only does ME/CFS affect multiple body systems and organs, but it does so with different and time-varying levels of severity and different patterns of comorbidities in different individuals, thereby producing a highly heterogeneous patient population [7,17–23]. This complexity represents a major challenge to the task of incriminating one underlying pathological mechanism. It is also possible that different causative molecular insults result in different subsequent clinical presentations and this could contribute towards heterogeneity in the disorder. Patient subtyping to manage this heterogeneity has been previously discussed in the field [20,23] and is lent credence by reproduced patterns of differential disease-associated gene expression [24–26], gene expression profiles concurrent with comorbid POTS [27], distinct DNA methylation profiles associated with quality of life scores and PEM [28], severity and frequency of physical or mental fatigue [29], or irritable bowel syndrome (IBS) comorbidity [30], which can be concurrent with specific changes to patient metabolism [31]. As timely, objective, and accurate diagnosis remains the most clear challenge facing the field, patient subtyping may be an important component of new diagnostic techniques and has seen early investigation with stratification-based severity scores [32] or cytokine co-expression patterns [33].

In summation, ME/CFS etiology has been difficult to pin down due to the combination of a diagnostic quagmire and the disorder's heterogeneous symptom presentation across multiple body systems. A traditional view has held that ME/CFS onset is often precipitated by some manner of bodily insult, commonly infection, however, the disorder is left without any known single causative pathogen to date. Given the heterogeneity of the patient population, this is unsurprising. It is possible that the initial pathological insult may not always be pathogen-mediated and could instead be instigated by alternative stresses of sufficient magnitude as to nudge homeostatic regulation loops into alternative stable states [34], and these varying modes of initial insult may contribute to the heterogeneity of ME/CFS clinical presentation.

Current research shows a tangible biomedical foundation underlying this clinical puzzle. Most of this evidence pertains to disturbed muscle function, metabolism, mitochondria, immunity, signaling, neurological, adrenal, and gut health. It is possible that these threads are together entangled as parts of an underlying molecular pathology reflecting a far-reaching homeostatic shift influencing each of these systems, perhaps differentially between individuals with varying clinical features. Furthermore, evidence of abnormalities affecting multiple systems is based on associations and the causal mechanisms responsible for the underlying pathology have yet to be determined. The following sections will address the current evidence for dysfunction across these systems in ME/CFS with specific examples of potential pathological interactions.

2. Abnormal Metabolism and Mitochondrial Function

The nature of the persistent fatigue and PEM experienced by patients renders the area of cellular energetics fertile ground for investigation. However, in the intervening years since early studies [35–37], mitochondria had been largely neglected in the field until their re-emergence as an area of interest during the last 10 years [9]. The recent interest in this area has since generated a basis to support some manner of both mitochondrial and broader metabolic dysfunction in ME/CFS.

2.1. Dysregulated Amino Acid Metabolism and Impaired Provision of TCA Cycle Substrate

This accumulation of evidence supporting dysregulated metabolism and mitochondrial energetics in ME/CFS has taken place across many experimental areas. There have been recent studies utilizing the metabolomics approach, which captures a quantitative snapshot of steady-state metabolite levels in a sample to infer underlying biochemical pathway modulation, typically achieved by either mass spectrometry (MS) or nuclear magnetic resonance (NMR) spectroscopy applications. The first of these studies used NMR to interrogate analytes within ME/CFS blood samples and reported decreases in glutamine and ornithine concentrations, suggesting abnormal amino acid metabolism linked to urea cycle dysregulation [38]. A subsequent study utilizing MS conversely reported an elevation in ornithine concentration with a decrease in citrulline, but this also suggests urea cycle dysregulation [6].

Subsequent work undertaken by the authors of the first study proposed that impaired glycolytic formation of pyruvate could be providing less downstream oxidized pyruvate derivatives to be used as substrate for the tricarboxylic acid (TCA) cycle [39]. Work by others suggested that instead of a reduction in the glycolytic pyruvate supply, a deficiency in pyruvate dehydrogenase (PDH) function may form a bottleneck for the provision of TCA cycle substrate [40]. These and the previous amino acid discrepancies could be due to differences in techniques (NMR vs. MS) and thus the range of detectable molecules. What could be taken from both lines of approach—supported by data from other similar studies [6,13,31] and one cell culture study [41]—is that there may be some manner of TCA cycle disturbance in ME/CFS, possibly one that is substrate supply-driven.

2.2. Inefficient ATP Synthesis and Abnormal Energy Stress Signaling

If the TCA cycle output of oxidative phosphorylation (OXPHOS) complex substrates is reduced by such a glycolysis [39] or PDH [40] defect, one might expect disturbances in cellular energy production in ME/CFS cells. There have been several studies which report a reduction of steady-state ATP levels [9,42,43], yet other studies have reported an elevation [44]. However, these steady-state measures do not provide information as to the metabolic flux (rates of production and depletion) of the molecule of interest. Real-time parameters of aerobic respiration and glycolysis can be measured in live cells by extracellular flux assays, which measure oxygen consumption rates (OCRs) and extracellular acidification rates (ECARs) using intact cells. Published studies of this type both found no significant difference in absolute ATP synthesis rates between the ME/CFS and control cells [41,45]. However, this does not necessarily mean that there is no ATP synthesis defect, since a defect/inefficiency in ATP synthesis could be offset by compensatory homeostatic mechanisms.

The homeostatic regulation of cellular energy metabolism is centered on two stress-sensing protein kinases, AMP-activated protein kinase (AMPK) [46] and target of rapamycin (TOR) [47], which play key, often mutually inhibitory, roles. If their activities are chronically dysregulated by metabolic abnormalities and energy insufficiencies in ME/CFS cells, they may be unable to respond to additional energy demand. This is supported by reports of AMPK in muscle cells from people with ME/CFS being unresponsive to stimulation by contraction-induced ATP depletion [43,48]. Such insensitivity could result from AMPK already being in an activated state in these cells, or to its inhibition by chronically hyperactivated TOR complex 1 (TORC1). Elevated TORC1 activity was recently observed in ME/CFS cells (lymphoblasts) and this was accompanied by inefficient mitochondrial ATP synthesis and abnormally high and presumably compensatory expression of mitochondrial proteins [41]. Elevated expression of mitochondrial proteins has also been found in other studies of patient saliva, lymphocytes, and platelets [41,49–51]. Furthermore, reduced creatine kinase (CK) levels in the serum of people with ME/CFS may suggest reduced cellular CK presence [15], which could contribute to inefficient ATP synthesis given the enzyme's roles in ATP homeostasis [52]. Despite the breadth of sample types tested that suggest dysregulated energy metabolism (serum, urine, feces, muscle, B cells, lymphoblasts), it remains to be directly demonstrated that the perturbation of the associated stress-sensing pathways is systemic and this should be an area of future investigation.

As noted above, glycolytic catabolism of glucose is a major supplier of acetyl coenzyme A (CoA) to the TCA cycle, and this can be assayed in intact cells by measuring the rate of acidification of the medium by cells provided with glucose as a substrate. This has been reported recently using natural killer (NK) cells from a small sample of six patients and six healthy controls [53]. Although the authors found no differences in aerobic respiration rates, they did observe a reduced glycolytic reserve in the ME/CFS cells. The glycolytic reserve is a measure of the excess capacity of glycolysis to meet cellular ATP demands when mitochondrial ATP synthesis by oxidative phosphorylation is inhibited. This small study reported individual O_2 consumption and extracellular acidification rates that were either negative or very small positive values, placing them at the threshold of reliable detection. This caveat also applies to heterogeneous peripheral blood mononuclear cell (PBMC) populations, which are commonly used for extracellular flux respirometry and have been previously employed in ME/CFS work [45]. This difficulty arises because peripheral blood lymphocytes are metabolically quiescent [54] and this not only makes metabolic rate assays technically difficult, but it may obscure differences in metabolism that would be apparent in actively metabolizing cells.

2.3. A Shift Towards Lipid Metabolism

The TCA cycle can also be provided with acetyl CoA produced by fatty acid beta-oxidation when glucose-derived sources are insufficient [55]. If the provision of substrate to the TCA cycle is indeed deficient in ME/CFS as previously suggested [31,39,40], a role for the compensatory elevation of fatty acid metabolism could be implicated in the disorder [41]. Fatty acid synthesis and beta-oxidation are regulated by both AMPK [56] and TORC1 [57]. AMPK promotes fatty acid beta-oxidation when activated by elevated ATP demand and promotes fatty acid biosynthesis when inactive, while TORC1 exerts the opposite effects. AMPK and TORC1 regulate each other in a complex reciprocal feedback network [58], so that it is also possible for scenarios to arise where both are simultaneously activated [59]. This raises the question: If both AMPK [43,48] and TORC1 [41] activities are elevated in ME/CFS cells, would we expect the rates of fatty acid catabolism to be increased or decreased? An answer may be found within the specific mechanisms of regulatory action of these pathways in lipid homeostasis. Activation of TORC1 promotes fatty acid biosynthesis by elevating the expression of gene products including acetyl-CoA carboxylase (ACC) through the upregulation of transcription factors Sterol Regulatory Element Binding Proteins 1 and 2 (SREBP-1 and SREBP-2) [60]. ACC activity results in an accumulation of malonyl CoA, which is a potent inhibitor of the mitochondrial import of fatty acids for beta oxidation. ACC, however, is a primary regulatory target of AMPK and is inactivated by phosphorylation when AMPK is activated [61]. In this way, the concurrent activation of AMPK and TORC1, if it does indeed occur in ME/CFS cells, may allow AMPK to constrain the effects of TORC1's upregulation of lipid-biosynthesis and downregulation of beta-oxidation. At the same time, both AMPK and TORC1 directly or indirectly induce the expression of diverse mitochondrial proteins, including those involved in fatty acid beta oxidation. The combined effects could be a steady state in which the cells have increased their use of beta oxidation relative to glycolysis as a supplier of acetyl CoA to the TCA cycle. Fatty acid oxidation is normally upregulated as a supplementary energy pathway during fasting or exercise as a response to reduced blood glucose concentration [62]. An increased reliance on fatty acid oxidation, even at rest, may therefore also contribute to the inability for people with ME/CFS to meet the elevated energy demands imposed by exertion. Such a switch to lipid oxidation can be mediated by elevated inflammation [63] and in combination with the pathological inflammation seen in patients [64] could be evidence of a pathological interaction between inflammation and metabolism in ME/CFS.

3. Disturbed Immunity, Signaling, and Inflammatory Pathways

3.1. NK Cells

The function of the immune system has been a focus of ME/CFS research for many years. Evidence for immune dysfunction in ME/CFS has largely been sought through study of NK cells, which are cytotoxic immune cells with roles in both the innate and adaptive immune responses. Multiple groups have reported reduced NK cell cytotoxicity or numbers [65–69] combined with concordant alterations to functional surface markers [70–72]. Conversely, other groups have reported increased cytotoxicity in combination with alterations to functional surface markers. For example, perforin, a glycoprotein used as a functional indicator of NK cell cytotoxicity due to its roles in NK cell mediated lysis [73,74], has been reported as upregulated [71], downregulated [65], or, along with every other assessed phenotypic parameter, unaltered in people with ME/CFS [75]. A recent, rigorous large-scale biobank study also found no significant differences in NK cell numbers, subtype composition, or assessed functional parameters [76]. In summation, NK research remains an area of active interest, but in light of conflicting findings, the role of NK cells in the disorder is still not well understood.

3.2. Calcium Signaling

Calcium signaling is crucial to immune cell function [77] and is tied to the mitochondria and endoplasmic reticulum as hubs of regulatory control and calcium storage [78]. Therefore, a disturbance to calcium signaling could contribute to pathological outcomes involving immune system or bioenergetic dysfunction, both of which have been implicated in ME/CFS. In addition to the previous evidence of altered surface proteins on NK cells from ME/CFS patients, a reduction in the expression of transient receptor potential melastatin 3 (TRPM3) calcium ion channels [79] has been reported in a subpopulation of ME/CFS NK cells [80–82]. The reason for the reduced expression of TRPM3 in these cells is unknown, but in other cell types, expression of TRPM3 is repressed by the activity of microRNA-204 (miR-204), encoded by intron 6 of the *TRPM3* gene [83]. However, miR-204 is not amongst the microRNAs whose expression is reportedly altered in ME/CFS patients [84].

Reduced expression of TRPM3 receptors would be expected to cause a reduction in Ca^{2+} responses to pregnenolone sulfate (PregS), a specific activating ligand for TRPM3 channels. However, the opposite was observed when Ca^{2+} levels were assayed by flow cytometry using Indo1, a Ca^{2+}-sensitive fluorescent dye in the TRPM3-depleted NK cells [80]. Subsequent studies using whole cell patch clamping, however, have reported a loss of PregS-stimulated Ca^{2+} responses [81,82].

3.3. Links to Mitochondrial Dysfunction

Cytosolic Ca^{2+} is a key element in the cell's extensive homeostatic networks, such that Ca^{2+} signals are regulated by and play regulatory roles in multiple processes in cells, including mitochondrial respiratory activity [85] as well as mitochondrial protein import [86] and the ion transport activity of TRPM3 itself [87], both of which are activated by Ca^{2+}-calmodulin. The mitochondria serve as both a source and a sink for cytosolic Ca^{2+} and the mitochondria interact closely with the endoplasmic reticulum at sites that mediate the exchange of lipids and Ca^{2+} signals [88]. The mitochondria thus form a hub of interaction between Ca^{2+} and other molecular signals that regulate mitochondrial function, such as AMPK and TORC1 activity. In NK cells specifically, where the calcium-signaling defect has been reported, TORC1 activity is required for both effector function and cytokine production [89–91] and it has been suggested that the development of NK cell antiviral memory is influenced by mitochondrial function [92]. The reports of altered NK effector function in ME/CFS could therefore also be related to abnormal mitochondrial function and TOR signaling. Disrupted intracellular signaling and mitochondrial function in ME/CFS have also been previously linked through myriad other pathways provoked by immune-inflammation and oxidative stress [93].

3.4. Inflammation

Chronic system-wide inflammation is thought to be central to ME/CFS in the clinical setting as it is associated with symptom severity [64], but the evidence demonstrating a role for specific pro-inflammatory cytokines is inconsistent. While there are indeed reports of the elevation of various pro-inflammatory cytokines in ME/CFS [33,71,94–99], which would tie in with the chronic inflammation in the clinical setting, these findings contrast with reports of reduced expression of pro-inflammatory agents, such as interleukin-8 or transforming growth factor-beta1 [100,101]. Consequently, evidence for the specific directional shift of individual cytokines has been previously summarized as largely inconsistent [102]. Despite these issues, cytokine expression has been previously associated with ME/CFS disease duration and may have value in aiding the stratification of patient cohorts [33,94]. One group has shown that a cohort of ME/CFS patients with leaky gut syndrome as a comorbidity may undergo significant symptom remission when the IgM and IgA immune responses are attenuated by treatment with anti-inflammatory and antioxidant medications [103,104]. This finding has contributed towards the potential link between gut hyperpermeability and inflammation in ME/CFS. Therefore, it is likely that dysregulated chronic inflammatory action by the immune system is an aspect of ME/CFS, despite inconsistent reports.

3.5. Autoimmunity

Autoimmunity in the condition is an area that remains little researched, and has been most recently summarized and presented as a hypothetical model for ME/CFS, with some ties to gut dysbiosis and aberrant metabolism [105]. Other autoimmune models for ME/CFS have been previously based on rituximab's role in B cell depletion as a possible therapeutic based on the promising outcomes of earlier studies [106,107]. This would be concordant with other reports of elevated naïve and transitional B cells in patients, which may suggest autoimmune tendencies [108]. However, a role for such B cell-mediated autoimmunity in the disorder is now challenged by the negative outcome of the more recent rituximab phase III clinical trial [109], which refutes the previous rituximab work. This may also indicate that autoimmunity only applies as a key pathomechanism in a small subset of patients who respond positively to rituximab treatment [110]. Other direct lines of evidence for autoimmune behavior in the disorder come from elevated autoantibody levels in sera [111], supported by the improvement of symptoms following autoantibody removal treatment [112], and abnormal IgM immune recognition of both microbial and human heat shock protein 60 in a subset of patients [113] or against phosphatidylinositol [114], despite the absence of an infective pathogen in each case.

4. Implications of Altered Gut Microbiota and Physiology

A disturbed gut microbiota [12,115–121] has been proposed to play a role in ME/CFS. This is accompanied by physiological gut abnormalities, such as impaired motility [122], elevated intestinal wall permeability [103,104,123,124], and IBS comorbidity [31,125,126], which has been proposed to comprise part of a ME/CFS subtype [30]. The implications of these disturbances could be far-reaching, since the intestinal microbiota both regulates [127,128] and is regulated by [129,130] the immune system. Additionally, many studies have demonstrated a link between the gut microbiota and host mitochondrial function or metabolism, with disturbances in one resulting in subsequent dysfunction in the other [131–136].

4.1. The Gut Microbiota and Metabolism

People with ME/CFS have been reported to present with gut microbiota disturbances and either metabolite variation [31,118] or mitochondrial dysfunction [116] and the two conditions could be linked. Sheedy et al. observed elevated Gram positive intestinal bacteria, which produce lactic acid that may lower the gut pH and lead to elevated gut permeability [137]. Furthermore, the translocation of these enteric lactic acid products into the bloodstream could contribute to the elevated lactate reported in the cerebrospinal fluid of ME/CFS patients [138–140] and in the blood of a subgroup of patients [141]. This contrasts with reports of reduced blood lactate as measured by H-NMR metabolomics [39], which suggests that lactic acidosis may only affect a subgroup of patients. If IBS comorbidity accompanied by gut dysbiosis and hyperpermeability is indeed a subtype of ME/CFS, the translocation of lactic acid produced by abnormally enriched Gram positive enteric bacteria in the affected individuals, rather than excessive production by the host metabolism, could explain this inconsistency.

4.2. Pathological Interactions between Gut Hyperpermeability and the Mitochondria

Broader implications for the immune system and mitochondrial function may come from reports of increased translocation of immunogenic bacterial secretions from the gut into the bloodstream, which in ME/CFS may be mediated by intestinal wall hyperpermeability in patients affected with IBS [104,142]. For example, the generation of excess free radicals, which occurs in the mitochondria [143], has been proposed to form part of a microbial defense mechanism [144–146], with enteric species, such as *Escherichia coli*, highly susceptible to the bactericidal properties of free radical derived reactive nitrogen species (RNS) [147]. Excess free radical generation not only results in the formation of RNS but also reactive oxygen species (ROS), whose production may be elevated in ME/CFS given the many reports of elevated oxidative stress in the disorder [148–153]. Therefore, excessive free radical generation as such an antimicrobial response to circulating antagonists of enteric origin could provide one explanation for the reports of elevated oxidative stress in the disorder. Such a response may indeed be elicited by the ordinarily commensal Gram negative bacteria *E. coli*, which, while also known to target the mitochondria by the secretion of other toxins [154,155], secretes immunogenic lipopolysaccharide (LPS). This endotoxin secretion is normally suppressed by the host microbiota at large [131], however, the composition of the host microbiota is reportedly altered in cases of ME/CFS [12,115–121]. Such a disturbance to the normal LPS secretion-suppressing host microbiota in ME/CFS and the presence of gut hyperpermeability may therefore not only lead to the synergistic amplification of bacterial toxin translocation into the blood and the consequent activation of inflammatory pathways [104,142], but may also expose body-wide mitochondria to circulating virulent factors produced by Gram negative antagonists, such as *E.coli*. This is supported by the increase in *E. coli* gut colonization reported in cases of IBS [156], which, again, can be an ME/CFS comorbidity.

4.3. The Gut–Brain Axis: Autonomic and Hormonal Dysregulation

Physiological stress, considered one predisposing factor for ME/CFS [157], has been suggested to play a role in modifying the gut microbiota in such a way that would reduce the numbers of *Bifidobacterium* and *Lactobacillus*, two genera responsible for the suppression of LPS-secreting commensal bacteria and has been implicated in this way in ME/CFS [158,159]. While the translocation of immunogenic LPS into the bloodstream is generally associated with body-wide inflammation [160,161], it may also lead to the elevation of proinflammatory elements and the stress hormone cortisol in the brain [162]. The transduction of immunogenic pathogen signals is but one aspect of the gut–brain axis, so it is pertinent to address the potential for broader gut-brain driven [163,164] or autonomic nervous dysregulation that may play a part in the disorder. Indeed, there is some evidence to support such dysregulation associated with vasomotor abnormalities [165] or mitochondrial Coenzyme Q10 deficiency associated with cardiovascular lesions [166]. There are relevant, respectively, to the ME/CFS comorbidity POTS, which likely involves vasomotor dysfunction [167], or to the cardinal symptom of chronic fatigue. Further, the linkage of cortisol-driven stress responses to the gut through the hypothalamic-pituitary-adrenal (HPA) axis [168] could be dysfunctional in ME/CFS due to the hypocortisolism previously suggested to play a role in the condition [169,170]. This possibility could weave another perturbed regulatory loop into the system, which may aid in perpetuating an altered homeostasis. This has been previously reviewed at length [171].

5. Multi-System Pathological Interactions

5.1. Exposure to Stressors and the Theoretical Homeostatic Perpetuation of a Disease State

The reported disturbances to ME/CFS metabolism have been linked to chronic activation of emergency cell survival mechanisms to cope with adverse conditions [7]. These adverse conditions could include energy stress, inflammation, HPA axis dysregulation, or pathogen exposure. They elicit a conserved homeostatic cell danger response [172] that could result in the cell shifting to an alternative resting steady state and contribute to ME/CFS pathology [34]. An alternative explanation would involve chronic ongoing exposure of cells to a causative insult. However, chronic pathogen exposure as the precipitating factor for such a response in ME/CFS seems unlikely, as theories of viral persistence have been thoroughly investigated and the evidence for chronic viral infection in ME/CFS is inconsistent [173].

Another feature of ME/CFS is the characteristic symptom heterogeneity. Patient histories suggest that the initial insult eliciting the shift to the ME/CFS state differs between individuals and so may dysregulate the underlying cellular stress signaling pathways in different ways. This could contribute to inconsistencies between various studies and highlights the need for sensitive diagnostics and patient stratification into recognizably different categories.

No matter the initial insult, each of the aforementioned possibilities can involve the interaction between chronic inflammation and immunological and mitochondrial dysfunction [99,174,175]. This is similar to theories previously presented by others pertaining to dysregulated homeostatic feedback loops [34]. Faced with a new challenge, such as the re-emergence of a dormant pathogen, over-exertion, or other stress depending on the tolerance of the individual, the affected pathways could again be perturbed, triggering a molecular cascade during bouts of PEM. In some patients, this may mimic the response to a recurrent infection regardless of whether the new trigger is pathogen-driven. Symptom flare-ups characteristic of ME/CFS may therefore result from antagonization of just one of the underlying nodes of a multi-system pathological web and a symptomatic body-wide cascade ensues.

For example, the elevated oxidative stress reported in the disorder [148–153] may be entangled with perturbed immune-inflammatory pathways [175–178], gut inflammation [158], and dysfunctional mitochondria. This may be exacerbated by other disturbances, such as the reported reduction in CK levels [15], which can lead to the absence of CK-mediated ROS suppression [179]. This raises the possibility of a vicious cycle of immunodysregulation and gut dysbiosis accompanied by poor physiological gut function [122] that contribute to the perpetuation of a chronic bowel disease state. Such an altered state could interact with the previously suggested HPA dysregulation [34] and contribute to the perpetuation of an alternative resting homeostasis.

5.2. Identifying Underlying Mechanisms

The earlier sections of this review have discussed the evidence for dysregulated biological mechanisms in ME/CFS patients at the molecular, cellular, tissue, organ, and whole body levels. These changes are summarized in Table 1 and together provide insights into potential underlying disease mechanisms.

Based on current biomedical literature, perturbations to the various systems listed in Table 1 are implicated in the underlying pathological mechanisms in ME/CFS. These phenomena are correlated clinically in that they appear in people with the disorder. However, the causal links between them are unknown and cannot be discerned purely on the basis of clinical correlation. There are many scenarios where more than one of the affected systems may exert pathological effects on another and vice versa. This complex and often reciprocal regulatory cross-talk between systems makes it difficult to distinguish cause from effect, so there is great need for the potential causal relationships to be addressed directly using appropriate experimental models.

Table 1. Brief summary of relevant reports contributing towards the biomedical basis of ME/CFS.

Area of Study	Brief Summary of Key Reports in ME/CFS
Metabolomics	• Multiple reports of disturbed amino acid metabolism [6,38–40,180]. • Dysregulated lipid metabolism [7,13,31,39], possible glycolysis impairment [39], possible PDH impairment [40], urea cycle dysregulation [6,38]. • Overall: TCA cycle substrate provision deficiency and reliance on alternative fuel sources.
Mitochondrial function	• Reduced [9] vs. elevated steady-state ATP levels [42,44,48] but resting ATP synthesis rates are normal [41,45]. • Complex V inefficient and compensated for by upregulation of supporting pathways [41].
Muscle activity	• Unresponsive AMPK and reduced glucose [43,48,141] and oxygen uptake [181].
Natural killer cells	• Overall inconsistent evidence—role mostly unknown [65–72].
Calcium signaling	• Evidence for impaired TRPM3 function [81,82].
Inflammation and cytokines	• Inconsistent molecular evidence [102,182], yet is likely to play a role based on clinical presentation and the many reported disturbances in related systems.
Autoimmunity	• Little researched, but proposed to form a subtype comorbid with IBS [114]. • Role for B cell-mediated autoimmunity challenged by negative outcome of rituximab trial [106,109,110].
B cells	• Linked to mitochondrial disturbances, subset proportions may vary [41,45,183].
Gut microbiota and physiology	• Widely reported disturbances to the gut microbiota [12,103,115–117,119,120,184] and gut hyperpermeability [103,123,124].
Autonomic and hormonal dysregulation	• Vasomotor abnormalities [165,185], hypocortisolism [169,170], broad HPA axis disturbance [186,187].

For example, the potential impact of gut hyperpermeability on body-wide mitochondrial function has been outlined in Section 4.2. However, the reverse may also take place. The differentiation, proliferation, and function of intestinal epithelial cells is known to depend upon normal mitochondrial function, with mitochondrial dysfunction resulting in subsequent hyperpermeability of the intestinal wall [188–190]. Therefore, it is impossible to distinguish cause from effect in this case with correlations alone. Similarly, changes in metabolite levels in ME/CFS have been associated with both IBS comorbidity [31] and alterations to intestinal flora composition [118]. However, it has not been experimentally shown whether the IBS is caused by host metabolic dysfunction or irregular metabolite production and excretion by an altered gut microbiota, or if the gut microflora and metabolic abnormalities are caused by the IBS.

The influence of the mitochondria upon the function of the immune system has similar implications. The mitochondria can partake in activation or suppression of inflammation indirectly by regulating autophagy, which in turn bears downstream regulatory consequences for the activation of inflammation [191]. Mitochondria also regulate elements of the innate immune system by the release of immunogenic ligands [178] and are important for immune cell effector function due to their classical roles in energy production and metabolism. Furthermore, immunological dysfunction is common in conditions which are primarily mitochondrial diseases [192]. This is an important consideration with regard to the gut microbiota since it, in turn, influences and is influenced by the function of the immune system and [128,163,193,194] immune cell population composition [195]. Therefore, changes to any one of the mitochondria, immune system, or gut may dysregulate the others, again emphasizing the importance of future research addressing cause–effect relationships.

6. Conclusions

ME/CFS is a heterogeneous condition that may encompass scenarios where uncertain, and possibly varying, underlying insults trigger body-wide molecular and cellular perturbations perpetuated by an alternative stable homeostatic states. Diagnostic advancement and the development of tools which objectively and accurately phenotype patients is therefore paramount for the development of mechanistic insight and effective therapeutics.

It is likely that the inflammation and immune dysfunction classically studied in ME/CFS are entangled with dysfunctional energetics, gut health, or autonomic and adrenal dysregulation. The evidence for metabolic and mitochondrial dysfunction indicates inefficient respiration, impaired provision of TCA cycle substrate, and metabolic shifts towards the utilization of alternative metabolites. Immune effector cell dysfunction, chronic inflammation, defective signaling, and elevated oxidative stress may interact with not only the dysfunctional energetics but also with abnormal gut physiology and microbiota composition. These effects on the gut may also tie back to mitochondrial function and vice versa. The reciprocal interactions between these affected systems and the varied clinical presentation of relevant symptoms between individuals make it difficult to postulate cause–effect relationships with confidence. Furthermore, while disturbances to this range of interconnected systems across the body have been demonstrated, in some cases concurrently, this body of research has historically relied upon correlations, which creates the urgent need for research utilizing direct experimental investigation of cause–effect relationships.

Author Contributions: D.M., writing—original draft preparation and editing; S.J.A. and P.R.F., writing—review and editing.

Funding: D.M. was the recipient of a La Trobe University Postgraduate Scholarship and Australian Government Research Training Program Fees Offset. This work was supported by generous patient donations and grants from the Judith Jane Mason & Harold Stannett Williams Memorial Foundation (Grant IDs: MAS2016F063, MAS2018F00026) and the McCusker Charitable Foundation.

Conflicts of Interest: The authors declare no conflict of interest.

References

1. Sharpe, M.C.; Archard, L.C.; Banatvala, J.E.; Borysiewicz, L.K.; Clare, A.W.; David, A.; Edwards, R.H.; Hawton, K.E.; Lambert, H.P.; Lane, R.J.; et al. A report—Chronic fatigue syndrome: Guidelines for research. *J. R. Soc. Med.* **1991**, *84*, 118–121. [CrossRef] [PubMed]
2. Fukuda, K.; Straus, S.E.; Hickie, I.; Sharpe, M.C.; Dobbins, J.G.; Komaroff, A. The chronic fatigue syndrome: A comprehensive approach to its definition and study. International Chronic Fatigue Syndrome Study Group. *Ann. Intern. Med.* **1994**, *121*, 953–959. [CrossRef] [PubMed]
3. Carruthers, B.M.; Jain, A.K.; De Meirleir, K.L.; Peterson, D.L.; Klimas, N.G.; Lerner, A.M.; Bested, A.C.; Flor-Henry, P.; Joshi, P.; Powles, A.C.; et al. Myalgic Encephalomyelitis/Chronic Fatigue Syndrome: Clinical Working Case Definition, Diagnostic and Treatment Protocols. *J. Chron. Fatigue Syndr.* **2003**, *11*, 7–36. [CrossRef]
4. Carruthers, B.M.; van de Sande, M.I.; De Meirleir, K.L.; Klimas, N.G.; Broderick, G.; Mitchell, T.; Staines, D.; Powles, A.C.; Speight, N.; Vallings, R.; et al. Myalgic encephalomyelitis: International Consensus Criteria. *J. Intern. Med.* **2011**, *270*, 327–338. [CrossRef] [PubMed]

5. Lidbury, B.A.; Kita, B.; Lewis, D.P.; Hayward, S.; Ludlow, H.; Hedger, M.P.; de Kretser, D.M. Activin B is a novel biomarker for chronic fatigue syndrome/myalgic encephalomyelitis (CFS/ME) diagnosis: A cross sectional study. *J. Transl. Med.* **2017**, *15*, 60. [CrossRef] [PubMed]
6. Yamano, E.; Sugimoto, M.; Hirayama, A.; Kume, S.; Yamato, M.; Jin, G.; Tajima, S.; Goda, N.; Iwai, K.; Fukuda, S.; et al. Index markers of chronic fatigue syndrome with dysfunction of TCA and urea cycles. *Sci. Rep.* **2016**, *6*, 34990. [CrossRef] [PubMed]
7. Naviaux, R.K.; Naviaux, J.C.; Li, K.; Bright, A.T.; Alaynick, W.A.; Wang, L.; Baxter, A.; Nathan, N.; Anderson, W.; Gordon, E. Metabolic features of chronic fatigue syndrome. *Proc. Natl. Acad. Sci. USA* **2016**, *113*, E5472–E5480. [CrossRef] [PubMed]
8. Brenu, E.W.; Ashton, K.J.; van Driel, M.; Staines, D.R.; Peterson, D.; Atkinson, G.M.; Marshall-Gradisnik, S.M. Cytotoxic lymphocyte microRNAs as prospective biomarkers for Chronic Fatigue Syndrome/Myalgic Encephalomyelitis. *J. Affect. Disord.* **2012**, *141*, 261–269. [CrossRef]
9. Myhill, S.; Booth, N.E.; McLaren-Howard, J. Chronic fatigue syndrome and mitochondrial dysfunction. *Int. J. Clin. Exp. Med.* **2009**, *2*, 1–16.
10. Booth, N.E.; Myhill, S.; McLaren-Howard, J. Mitochondrial dysfunction and the pathophysiology of Myalgic Encephalomyelitis/Chronic Fatigue Syndrome (ME/CFS). *Int. J. Clin. Exp. Med.* **2012**, *5*, 208–220.
11. Myhill, S.; Booth, N.E.; McLaren-Howard, J. Targeting mitochondrial dysfunction in the treatment of Myalgic Encephalomyelitis/Chronic Fatigue Syndrome (ME/CFS)-a clinical audit. *Int. J. Clin. Exp. Med.* **2013**, *6*, 1–15.
12. Giloteaux, L.; Goodrich, J.K.; Walters, W.A.; Levine, S.M.; Ley, R.E.; Hanson, M.R. Reduced diversity and altered composition of the gut microbiome in individuals with myalgic encephalomyelitis/chronic fatigue syndrome. *Microbiome* **2016**, *4*, 30. [CrossRef]
13. Germain, A.; Ruppert, D.; Levine, S.M.; Hanson, M.R. Metabolic profiling of a myalgic encephalomyelitis/chronic fatigue syndrome discovery cohort reveals disturbances in fatty acid and lipid metabolism. *Mol. Biosyst.* **2017**, *13*, 371–379. [CrossRef] [PubMed]
14. Esfandyarpour, R.; Kashi, A.; Nemat-Gorgani, M.; Wilhelmy, J.; Davis, R.W. A nanoelectronics-blood-based diagnostic biomarker for myalgic encephalomyelitis/chronic fatigue syndrome (ME/CFS). *Proc. Natl. Acad. Sci. USA* **2019**. [CrossRef]
15. Nacul, L.; de Barros, B.; Kingdon, C.C.; Cliff, J.M.; Clark, T.G.; Mudie, K.; Dockrell, H.M.; Lacerda, E.M. Evidence of Clinical Pathology Abnormalities in People with Myalgic Encephalomyelitis/Chronic Fatigue Syndrome (ME/CFS) from an Analytic Cross-Sectional Study. *Diagnostics* **2019**, *9*, 41. [CrossRef]
16. Nacul, L.C.; Mudie, K.; Kingdon, C.C.; Clark, T.G.; Lacerda, E.M. Hand Grip Strength as a Clinical Biomarker for ME/CFS and Disease Severity. *Front. Neurol.* **2018**, *9*, 992. [CrossRef]
17. DeLuca, J.; Johnson, S.K.; Ellis, S.P.; Natelson, B.H. Sudden vs gradual onset of chronic fatigue syndrome differentiates individuals on cognitive and psychiatric measures. *J. Psychiatr. Res.* **1997**, *31*, 83–90. [CrossRef]
18. Lane, R.J.; Barrett, M.C.; Taylor, D.J.; Kemp, G.J.; Lodi, R. Heterogeneity in chronic fatigue syndrome: Evidence from magnetic resonance spectroscopy of muscle. *Neuromuscul. Disord.* **1998**, *8*, 204–209. [CrossRef]
19. Afari, N.; Buchwald, D. Chronic fatigue syndrome: A review. *Am. J. Psychiatry* **2003**, *160*, 221–236. [CrossRef]
20. Jason, L.A.; Corradi, K.; Torres-Harding, S.; Taylor, R.R.; King, C. Chronic fatigue syndrome: The need for subtypes. *Neuropsychol. Rev.* **2005**, *15*, 29–58. [CrossRef]
21. Morris, G.; Maes, M. Case definitions and diagnostic criteria for Myalgic Encephalomyelitis and Chronic fatigue Syndrome: From clinical-consensus to evidence-based case definitions. *Neuroendocrinol. Lett.* **2013**, *34*, 185–199. [PubMed]
22. Hardcastle, S.L.; Brenu, E.W.; Johnston, S.; Nguyen, T.; Huth, T.; Ramos, S.; Staines, D.; Marshall-Gradisnik, S. Longitudinal analysis of immune abnormalities in varying severities of Chronic Fatigue Syndrome/Myalgic Encephalomyelitis patients. *J. Transl. Med.* **2015**, *13*, 299. [CrossRef] [PubMed]
23. Maclachlan, L.; Watson, S.; Gallagher, P.; Finkelmeyer, A.; Jason, L.A.; Sunnquist, M.; Newton, J.L. Are current chronic fatigue syndrome criteria diagnosing different disease phenotypes? *PLoS ONE* **2017**, *12*, e0186885. [CrossRef] [PubMed]
24. Kerr, J.R.; Petty, R.; Burke, B.; Gough, J.; Fear, D.; Sinclair, L.I.; Mattey, D.L.; Richards, S.C.; Montgomery, J.; Baldwin, D.A.; et al. Gene expression subtypes in patients with chronic fatigue syndrome/myalgic encephalomyelitis. *J. Infect. Dis.* **2008**, *197*, 1171–1184. [CrossRef] [PubMed]

25. Kerr, J.R.; Burke, B.; Petty, R.; Gough, J.; Fear, D.; Mattey, D.L.; Axford, J.S.; Dalgleish, A.G.; Nutt, D.J. Seven genomic subtypes of chronic fatigue syndrome/myalgic encephalomyelitis: A detailed analysis of gene networks and clinical phenotypes. *J. Clin. Pathol.* **2008**, *61*, 730–739. [CrossRef] [PubMed]
26. Zhang, L.; Gough, J.; Christmas, D.; Mattey, D.L.; Richards, S.C.; Main, J.; Enlander, D.; Honeybourne, D.; Ayres, J.G.; Nutt, D.J.; et al. Microbial infections in eight genomic subtypes of chronic fatigue syndrome/myalgic encephalomyelitis. *J. Clin. Pathol.* **2010**, *63*, 156–164. [CrossRef] [PubMed]
27. Light, K.C.; Agarwal, N.; Iacob, E.; White, A.T.; Kinney, A.Y.; VanHaitsma, T.A.; Aizad, H.; Hughen, R.W.; Bateman, L.; Light, A.R. Differing leukocyte gene expression profiles associated with fatigue in patients with prostate cancer versus chronic fatigue syndrome. *Psychoneuroendocrinology* **2013**, *38*, 2983–2995. [CrossRef]
28. De Vega, W.C.; Erdman, L.; Vernon, S.D.; Goldenberg, A.; McGowan, P.O. Integration of DNA methylation & health scores identifies subtypes in myalgic encephalomyelitis/chronic fatigue syndrome. *Epigenomics* **2018**, *10*, 539–557. [CrossRef]
29. Jason, L.A.; Boulton, A.; Porter, N.S.; Jessen, T.; Njoku, M.G.; Friedberg, F. Classification of myalgic encephalomyelitis/chronic fatigue syndrome by types of fatigue. *Behav. Med.* **2010**, *36*, 24–31. [CrossRef]
30. Maes, M.; Leunis, J.C.; Geffard, M.; Berk, M. Evidence for the existence of Myalgic Encephalomyelitis/Chronic Fatigue Syndrome (ME/CFS) with and without abdominal discomfort (irritable bowel) syndrome. *Neuroendocrinol. Lett.* **2014**, *35*, 445–453.
31. Nagy-Szakal, D.; Barupal, D.K.; Lee, B.; Che, X.; Williams, B.L.; Kahn, E.J.R.; Ukaigwe, J.E.; Bateman, L.; Klimas, N.G.; Komaroff, A.L.; et al. Insights into myalgic encephalomyelitis/chronic fatigue syndrome phenotypes through comprehensive metabolomics. *Sci. Rep.* **2018**, *8*, 10056. [CrossRef]
32. Richardson, A.M.; Lewis, D.P.; Kita, B.; Ludlow, H.; Groome, N.P.; Hedger, M.P.; de Kretser, D.M.; Lidbury, B.A. Weighting of orthostatic intolerance time measurements with standing difficulty score stratifies ME/CFS symptom severity and analyte detection. *J. Transl. Med.* **2018**, *16*, 97. [CrossRef]
33. Russell, L.; Broderick, G.; Taylor, R.; Fernandes, H.; Harvey, J.; Barnes, Z.; Smylie, A.; Collado, F.; Balbin, E.G.; Katz, B.Z.; et al. Illness progression in chronic fatigue syndrome: A shifting immune baseline. *BMC Immunol.* **2016**, *17*, 3. [CrossRef]
34. Craddock, T.J.; Fritsch, P.; Rice, M.A., Jr.; del Rosario, R.M.; Miller, D.B.; Fletcher, M.A.; Klimas, N.G.; Broderick, G. A role for homeostatic drive in the perpetuation of complex chronic illness: Gulf War Illness and chronic fatigue syndrome. *PLoS ONE* **2014**, *9*, e84839. [CrossRef]
35. Behan, W.M.; More, I.A.; Behan, P.O. Mitochondrial abnormalities in the postviral fatigue syndrome. *Acta Neuropathol.* **1991**, *83*, 61–65. [CrossRef]
36. Barnes, P.R.; Taylor, D.J.; Kemp, G.J.; Radda, G.K. Skeletal muscle bioenergetics in the chronic fatigue syndrome. *J. Neurol. Neurosurg. Psychiatry* **1993**, *56*, 679–683. [CrossRef]
37. McCully, K.K.; Natelson, B.H.; Iotti, S.; Sisto, S.; Leigh, J.S., Jr. Reduced oxidative muscle metabolism in chronic fatigue syndrome. *Muscle Nerve* **1996**, *19*, 621–625. [CrossRef]
38. Armstrong, C.W.; McGregor, N.R.; Sheedy, J.R.; Buttfield, I.; Butt, H.L.; Gooley, P.R. NMR metabolic profiling of serum identifies amino acid disturbances in chronic fatigue syndrome. *Clin. Chim. Acta* **2012**, *413*, 1525–1531. [CrossRef]
39. Armstrong, C.W.; McGregor, N.R.; Lewis, D.; Butt, H.; Gooley, P.R. Metabolic profiling reveals anomalous energy metabolism and oxidative stress pathways in chronic fatigue syndrome patients. *Metabolomics* **2015**, *11*, 1626–1639. [CrossRef]
40. Fluge, O.; Mella, O.; Bruland, O.; Risa, K.; Dyrstad, S.E.; Alme, K.; Rekeland, I.G.; Sapkota, D.; Rosland, G.V.; Fossa, A.; et al. Metabolic profiling indicates impaired pyruvate dehydrogenase function in myalgic encephalopathy/chronic fatigue syndrome. *JCI Insight* **2016**, *1*, e89376. [CrossRef]
41. Missailidis, D.; Annesley, S.J.; Allan, C.Y.; Sanislav, O.; Lidbury, B.A.; Lewis, D.P.; Fisher, P.R. An isolated Complex V defect and dysregulated mitochondrial function in immortalized lymphocytes from ME/CFS patients. **2019**. submitted.
42. Castro-Marrero, J.; Cordero, M.D.; Saez-Francas, N.; Jimenez-Gutierrez, C.; Aguilar-Montilla, F.J.; Aliste, L.; Alegre-Martin, J. Could mitochondrial dysfunction be a differentiating marker between chronic fatigue syndrome and fibromyalgia? *Antioxid. Redox Signal.* **2013**, *19*, 1855–1860. [CrossRef] [PubMed]
43. Brown, A.E.; Dibnah, B.; Fisher, E.; Newton, J.L.; Walker, M. Pharmacological activation of AMPK and glucose uptake in cultured human skeletal muscle cells from patients with ME/CFS. *Biosci. Rep.* **2018**, *38*. [CrossRef] [PubMed]

44. Lawson, N.; Hsieh, C.H.; March, D.; Wang, X. Elevated Energy Production in Chronic Fatigue Syndrome Patients. *J. Nat. Sci.* **2016**, *2*, e221.
45. Tomas, C.; Brown, A.; Strassheim, V.; Elson, J.L.; Newton, J.; Manning, P. Cellular bioenergetics is impaired in patients with chronic fatigue syndrome. *PLoS ONE* **2017**, *12*, e0186802. [CrossRef] [PubMed]
46. Hardie, D.G.; Carling, D. The AMP-activated protein kinase-fuel gauge of the mammalian cell? *Eur. J. Biochem.* **1997**, *246*, 259–273. [CrossRef]
47. Ma, X.M.; Blenis, J. Molecular mechanisms of mTOR-mediated translational control. *Nat. Rev. Mol. Cell Biol.* **2009**, *10*, 307–318. [CrossRef]
48. Brown, A.E.; Jones, D.E.; Walker, M.; Newton, J.L. Abnormalities of AMPK activation and glucose uptake in cultured skeletal muscle cells from individuals with chronic fatigue syndrome. *PLoS ONE* **2015**, *10*, e0122982. [CrossRef]
49. Ciregia, F.; Kollipara, L.; Giusti, L.; Zahedi, R.P.; Giacomelli, C.; Mazzoni, M.R.; Giannaccini, G.; Scarpellini, P.; Urbani, A.; Sickmann, A.; et al. Bottom-up proteomics suggests an association between differential expression of mitochondrial proteins and chronic fatigue syndrome. *Transl. Psychiatry* **2016**, *6*, e904. [CrossRef]
50. Kaushik, N.; Fear, D.; Richards, S.C.; McDermott, C.R.; Nuwaysir, E.F.; Kellam, P.; Harrison, T.J.; Wilkinson, R.J.; Tyrrell, D.A.; Holgate, S.T.; et al. Gene expression in peripheral blood mononuclear cells from patients with chronic fatigue syndrome. *J. Clin. Pathol.* **2005**, *58*, 826–832. [CrossRef]
51. Vernon, S.D.; Whistler, T.; Cameron, B.; Hickie, I.B.; Reeves, W.C.; Lloyd, A. Preliminary evidence of mitochondrial dysfunction associated with post-infective fatigue after acute infection with Epstein Barr virus. *BMC Infect. Dis.* **2006**, *6*, 15. [CrossRef] [PubMed]
52. Wallimann, T.; Wyss, M.; Brdiczka, D.; Nicolay, K.; Eppenberger, H.M. Intracellular compartmentation, structure and function of creatine kinase isoenzymes in tissues with high and fluctuating energy demands: The "phosphocreatine circuit" for cellular energy homeostasis. *Biochem. J.* **1992**, *28*, 21–40. [CrossRef] [PubMed]
53. Nguyen, T.; Staines, D.; Johnston, S.; Marshall-Gradisnik, S. Reduced glycolytic reserve in isolated natural killer cells from Myalgic encephalomyelitis/chronic fatigue syndrome patients: A preliminary investigation. *Asian Pac. J. Allergy Immunol.* **2018**. [CrossRef]
54. Gardiner, C.M.; Finlay, D.K. What Fuels Natural Killers? Metabolism and NK Cell Responses. *Front. Immunol.* **2017**, *8*, 367. [CrossRef] [PubMed]
55. Abdel-aleem, S.; Nada, M.A.; Sayed-Ahmed, M.; Hendrickson, S.C.; St Louis, J.; Walthall, H.P.; Lowe, J.E. Regulation of fatty acid oxidation by acetyl-CoA generated from glucose utilization in isolated myocytes. *J. Mol. Cell. Cardiol.* **1996**, *28*, 825–833. [CrossRef] [PubMed]
56. Hardie, D.G.; Pan, D.A. Regulation of fatty acid synthesis and oxidation by the AMP-activated protein kinase. *Biochem. Soc. Trans.* **2002**, *30*, 1064–1070. [CrossRef] [PubMed]
57. Laplante, M.; Sabatini, D.M. mTOR signaling in growth control and disease. *Cell* **2012**, *149*, 274–293. [CrossRef] [PubMed]
58. Hindupur, S.K.; Gonzalez, A.; Hall, M.N. The opposing actions of target of rapamycin and AMP-activated protein kinase in cell growth control. *Cold Spring Harb. Perspect. Biol.* **2015**, *7*, a019141. [CrossRef]
59. Dalle Pezze, P.; Ruf, S.; Sonntag, A.G.; Langelaar-Makkinje, M.; Hall, P.; Heberle, A.M.; Razquin Navas, P.; van Eunen, K.; Tolle, R.C.; Schwarz, J.J.; et al. A systems study reveals concurrent activation of AMPK and mTOR by amino acids. *Nat. Commun.* **2016**, *7*, 13254. [CrossRef]
60. Horton, J.D.; Shah, N.A.; Warrington, J.A.; Anderson, N.N.; Park, S.W.; Brown, M.S.; Goldstein, J.L. Combined analysis of oligonucleotide microarray data from transgenic and knockout mice identifies direct SREBP target genes. *Proc. Natl. Acad. Sci. USA* **2003**, *100*, 12027–12032. [CrossRef]
61. Winder, W.W.; Hardie, D.G. Inactivation of acetyl-CoA carboxylase and activation of AMP-activated protein kinase in muscle during exercise. *Am. J. Physiol.* **1996**, *270*, E299–E304. [CrossRef]
62. Bartlett, K.; Eaton, S. Mitochondrial beta-oxidation. *Eur. J. Biochem.* **2004**, *271*, 462–469. [CrossRef] [PubMed]
63. Liu, T.F.; Vachharajani, V.T.; Yoza, B.K.; McCall, C.E. NAD+-dependent sirtuin 1 and 6 proteins coordinate a switch from glucose to fatty acid oxidation during the acute inflammatory response. *J. Biol. Chem.* **2012**, *287*, 25758–25769. [CrossRef] [PubMed]
64. Komaroff, A.L. Inflammation correlates with symptoms in chronic fatigue syndrome. *Proc. Natl. Acad. Sci. USA* **2017**, *114*, 8914–8916. [CrossRef] [PubMed]

65. Maher, K.J.; Klimas, N.G.; Fletcher, M.A. Chronic fatigue syndrome is associated with diminished intracellular perforin. *Clin. Exp. Immunol.* **2005**, *142*, 505–511. [CrossRef]
66. Fletcher, M.A.; Zeng, X.R.; Maher, K.; Levis, S.; Hurwitz, B.; Antoni, M.; Broderick, G.; Klimas, N.G. Biomarkers in chronic fatigue syndrome: Evaluation of natural killer cell function and dipeptidyl peptidase IV/CD26. *PLoS ONE* **2010**, *5*, e10817. [CrossRef] [PubMed]
67. Marshall-Gradisnik, S.; Huth, T.; Chacko, A.; Johnston, S.; Smith, P.; Staines, D. Natural killer cells and single nucleotide polymorphisms of specific ion channels and receptor genes in myalgic encephalomyelitis/chronic fatigue syndrome. *Appl. Clin. Genet.* **2016**, *9*, 39–47. [CrossRef]
68. Lorusso, L.; Mikhaylova, S.V.; Capelli, E.; Ferrari, D.; Ngonga, G.K.; Ricevuti, G. Immunological aspects of chronic fatigue syndrome. *Autoimmun. Rev.* **2009**, *8*, 287–291. [CrossRef]
69. Barker, E.; Fujimura, S.F.; Fadem, M.B.; Landay, A.L.; Levy, J.A. Immunologic abnormalities associated with chronic fatigue syndrome. *Clin. Infect. Dis.* **1994**, *18*, S136–S141. [CrossRef]
70. Tirelli, U.; Marotta, G.; Improta, S.; Pinto, A. Immunological abnormalities in patients with chronic fatigue syndrome. *Scand. J. Immunol.* **1994**, *40*, 601–608. [CrossRef]
71. Brenu, E.W.; van Driel, M.L.; Staines, D.R.; Ashton, K.J.; Ramos, S.B.; Keane, J.; Klimas, N.G.; Marshall-Gradisnik, S.M. Immunological abnormalities as potential biomarkers in Chronic Fatigue Syndrome/Myalgic Encephalomyelitis. *J. Transl. Med.* **2011**, *9*, 81. [CrossRef]
72. Klimas, N.G.; Salvato, F.R.; Morgan, R.; Fletcher, M.A. Immunologic abnormalities in chronic fatigue syndrome. *J. Clin. Microbiol.* **1990**, *28*, 1403–1410.
73. Kawasaki, A.; Shinkai, Y.; Kuwana, Y.; Furuya, A.; Iigo, Y.; Hanai, N.; Itoh, S.; Yagita, H.; Okumura, K. Perforin, a pore-forming protein detectable by monoclonal antibodies, is a functional marker for killer cells. *Int. Immunol.* **1990**, *2*, 677–684. [CrossRef]
74. Osinska, I.; Popko, K.; Demkow, U. Perforin: An important player in immune response. *Cent. Eur. J. Immunol.* **2014**, *39*, 109–115. [CrossRef]
75. Theorell, J.; Bileviciute-Ljungar, I.; Tesi, B.; Schlums, H.; Johnsgaard, M.S.; Asadi-Azarbaijani, B.; Bolle Strand, E.; Bryceson, Y.T. Unperturbed Cytotoxic Lymphocyte Phenotype and Function in Myalgic Encephalomyelitis/Chronic Fatigue Syndrome Patients. *Front. Immunol.* **2017**, *8*, 723. [CrossRef]
76. Cliff, J.M.; King, E.C.; Lee, J.S.; Sepulveda, N.; Wolf, A.S.; Kingdon, C.; Bowman, E.; Dockrell, H.M.; Nacul, L.; Lacerda, E.; et al. Cellular Immune Function in Myalgic Encephalomyelitis/Chronic Fatigue Syndrome (ME/CFS). *Front. Immunol.* **2019**, *10*, 796. [CrossRef]
77. Vig, M.; Kinet, J.-P. Calcium signalling in immune cells. *Nat. Immunol.* **2009**, *10*, 21–27. [CrossRef]
78. Rizzuto, R.; De Stefani, D.; Raffaello, A.; Mammucari, C. Mitochondria as sensors and regulators of calcium signalling. *Nat. Rev. Mol. Cell Biol.* **2012**, *13*, 566–578. [CrossRef]
79. Grimm, C.; Kraft, R.; Sauerbruch, S.; Schultz, G.; Harteneck, C. Molecular and functional characterization of the melastatin-related cation channel TRPM3. *J. Biol. Chem.* **2003**, *278*, 21493–21501. [CrossRef]
80. Nguyen, T.; Johnston, S.; Clarke, L.; Smith, P.; Staines, D.; Marshall-Gradisnik, S. Impaired calcium mobilization in natural killer cells from chronic fatigue syndrome/myalgic encephalomyelitis patients is associated with transient receptor potential melastatin 3 ion channels. *Clin. Exp. Immunol.* **2017**, *187*, 284–293. [CrossRef]
81. Cabanas, H.; Muraki, K.; Eaton, N.; Balinas, C.; Staines, D.; Marshall-Gradisnik, S. Loss of Transient Receptor Potential Melastatin 3 ion channel function in natural killer cells from Chronic Fatigue Syndrome/Myalgic Encephalomyelitis patients. *Mol. Med.* **2018**, *24*, 44. [CrossRef] [PubMed]
82. Cabanas, H.; Muraki, K.; Balinas, C.; Eaton-Fitch, N.; Staines, D.; Marshall-Gradisnik, S. Validation of impaired Transient Receptor Potential Melastatin 3 ion channel activity in natural killer cells from Chronic Fatigue Syndrome/ Myalgic Encephalomyelitis patients. *Mol. Med.* **2019**, *25*, 14. [CrossRef]
83. Cost, N.G.; Czyzyk-Krzeska, M.F. Regulation of autophagy by two products of one gene: TRPM3 and miR-204. *Mol. Cell. Oncol.* **2015**, *2*, e1002712. [CrossRef] [PubMed]
84. Almenar-Perez, E.; Sanchez-Fito, T.; Ovejero, T.; Nathanson, L.; Oltra, E. Impact of Polypharmacy on Candidate Biomarker miRNomes for the Diagnosis of Fibromyalgia and Myalgic Encephalomyelitis/Chronic Fatigue Syndrome: Striking Back on Treatments. *Pharmaceutics* **2019**, *11*, 126. [CrossRef]
85. Tepikin, A.V. Mitochondrial junctions with cellular organelles: Ca^{2+} signalling perspective. *Pflugers Arch.* **2018**, *470*, 1181–1192. [CrossRef] [PubMed]

86. Aich, A.; Shaha, C. Novel role of calmodulin in regulating protein transport to mitochondria in a unicellular eukaryote. *Mol. Cell. Biol.* **2013**, *33*, 4579–4593. [CrossRef] [PubMed]
87. Przibilla, J.; Dembla, S.; Rizun, O.; Lis, A.; Jung, M.; Oberwinkler, J.; Beck, A.; Philipp, S.E. Ca^{2+}-dependent regulation and binding of calmodulin to multiple sites of Transient Receptor Potential Melastatin 3 (TRPM3) ion channels. *Cell Calcium* **2018**, *73*, 40–52. [CrossRef] [PubMed]
88. Szymanski, J.; Janikiewicz, J.; Michalska, B.; Patalas-Krawczyk, P.; Perrone, M.; Ziolkowski, W.; Duszynski, J.; Pinton, P.; Dobrzyn, A.; Wieckowski, M.R. Interaction of Mitochondria with the Endoplasmic Reticulum and Plasma Membrane in Calcium Homeostasis, Lipid Trafficking and Mitochondrial Structure. *Int. J. Mol. Sci.* **2017**, *18*, 1576. [CrossRef]
89. Donnelly, R.P.; Loftus, R.M.; Keating, S.E.; Liou, K.T.; Biron, C.A.; Gardiner, C.M.; Finlay, D.K. mTORC1-dependent metabolic reprogramming is a prerequisite for NK cell effector function. *J. Immunol.* **2014**, *193*, 4477–4484. [CrossRef]
90. Viel, S.; Marcais, A.; Guimaraes, F.S.; Loftus, R.; Rabilloud, J.; Grau, M.; Degouve, S.; Djebali, S.; Sanlaville, A.; Charrier, E.; et al. TGF-beta inhibits the activation and functions of NK cells by repressing the mTOR pathway. *Sci. Signal.* **2016**, *9*, ra19. [CrossRef]
91. Salmond, R.J.; Mirchandani, A.S.; Besnard, A.G.; Bain, C.C.; Thomson, N.C.; Liew, F.Y. IL-33 induces innate lymphoid cell-mediated airway inflammation by activating mammalian target of rapamycin. *J. Allergy Clin. Immunol.* **2012**, *130*, 1159–1166.e1156. [CrossRef] [PubMed]
92. Wagner, J.A.; Fehniger, T.A. Memory NK Cells Take Out the (Mitochondrial) Garbage. *Immunity* **2015**, *43*, 218–220. [CrossRef] [PubMed]
93. Morris, G.; Maes, M. Oxidative and Nitrosative Stress and Immune-Inflammatory Pathways in Patients with Myalgic Encephalomyelitis (ME)/Chronic Fatigue Syndrome (CFS). *Curr. Neuropharmacol.* **2014**, *12*, 168–185. [CrossRef] [PubMed]
94. Hornig, M.; Montoya, J.G.; Klimas, N.G.; Levine, S.; Felsenstein, D.; Bateman, L.; Peterson, D.L.; Gottschalk, C.G.; Schultz, A.F.; Che, X.; et al. Distinct plasma immune signatures in ME/CFS are present early in the course of illness. *Sci. Adv.* **2015**, *1*. [CrossRef] [PubMed]
95. Maes, M.; Twisk, F.N.; Ringel, K. Inflammatory and cell-mediated immune biomarkers in myalgic encephalomyelitis/chronic fatigue syndrome and depression: Inflammatory markers are higher in myalgic encephalomyelitis/chronic fatigue syndrome than in depression. *Psychother. Psychosom.* **2012**, *81*, 286–295. [CrossRef] [PubMed]
96. Milrad, S.F.; Hall, D.L.; Jutagir, D.R.; Lattie, E.G.; Ironson, G.H.; Wohlgemuth, W.; Nunez, M.V.; Garcia, L.; Czaja, S.J.; Perdomo, D.M.; et al. Poor sleep quality is associated with greater circulating pro-inflammatory cytokines and severity and frequency of chronic fatigue syndrome/myalgic encephalomyelitis (CFS/ME) symptoms in women. *J. NeuroImmunol.* **2017**, *303*, 43–50. [CrossRef] [PubMed]
97. Montoya, J.G.; Holmes, T.H.; Anderson, J.N.; Maecker, H.T.; Rosenberg-Hasson, Y.; Valencia, I.J.; Chu, L.; Younger, J.W.; Tato, C.M.; Davis, M.M. Cytokine signature associated with disease severity in chronic fatigue syndrome patients. *Proc. Natl. Acad. Sci. USA* **2017**, *114*, E7150–E7158. [CrossRef] [PubMed]
98. Peterson, D.; Brenu, E.W.; Gottschalk, G.; Ramos, S.; Nguyen, T.; Staines, D.; Marshall-Gradisnik, S. Cytokines in the cerebrospinal fluids of patients with chronic fatigue syndrome/myalgic encephalomyelitis. *Mediat. Inflamm.* **2015**, *2015*, 929720. [CrossRef]
99. Maes, M.; Twisk, F.N.; Kubera, M.; Ringel, K. Evidence for inflammation and activation of cell-mediated immunity in Myalgic Encephalomyelitis/Chronic Fatigue Syndrome (ME/CFS): Increased interleukin-1, tumor necrosis factor-alpha, PMN-elastase, lysozyme and neopterin. *J. Affect. Disord.* **2012**, *136*, 933–939. [CrossRef]
100. Tomoda, A.; Joudoi, T.; Rabab, E.M.; Matsumoto, T.; Park, T.H.; Miike, T. Cytokine production and modulation: Comparison of patients with chronic fatigue syndrome and normal controls. *Psychiatry Res.* **2005**, *134*, 101–104. [CrossRef]
101. Fletcher, M.A.; Zeng, X.R.; Barnes, Z.; Levis, S.; Klimas, N.G. Plasma cytokines in women with chronic fatigue syndrome. *J. Transl. Med.* **2009**, *7*, 96. [CrossRef]
102. Mensah, F.K.F.; Bansal, A.S.; Ford, B.; Cambridge, G. Chronic fatigue syndrome and the immune system: Where are we now? *Neurophysiol. Clin.* **2017**, *47*, 131–138. [CrossRef]

103. Maes, M.; Coucke, F.; Leunis, J.C. Normalization of the increased translocation of endotoxin from gram negative enterobacteria (leaky gut) is accompanied by a remission of chronic fatigue syndrome. *Neuroendocrinol. Lett.* **2007**, *28*, 739–744.
104. Maes, M.; Leunis, J.C. Normalization of leaky gut in chronic fatigue syndrome (CFS) is accompanied by a clinical improvement: Effects of age, duration of illness and the translocation of LPS from gram-negative bacteria. *Neuroendocrinol. Lett.* **2008**, *29*, 902–910.
105. Blomberg, J.; Gottfries, C.G.; Elfaitouri, A.; Rizwan, M.; Rosen, A. Infection Elicited Autoimmunity and Myalgic Encephalomyelitis/Chronic Fatigue Syndrome: An Explanatory Model. *Front. Immunol.* **2018**, *9*, 229. [CrossRef]
106. Fluge, O.; Risa, K.; Lunde, S.; Alme, K.; Rekeland, I.G.; Sapkota, D.; Kristoffersen, E.K.; Sorland, K.; Bruland, O.; Dahl, O.; et al. B-Lymphocyte Depletion in Myalgic Encephalopathy/Chronic Fatigue Syndrome. An Open-Label Phase II Study with Rituximab Maintenance Treatment. *PLoS ONE* **2015**, *10*, e0129898. [CrossRef]
107. Fluge, O.; Mella, O. Clinical impact of B-cell depletion with the anti-CD20 antibody rituximab in chronic fatigue syndrome: A preliminary case series. *BMC Neurol.* **2009**, *9*, 28. [CrossRef]
108. Bradley, A.S.; Ford, B.; Bansal, A.S. Altered functional B cell subset populations in patients with chronic fatigue syndrome compared to healthy controls. *Clin. Exp. Immunol.* **2013**, *172*, 73–80. [CrossRef]
109. Fluge, O.; Rekeland, I.G.; Lien, K.; Thurmer, H.; Borchgrevink, P.C.; Schafer, C.; Sorland, K.; Assmus, J.; Ktoridou-Valen, I.; Herder, I.; et al. B-Lymphocyte Depletion in Patients with Myalgic Encephalomyelitis/Chronic Fatigue Syndrome: A Randomized, Double-Blind, Placebo-Controlled Trial. *Ann. Intern. Med.* **2019**. [CrossRef]
110. Rekeland, I.G.; Fluge, O.; Alme, K.; Risa, K.; Sorland, K.; Mella, O.; de Vries, A.; Schjott, J. Rituximab Serum Concentrations and Anti-Rituximab Antibodies During B-Cell Depletion Therapy for Myalgic Encephalopathy/Chronic Fatigue Syndrome. *Clin. Ther.* **2018**. [CrossRef]
111. Loebel, M.; Grabowski, P.; Heidecke, H.; Bauer, S.; Hanitsch, L.G.; Wittke, K.; Meisel, C.; Reinke, P.; Volk, H.D.; Fluge, O.; et al. Antibodies to beta adrenergic and muscarinic cholinergic receptors in patients with Chronic Fatigue Syndrome. *Brain Behav. Immun.* **2016**, *52*, 32–39. [CrossRef]
112. Scheibenbogen, C.; Loebel, M.; Freitag, H.; Krueger, A.; Bauer, S.; Antelmann, M.; Doehner, W.; Scherbakov, N.; Heidecke, H.; Reinke, P.; et al. Immunoadsorption to remove ss2 adrenergic receptor antibodies in Chronic Fatigue Syndrome CFS/ME. *PLoS ONE* **2018**, *13*, e0193672. [CrossRef]
113. Elfaitouri, A.; Herrmann, B.; Bolin-Wiener, A.; Wang, Y.; Gottfries, C.G.; Zachrisson, O.; Pipkorn, R.; Ronnblom, L.; Blomberg, J. Epitopes of microbial and human heat shock protein 60 and their recognition in myalgic encephalomyelitis. *PLoS ONE* **2013**, *8*, e81155. [CrossRef]
114. Maes, M.; Mihaylova, I.; Leunis, J.C. Increased serum IgM antibodies directed against phosphatidyl inositol (Pi) in chronic fatigue syndrome (CFS) and major depression: Evidence that an IgM-mediated immune response against Pi is one factor underpinning the comorbidity between both CFS and depression. *Neuroendocrinol. Lett.* **2007**, *28*, 861–867.
115. Butt, H.L.; Dunstan, R.; McGregor, N.R.; Roberts, T.K. Bacterial colonosis in patients with persistent fatigue. In Proceedings of the AHMF International Clinical and Scientific Conference, Sydney, Australia, 1–2 December 2001.
116. Sheedy, J.R.; Wettenhall, R.E.; Scanlon, D.; Gooley, P.R.; Lewis, D.P.; McGregor, N.; Stapleton, D.I.; Butt, H.L.; de Meirleir, K.L. Increased d-lactic Acid intestinal bacteria in patients with chronic fatigue syndrome. *In Vivo* **2009**, *23*, 621–628.
117. Jackson, M.L.; Butt, H.; Ball, M.; Lewis, D.P.; Bruck, D. Sleep quality and the treatment of intestinal microbiota imbalance in Chronic Fatigue Syndrome: A pilot study. *Sleep Sci.* **2015**, *8*, 124–133. [CrossRef]
118. Armstrong, C.W.; McGregor, N.R.; Lewis, D.P.; Butt, H.L.; Gooley, P.R. The association of fecal microbiota and fecal, blood serum and urine metabolites in myalgic encephalomyelitis/chronic fatigue syndrome. *Metabolomics* **2017**, *13*, 8. [CrossRef]
119. Fremont, M.; Coomans, D.; Massart, S.; De Meirleir, K. High-throughput 16S rRNA gene sequencing reveals alterations of intestinal microbiota in myalgic encephalomyelitis/chronic fatigue syndrome patients. *Anaerobe* **2013**, *22*, 50–56. [CrossRef]

120. Shukla, S.K.; Cook, D.; Meyer, J.; Vernon, S.D.; Le, T.; Clevidence, D.; Robertson, C.E.; Schrodi, S.J.; Yale, S.; Frank, D.N. Changes in Gut and Plasma Microbiome following Exercise Challenge in Myalgic Encephalomyelitis/Chronic Fatigue Syndrome (ME/CFS). *PLoS ONE* **2015**, *10*, e0145453. [CrossRef]
121. Rao, A.V.; Bested, A.C.; Beaulne, T.M.; Katzman, M.A.; Iorio, C.; Berardi, J.M.; Logan, A.C. A randomized, double-blind, placebo-controlled pilot study of a probiotic in emotional symptoms of chronic fatigue syndrome. *Gut Pathog.* **2009**, *1*, 6. [CrossRef]
122. Burnet, R.B.; Chatterton, B.E. Gastric emptying is slow in chronic fatigue syndrome. *BMC Gastroenterol.* **2004**, *4*, 32. [CrossRef]
123. Morris, G.; Berk, M.; Carvalho, A.F.; Caso, J.R.; Sanz, Y.; Maes, M. The Role of Microbiota and Intestinal Permeability in the Pathophysiology of Autoimmune and Neuroimmune Processes with an Emphasis on Inflammatory Bowel Disease Type 1 Diabetes and Chronic Fatigue Syndrome. *Curr. Pharm. Des.* **2016**, *22*, 6058–6075. [CrossRef]
124. Maes, M.; Mihaylova, I.; Leunis, J.C. Increased serum IgA and IgM against LPS of enterobacteria in chronic fatigue syndrome (CFS): Indication for the involvement of gram-negative enterobacteria in the etiology of CFS and for the presence of an increased gut-intestinal permeability. *J. Affect. Disord.* **2007**, *99*, 237–240. [CrossRef]
125. Aaron, L.A.; Burke, M.M.; Buchwald, D. Overlapping conditions among patients with chronic fatigue syndrome, fibromyalgia, and temporomandibular disorder. *Arch. Intern. Med.* **2000**, *160*, 221–227. [CrossRef]
126. Tsai, S.Y.; Chen, H.J.; Lio, C.F.; Kuo, C.F.; Kao, A.C.; Wang, W.S.; Yao, W.C.; Chen, C.; Yang, T.Y. Increased risk of chronic fatigue syndrome in patients with inflammatory bowel disease: A population-based retrospective cohort study. *J. Transl. Med.* **2019**, *17*, 55. [CrossRef]
127. Grainger, J.; Daw, R.; Wemyss, K. Systemic instruction of cell-mediated immunity by the intestinal microbiome. *F1000Research* **2018**, *7*. [CrossRef]
128. Brown, R.L.; Clarke, T.B. The regulation of host defences to infection by the microbiota. *Immunology* **2017**, *150*, 1–6. [CrossRef]
129. Neumann, C.; Blume, J.; Roy, U.; Teh, P.P.; Vasanthakumar, A.; Beller, A.; Liao, Y.; Heinrich, F.; Arenzana, T.L.; Hackney, J.A.; et al. c-Maf-dependent Treg cell control of intestinal TH17 cells and IgA establishes host-microbiota homeostasis. *Nat. Immunol.* **2019**, *20*, 471–481. [CrossRef]
130. Nakajima, A.; Vogelzang, A.; Maruya, M.; Miyajima, M.; Murata, M.; Son, A.; Kuwahara, T.; Tsuruyama, T.; Yamada, S.; Matsuura, M.; et al. IgA regulates the composition and metabolic function of gut microbiota by promoting symbiosis between bacteria. *J. Exp. Med.* **2018**, *215*, 2019–2034. [CrossRef]
131. Kaliannan, K.; Wang, B.; Li, X.Y.; Kim, K.J.; Kang, J.X. A host-microbiome interaction mediates the opposing effects of omega-6 and omega-3 fatty acids on metabolic endotoxemia. *Sci. Rep.* **2015**, *5*, 11276. [CrossRef]
132. Clark, A.; Mach, N. The Crosstalk between the Gut Microbiota and Mitochondria during Exercise. *Front. Physiol.* **2017**, *8*, 319. [CrossRef]
133. Bretin, A.; Gewirtz, A.T.; Chassaing, B. Microbiota and metabolism: what's new in 2018? *Am. J. Physiol. Endocrinol. Metab* **2018**, *315*, E1–E6. [CrossRef]
134. Janssen, A.W.; Kersten, S. The role of the gut microbiota in metabolic health. *FASEB J.* **2015**, *29*, 3111–3123. [CrossRef]
135. Chambers, E.S.; Preston, T.; Frost, G.; Morrison, D.J. Role of Gut Microbiota-Generated Short-Chain Fatty Acids in Metabolic and Cardiovascular Health. *Curr. Nutr. Rep.* **2018**, *7*, 198–206. [CrossRef]
136. Saint-Georges-Chaumet, Y.; Edeas, M. Microbiota-mitochondria inter-talk: Consequence for microbiota-host interaction. *Pathog. Dis.* **2016**, *74*, ftv096. [CrossRef]
137. Henriksson, A.E.; Tagesson, C.; Uribe, A.; Uvnas-Moberg, K.; Nord, C.E.; Gullberg, R.; Johansson, C. Effects of prostaglandin E2 on disease activity, gastric secretion and intestinal permeability, and morphology in patients with rheumatoid arthritis. *Ann. Rheum. Dis.* **1988**, *47*, 620–627. [CrossRef]
138. Mathew, S.J.; Mao, X.; Keegan, K.A.; Levine, S.M.; Smith, E.L.; Heier, L.A.; Otcheretko, V.; Coplan, J.D.; Shungu, D.C. Ventricular cerebrospinal fluid lactate is increased in chronic fatigue syndrome compared with generalized anxiety disorder: An in vivo 3.0 T ^{1}H MRS imaging study. *NMR Biomed.* **2009**, *22*, 251–258. [CrossRef]
139. Murrough, J.W.; Mao, X.; Collins, K.A.; Kelly, C.; Andrade, G.; Nestadt, P.; Levine, S.M.; Mathew, S.J.; Shungu, D.C. Increased ventricular lactate in chronic fatigue syndrome measured by 1H MRS imaging at 3.0 T. II: Comparison with major depressive disorder. *NMR Biomed.* **2010**, *23*, 643–650. [CrossRef]

140. Shungu, D.C.; Weiduschat, N.; Murrough, J.W.; Mao, X.; Pillemer, S.; Dyke, J.P.; Medow, M.S.; Natelson, B.H.; Stewart, J.M.; Mathew, S.J. Increased ventricular lactate in chronic fatigue syndrome. III. Relationships to cortical glutathione and clinical symptoms implicate oxidative stress in disorder pathophysiology. *NMR Biomed.* **2012**, *25*, 1073–1087. [CrossRef]
141. Rutherford, G.; Manning, P.; Newton, J.L. Understanding Muscle Dysfunction in Chronic Fatigue Syndrome. *J. Aging Res.* **2016**, *2016*, 2497348. [CrossRef]
142. Maes, M.; Twisk, F.N.; Kubera, M.; Ringel, K.; Leunis, J.C.; Geffard, M. Increased IgA responses to the LPS of commensal bacteria is associated with inflammation and activation of cell-mediated immunity in chronic fatigue syndrome. *J. Affect. Disord.* **2012**, *136*, 909–917. [CrossRef] [PubMed]
143. Cadenas, E.; Davies, K.J. Mitochondrial free radical generation, oxidative stress, and aging. *Free Radic. Biol. Med.* **2000**, *29*, 222–230. [CrossRef]
144. Naviaux, R.K. Oxidative shielding or oxidative stress? *J. Pharmacol. Exp. Ther.* **2012**, *342*, 608–618. [CrossRef] [PubMed]
145. Ghosh, S.; Dai, C.; Brown, K.; Rajendiran, E.; Makarenko, S.; Baker, J.; Ma, C.; Halder, S.; Montero, M.; Ionescu, V.A.; et al. Colonic microbiota alters host susceptibility to infectious colitis by modulating inflammation, redox status, and ion transporter gene expression. *Am. J. Physiol. Gastrointest. Liver Physiol.* **2011**, *301*, G39–G49. [CrossRef]
146. Abuaita, B.H.; Schultz, T.L.; O'Riordan, M.X. Mitochondria-Derived Vesicles Deliver Antimicrobial Reactive Oxygen Species to Control Phagosome-Localized Staphylococcus aureus. *Cell Host Microbe* **2018**, *24*, 625–636. [CrossRef]
147. Hurst, J.K.; Lymar, S.V. Toxicity of peroxynitrite and related reactive nitrogen species toward Escherichia coli. *Chem. Res. Toxicol.* **1997**, *10*, 802–810. [CrossRef]
148. Vecchiet, L.; Montanari, G.; Pizzigallo, E.; Iezzi, S.; de Bigontina, P.; Dragani, L.; Vecchiet, J.; Giamberardino, M.A. Sensory characterization of somatic parietal tissues in humans with chronic fatigue syndrome. *Neurosci. Lett.* **1996**, *208*, 117–120. [CrossRef]
149. Vecchiet, J.; Cipollone, F.; Falasca, K.; Mezzetti, A.; Pizzigallo, E.; Bucciarelli, T.; De Laurentis, S.; Affaitati, G.; De Cesare, D.; Giamberardino, M.A. Relationship between musculoskeletal symptoms and blood markers of oxidative stress in patients with chronic fatigue syndrome. *Neurosci. Lett.* **2003**, *335*, 151–154. [CrossRef]
150. Kennedy, G.; Spence, V.A.; McLaren, M.; Hill, A.; Underwood, C.; Belch, J.J. Oxidative stress levels are raised in chronic fatigue syndrome and are associated with clinical symptoms. *Free Radic. Biol. Med.* **2005**, *39*, 584–589. [CrossRef]
151. Jammes, Y.; Steinberg, J.G.; Mambrini, O.; Bregeon, F.; Delliaux, S. Chronic fatigue syndrome: Assessment of increased oxidative stress and altered muscle excitability in response to incremental exercise. *J. Intern. Med.* **2005**, *257*, 299–310. [CrossRef] [PubMed]
152. Jammes, Y.; Steinberg, J.G.; Delliaux, S. Chronic fatigue syndrome: Acute infection and history of physical activity affect resting levels and response to exercise of plasma oxidant/antioxidant status and heat shock proteins. *J. Intern. Med.* **2012**, *272*, 74–84. [CrossRef] [PubMed]
153. Polli, A.; Van Oosterwijck, J.; Nijs, J.; Marusic, U.; De Wandele, I.; Paul, L.; Meeus, M.; Moorkens, G.; Lambrecht, L.; Ickmans, K. Relationship Between Exercise-induced Oxidative Stress Changes and Parasympathetic Activity in Chronic Fatigue Syndrome: An Observational Study in Patients and Healthy Subjects. *Clin. Ther.* **2019**. [CrossRef] [PubMed]
154. Papatheodorou, P.; Domanska, G.; Oxle, M.; Mathieu, J.; Selchow, O.; Kenny, B.; Rassow, J. The enteropathogenic Escherichia coli (EPEC) Map effector is imported into the mitochondrial matrix by the TOM/Hsp70 system and alters organelle morphology. *Cell. Microbiol.* **2006**, *8*, 677–689. [CrossRef] [PubMed]
155. Crane, J.K.; McNamara, B.P.; Donnenberg, M.S. Role of EspF in host cell death induced by enteropathogenic Escherichia coli. *Cell. MicroBiol.* **2001**, *3*, 197–211. [CrossRef] [PubMed]
156. Swidsinski, A.; Ladhoff, A.; Pernthaler, A.; Swidsinski, S.; Loening-Baucke, V.; Ortner, M.; Weber, J.; Hoffmann, U.; Schreiber, S.; Dietel, M.; et al. Mucosal flora in inflammatory bowel disease. *Gastroenterology* **2002**, *122*, 44–54. [CrossRef] [PubMed]
157. Nater, U.M.; Maloney, E.; Heim, C.; Reeves, W.C. Cumulative life stress in chronic fatigue syndrome. *Psychiatry Res.* **2011**, *189*, 318–320. [CrossRef] [PubMed]

158. Lakhan, S.E.; Kirchgessner, A. Gut inflammation in chronic fatigue syndrome. *Nutr. Metab.* **2010**, *7*, 79. [CrossRef] [PubMed]
159. Gaab, J.; Rohleder, N.; Heitz, V.; Engert, V.; Schad, T.; Schurmeyer, T.H.; Ehlert, U. Stress-induced changes in LPS-induced pro-inflammatory cytokine production in chronic fatigue syndrome. *Psychoneuroendocrinology* **2005**, *30*, 188–198. [CrossRef] [PubMed]
160. Cani, P.D.; Possemiers, S.; Van de Wiele, T.; Guiot, Y.; Everard, A.; Rottier, O.; Geurts, L.; Naslain, D.; Neyrinck, A.; Lambert, D.M.; et al. Changes in gut microbiota control inflammation in obese mice through a mechanism involving GLP-2-driven improvement of gut permeability. *Gut* **2009**, *58*, 1091–1103. [CrossRef] [PubMed]
161. Martich, G.D.; Boujoukos, A.J.; Suffredini, A.F. Response of man to endotoxin. *Immunobiology* **1993**, *187*, 403–416. [CrossRef]
162. Nordgreen, J.; Munsterhjelm, C.; Aae, F.; Popova, A.; Boysen, P.; Ranheim, B.; Heinonen, M.; Raszplewicz, J.; Piepponen, P.; Lervik, A.; et al. The effect of lipopolysaccharide (LPS) on inflammatory markers in blood and brain and on Behav. ior in individually-housed pigs. *Physiol. Behav.* **2018**, *195*, 98–111. [CrossRef] [PubMed]
163. Carabotti, M.; Scirocco, A.; Maselli, M.A.; Severi, C. The gut-brain axis: Interactions between enteric microbiota, central and enteric nervous systems. *Ann. Gastroenterol.* **2015**, *28*, 203–209. [PubMed]
164. Furness, J.B. The enteric nervous system: Normal functions and enteric neuropathies. *Neurogastroenterol. Motil.* **2008**, *20* (Suppl. 1), 32–38. [CrossRef] [PubMed]
165. Barnden, L.R.; Kwiatek, R.; Crouch, B.; Burnet, R.; Del Fante, P. Autonomic correlations with MRI are abnormal in the brainstem vasomotor centre in Chronic Fatigue Syndrome. *Neuroimage Clin.* **2016**, *11*, 530–537. [CrossRef] [PubMed]
166. Maes, M.; Mihaylova, I.; Kubera, M.; Uytterhoeven, M.; Vrydags, N.; Bosmans, E. Coenzyme Q10 deficiency in myalgic encephalomyelitis/chronic fatigue syndrome (ME/CFS) is related to fatigue, autonomic and neurocognitive symptoms and is another risk factor explaining the early mortality in ME/CFS due to cardiovascular disorder. *NeuroEndocrinol. Lett.* **2009**, *30*, 470–476. [PubMed]
167. Freitas, J.; Santos, R.; Azevedo, E.; Costa, O.; Carvalho, M.; de Freitas, A.F. Reversible sympathetic vasomotor dysfunction in POTS patients. *Rev. Port. Cardiol.* **2000**, *19*, 1163–1170. [PubMed]
168. Tsigos, C.; Chrousos, G.P. Hypothalamic-pituitary-adrenal axis, neuroendocrine factors and stress. *J. Psychosom. Res.* **2002**, *53*, 865–871. [CrossRef]
169. Tak, L.M.; Cleare, A.J.; Ormel, J.; Manoharan, A.; Kok, I.C.; Wessely, S.; Rosmalen, J.G. Meta-analysis and meta-regression of hypothalamic-pituitary-adrenal axis activity in functional somatic disorders. *Biol. Psychol.* **2011**, *87*, 183–194. [CrossRef]
170. Poteliakhoff, A. Adrenocortical activity and some clinical findings in acute and chronic fatigue. *J. Psychosom. Res.* **1981**, *25*, 91–95. [CrossRef]
171. Tomas, C.; Newton, J.; Watson, S. A review of hypothalamic-pituitary-adrenal axis function in chronic fatigue syndrome. *ISRN Neurosci.* **2013**, *2013*, 784520. [CrossRef]
172. Naviaux, R.K. Metabolic features of the cell danger response. *Mitochondrion* **2014**, *16*, 7–17. [CrossRef] [PubMed]
173. Rasa, S.; Nora-Krukle, Z.; Henning, N.; Eliassen, E.; Shikova, E.; Harrer, T.; Scheibenbogen, C.; Murovska, M.; Prusty, B.K.; the European Network on ME/CFS. Chronic viral infections in myalgic encephalomyelitis/chronic fatigue syndrome (ME/CFS). *J. Transl. Med.* **2018**, *16*, 268. [CrossRef] [PubMed]
174. Lacourt, T.E.; Vichaya, E.G.; Chiu, G.S.; Dantzer, R.; Heijnen, C.J. The High Costs of Low-Grade Inflammation: Persistent Fatigue as a Consequence of Reduced Cellular-Energy Availability and Non-adaptive Energy Expenditure. *Front. Behav. NeuroSci.* **2018**, *12*, 78. [CrossRef] [PubMed]
175. Morris, G.; Maes, M. Mitochondrial dysfunctions in myalgic encephalomyelitis/chronic fatigue syndrome explained by activated immuno-inflammatory, oxidative and nitrosative stress pathways. *Metab. Brain Dis.* **2014**, *29*, 19–36. [CrossRef] [PubMed]
176. Meeus, M.; Nijs, J.; Hermans, L.; Goubert, D.; Calders, P. The role of mitochondrial dysfunctions due to oxidative and nitrosative stress in the chronic pain or chronic fatigue syndromes and fibromyalgia patients: Peripheral and central mechanisms as therapeutic targets? *Expert Opin. Ther. Targets* **2013**, *17*, 1081–1089. [CrossRef] [PubMed]
177. Van Horssen, J.; van Schaik, P.; Witte, M. Inflammation and mitochondrial dysfunction: A vicious circle in neurodegenerative disorders? *Neurosci. Lett.* **2017**. [CrossRef] [PubMed]

178. Kolmychkova, K.I.; Zhelankin, A.V.; Karagodin, V.P.; Orekhov, A.N. Mitochondria and inflammation. *Patol. Fiziol. Eksp. Ter.* **2016**, *60*, 114–121. [PubMed]
179. Meyer, L.E.; Machado, L.B.; Santiago, A.P.; da-Silva, W.S.; De Felice, F.G.; Holub, O.; Oliveira, M.F.; Galina, A. Mitochondrial creatine kinase activity prevents reactive oxygen species generation: Antioxidant role of mitochondrial kinase-dependent ADP re-cycling activity. *J. Biol. Chem.* **2006**, *281*, 37361–37371. [CrossRef]
180. Armstrong, C.W.; McGregor, N.R.; Butt, H.L.; Gooley, P.R. Metabolism in chronic fatigue syndrome. *Adv. Clin. Chem.* **2014**, *66*, 121–172.
181. Vermeulen, R.C.; Vermeulen van Eck, I.W. Decreased oxygen extraction during cardiopulmonary exercise test in patients with chronic fatigue syndrome. *J. Transl. Med.* **2014**, *12*, 20. [CrossRef]
182. Blundell, S.; Ray, K.K.; Buckland, M.; White, P.D. Chronic fatigue syndrome and circulating cytokines: A systematic review. *Brain Behav. Immun.* **2015**, *50*, 186–195. [CrossRef] [PubMed]
183. Mensah, F.F.K.; Armstrong, C.W.; Reddy, V.; Bansal, A.S.; Berkovitz, S.; Leandro, M.J.; Cambridge, G. CD24 Expression and B Cell Maturation Shows a Novel Link with Energy Metabolism: Potential Implications for Patients with Myalgic Encephalomyelitis/Chronic Fatigue Syndrome. *Front. Immunol.* **2018**, *9*, 2421. [CrossRef] [PubMed]
184. Mandarano, A.H.; Giloteaux, L.; Keller, B.A.; Levine, S.M.; Hanson, M.R. Eukaryotes in the gut microbiota in myalgic encephalomyelitis/chronic fatigue syndrome. *PeerJ* **2018**, *6*, e4282. [CrossRef] [PubMed]
185. Allen, J.; Murray, A.; Di Maria, C.; Newton, J.L. Chronic fatigue syndrome and impaired peripheral pulse characteristics on orthostasis—A new potential diagnostic biomarker. *Physiol. Meas.* **2012**, *33*, 231–241. [CrossRef] [PubMed]
186. Demitrack, M.A.; Dale, J.K.; Straus, S.E.; Laue, L.; Listwak, S.J.; Kruesi, M.J.; Chrousos, G.P.; Gold, P.W. Evidence for impaired activation of the hypothalamic-pituitary-adrenal axis in patients with chronic fatigue syndrome. *J. Clin. Endocrinol. Metab.* **1991**, *73*, 1224–1234. [CrossRef] [PubMed]
187. Papadopoulos, A.S.; Cleare, A.J. Hypothalamic-pituitary-adrenal axis dysfunction in chronic fatigue syndrome. *Nat. Rev. Endocrinol.* **2011**, *8*, 22–32. [CrossRef] [PubMed]
188. Berger, E.; Rath, E.; Yuan, D.; Waldschmitt, N.; Khaloian, S.; Allgauer, M.; Staszewski, O.; Lobner, E.M.; Schottl, T.; Giesbertz, P.; et al. Mitochondrial function controls intestinal epithelial stemness and proliferation. *Nat. Commun.* **2016**, *7*, 13171. [CrossRef]
189. Novak, E.A.; Mollen, K.P. Mitochondrial dysfunction in inflammatory bowel disease. *Front. Cell Dev. Biol.* **2015**, *3*, 62. [CrossRef]
190. Madsen, K.L.; Yanchar, N.L.; Sigalet, D.L.; Reigel, T.; Fedorak, R.N. FK506 increases permeability in rat intestine by inhibiting mitochondrial function. *Gastroenterology* **1995**, *109*, 107–114. [CrossRef]
191. Green, D.R.; Galluzzi, L.; Kroemer, G. Mitochondria and the autophagy-inflammation-cell death axis in organismal aging. *Science* **2011**, *333*, 1109–1112. [CrossRef]
192. Walker, M.A.; Volpi, S.; Sims, K.B.; Walter, J.E.; Traggiai, E. Powering the immune system: Mitochondria in immune function and deficiency. *J. Immunol. Res.* **2014**, *2014*, 164309. [CrossRef]
193. Belkaid, Y.; Hand, T.W. Role of the microbiota in immunity and inflammation. *Cell* **2014**, *157*, 121–141. [CrossRef]
194. Wu, H.J.; Wu, E. The role of gut microbiota in immune homeostasis and autoimmunity. *Gut Microbes* **2012**, *3*, 4–14. [CrossRef]
195. Kamada, N.; Nunez, G. Role of the gut microbiota in the development and function of lymphoid cells. *J. Immunol.* **2013**, *190*, 1389–1395. [CrossRef]

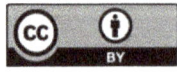

© 2019 by the authors. Licensee MDPI, Basel, Switzerland. This article is an open access article distributed under the terms and conditions of the Creative Commons Attribution (CC BY) license (http://creativecommons.org/licenses/by/4.0/).

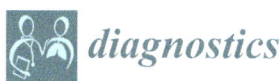

Commentary

Current Research Provides Insight into the Biological Basis and Diagnostic Potential for Myalgic Encephalomyelitis/Chronic Fatigue Syndrome (ME/CFS)

Eiren Sweetman [1], Alex Noble [1], Christina Edgar [1], Angus Mackay [1], Amber Helliwell [1], Rosamund Vallings [2], Margaret Ryan [3] and Warren Tate [1],*

1. Department of Biochemistry, University of Otago, Dunedin 9016, New Zealand
2. Howick Health and Medical Centre, Auckland 2014, New Zealand
3. Department of Anatomy, University of Otago, Dunedin 9016, New Zealand
* Correspondence: warren.tate@otago.ac.nz

Received: 30 May 2019; Accepted: 3 July 2019; Published: 10 July 2019

Abstract: Myalgic encephalomyelitis/chronic fatigue syndrome (ME/CFS) is a severe fatigue illness that occurs most commonly following a viral infection, but other physiological triggers are also implicated. It has a profound long-term impact on the life of the affected person. ME/CFS is diagnosed primarily by the exclusion of other fatigue illnesses, but the availability of multiple case definitions for ME/CFS has complicated diagnosis for clinicians. There has been ongoing controversy over the nature of ME/CFS, but a recent detailed report from the Institute of Medicine (Academy of Sciences, USA) concluded that ME/CFS is a medical, not psychiatric illness. Importantly, aspects of the biological basis of the ongoing disease have been revealed over the last 2–3 years that promise new leads towards an effective clinical diagnostic test that may have a general application. Our detailed molecular studies with a preclinical study of ME/CFS patients, along with the complementary research of others, have reported an elevation of inflammatory and immune processes, ongoing neuro-inflammation, and decreases in general metabolism and mitochondrial function for energy production in ME/CFS, which contribute to the ongoing remitting/relapsing etiology of the illness. These biological changes have generated potential molecular biomarkers for use in diagnostic ME/CFS testing.

Keywords: myalgic encephalomyelitis; chronic fatigue syndrome; diagnostic biomarker; inflammation and immunity; metabolism; mitochondria; circadian rhythm; neuro-inflammation

---

1. Introduction

Myalgic Encephalomyelitis/Chronic Fatigue Syndrome (ME/CFS): A Significant Global Health Problem

The reported worldwide prevalence of ME/CFS varies from 0.4–2.6% of the population among countries and cultures [1], making it significantly more prevalent than other fatigue illnesses, such as multiple sclerosis, with, for example, up to ~240,000 Australians [2] and ~20,000 New Zealanders [3] affected with ME/CFS compared to ~25,000 and ~4000 respectively with multiple sclerosis. The first recognition of ME/CFS in New Zealand dates from an outbreak in a small rural town, Tapanui, in 1983, with an unexplained flu-like illness given the name 'Tapanui flu' [4], which was later classified as ME/CFS [5]. Similar outbreaks have been reported in isolated communities around the world since the 1930s [6]. A 2013 meta-analysis [7] found that ME/CFS prevalence from self-reporting assessment was 3.28% (95% Confidence Interval (CI): 2.24–4.33) but by clinical assessment was only 0.76% (95% CI: 0.23–1.29), using the 1994 Fukuda clinical case definition [8]. This discrepancy in prevalence highlights the importance of an understanding of the disease by health practitioners, and the use of clinically consistent diagnostic criteria for ME/CFS.

2. Clinical Characteristics of ME/CFS

Since ME/CFS has as yet no conclusive diagnostic laboratory test, and an ill-defined pathophysiology [9], there has been a diverse range of opinions as to the precise nature of the disease among health professionals and throughout wider society. This confusion surrounding the ME/CFS diagnosis among health practitioners worldwide has meant that patients and families are often without the support of their healthcare system and social support systems. A diagnostic molecular biomarker, tool, or accessible procedure specific for ME/CFS, that is readily transferable to diagnostic laboratories for routine tests on community-wide patient samples, is urgently needed.

Onset of ME/CFS frequently follows an acute viral infection or period of stress [1], but more gradual onset can occur, with the complex of symptoms developing over a period of weeks or months [10]. Many unique 'outbreaks' of an ME/CFS-like disease are recorded, suggesting it can arise from the spread of an initiating infectious agent. Certainly, ME/CFS is commonly self-reported following a glandular fever episode from Epstein Barr virus infection [11–14]. Twin studies indicate a genetic susceptibility for ME/CFS, with a higher rate of fatigue concordance in monozygotic twins than dizygotic twins [15–17]. In susceptible people, a diverse range of initiating agents can produce the same physiological 'shock' that precipitates progression into the life-long condition of ME/CFS [18]. Apart from viruses, factors such as toxins or agricultural chemicals like organophosphates, and physiological stressors, such as vaccinations [11,18], can precipitate the illness [11–13]. A recent publication examined 19 cases of patients diagnosed with either ME/CFS or fibromyalgia following hepatitis B vaccination, concluding that, in some cases, both of the illnesses could be temporally related to immunisation as part of autoimmune (auto-inflammatory) syndromes induced by adjuvants (ASIA) [19]. ME/CFS affects people of all ages and within all socio-economic groups, but it is more common in women (reported to be a ratio between 2:1 to 6:1, female to male) [11–13]. The defining symptom of ME/CFS is persistent, debilitating fatigue, lasting beyond six months. Most clinical diagnostic criteria describe this as physical and mental and disabling, usually of acute onset. It is significantly exacerbated by exercise, and mental or emotional exertion (post-exertional malaise), and is not alleviated by rest [6,14,20]. A myriad of flu-like and respiratory symptoms, cognitive impairment, tender lymph nodes, muscle and joint pain (myalgia), severe headaches, new allergies, severely disturbed sleep patterns with un-refreshing sleep, and mood changes are commonly experienced [6,14,20]. Multi-system co-morbidities, for example, POTS (postural orthostatic tachycardia syndrome), depression, and irritable bowel syndrome are often found [20,21]. Nevertheless, the severity and the range of ME/CFS symptoms can vary, with three in every four patients progressing from an extended acute phase to a chronic state of ongoing debilitating illness that still requires dramatic lifestyle changes to manage the frequency of severe relapses [14]. It is claimed that only about 5% of ME/CFS patients will return to their previous state of health and well-being [22], therefore for most of those affected it is a life-long disease.

3. Clinical Case Definitions

At present, a formal diagnosis is given only after eliminating all other diseases with similar symptoms, and with the presence of a range of self-reported symptoms fitting within defined sets of clinical criteria [9,11,12,20,21]. The difficulty for both patients and health practitioners has been that over 20 different case definitions or diagnostic criteria for ME/CFS exist [23]. Since the underlying pathophysiology of ME/CFS is still largely unknown, there is no gold standard against which to assess the effectiveness of each case definition. The 1994 Fukuda diagnostic criteria [8] developed by the Centre for Disease Control in the USA, is most commonly used by researchers and clinicians [1], yet it does not include the core defining symptoms of post-exertional malaise and neurocognitive disturbances, nor does it exclude patients whose symptoms may originate from a psychiatric disorder. The Canadian Consensus Criteria (CCC) [24] developed in 2003 by an international

ME/CFS expert group was a significant improvement as it highlighted post-exertional malaise as a core symptom, along with fatigue, sleep dysfunction and pain. Additionally, neurological/cognitive and autonomic/neuroendocrine/immune symptom groups were included. In 2011, the 'International Consensus Criteria' were formulated as a refinement of the CCC, putting emphasis on inflammation and neuropathology and focusing on neurological disturbance, immune/gastrointestinal, and energy impairments [20]. These criteria have yet to be generally accepted, and they may be selective for a subset of ME/CFS patients only.

To redress the confusion created by so many case definitions, a clinical guideline IACFS/ME primer for General Health Practitioners (GPs) was developed in 2012 by a panel of experts from the International Association for Chronic Fatigue Syndrome/Myalgic Encephalomyelitis (IACFS/ME) [21]. This included commonly used clinical guidelines, but showed considerable variation in symptoms and co-morbidities from those based on individual case definitions [25]. A detailed review of the criteria used to diagnose ME/CFS was released in 2015 by the Institute of Medicine (IOM) of the Academy of Sciences USA [6] along with a simplified core set of diagnostic criteria. The IOM report acknowledged that the stigma associated with a diagnosis of ME/CFS is largely due to both the lack of knowledge of the disease and the lack of acknowledgement of it as a distinct disease. Most importantly, the report stressed that based on all the available evidence, ME/CFS is a medical and not a psychiatric illness [6]. In our view, the Canadian Consensus Criteria (CCC) [24] are the best available definitions for both clinical diagnosis and for preclinical patient research studies.

4. Physiological Cause of ME/CFS and Current Treatments

To date, treatments for ME/CFS have targeted specific symptoms, such as sleep disruption, fatigue, muscle pain and emotional disturbance [11]. While the underlying primary physiological deficit in ME/CFS is still unknown, many differences in physiology and metabolism between ME/CFS patients and healthy controls have now been discovered in the last 2–3 years, enabling some understanding of the biological basis for the severely compromised health of ME/CFS patients. The research has highlighted areas for potential treatment. As ME/CFS patients have a significant immunological dysfunction, intravenous immunoglobulin therapy, interferon and ampligen, have been explored, but as yet with no conclusive outcomes [1]. Antidepressants, anti-allergy drugs, vitamin and mineral supplementation, and non-steroidal anti-inflammatory drugs have all been trialed among patient groups with mixed results [11,26]. A chance finding of remission of ME/CFS symptoms in a patient within a group undergoing cytotoxic treatment for Hodgkin's Lymphoma resulted in the hypothesis that B-cell depletion might provide a potentially effective treatment for ME/CFS [27]. Subsequent trials with ME/CFS patients using a monoclonal anti-CD20 antibody targeting a B-cell surface protein, Rituximab, seemed highly promising [28,29]. Disappointingly, however, the multicentre phase III trial ultimately was less successful [30]. Most recently, a phase II trial of a mixture of the Central Nervous System (CNS) stimulant Ritalin (methylphenidate hydrochloride) and mitochondrial support nutrients (KPAX002) [31] suggested that there was a trend towards improvement in fatigue. Two behavioural interventions, graded exercise therapy (GET) and cognitive behavioural therapy (CBT), have been controversial treatments for ME/CFS [11]. GET focuses on gradually increasing physical activity over time, but it has had limited success and often exacerbates the characteristic 'exercise intolerance' or post-exertional malaise of ME/CFS, as well as other symptoms. CBT by contrast is a psychotherapy approach that encourages patients to analyse their symptoms and develop strategies to function around them. Undoubtedly this approach has benefitted some patients in managing and living with their disease. A large-scale 'Pacing, graded Activity, and Cognitive behaviour therapy; a randomised Evaluation' (PACE) study incorporating these strategies in the UK was claimed to show a favourable response with both GET and CBT interventions together [32], but the method of analysis and thereby the conclusions have been strongly criticised [33], particularly in a special issue in 2017 of the Journal of Health Psychology [34].

5. Biomarkers Leading to a Diagnostic Test

As there is no single molecular biomarker test for ME/CFS, there are long delays and high costs involved in the diagnostic process, with increased potential for misdiagnosis, all of which fundamentally impedes patient care. Many potential diagnostic biomarkers have been identified by researchers—almost all of which indicate the involvement of improper immune function, inflammation, and signs of autoimmunity, e.g., differences in cytokine profiles, natural killer (NK) cell function, or responsiveness of T-cells, in ME/CFS. To date, research into clinically useful diagnostic biomarker identification for ME/CFS has been limited generally to small cohorts (with study sizes frequently <10, and rarely with validation in larger cohorts above $n = 40$). A further limitation to biomarker discovery is the lack of any comprehensive follow-up studies of potential biomarkers with different ME/CFS patient groups, or comparing ME/CFS with other similarly presenting illnesses. Another important factor obstructing biomarker discovery is the use of different diagnostic criteria from the many available to define the ME/CFS patient group, preventing meaningful comparisons between studies. While the majority of research groups do use the 1994 Fukuda criteria, as discussed earlier, the Fukuda criteria may confound clinical or diagnostic biomarker studies as it imprecisely defines ME/CFS symptomology and fails to exclude patients with a psychiatric disorder. The lack of follow-up studies, or failure to validate the results of an original study, has meant that potential biomarkers have rarely progressed to clinical trials.

Despite these significant handicaps to diagnostic research, exciting recent studies have emerged that seem to have considerable promise for further development into a general accessible diagnostic test. Nanoneedle bioarray technology, developed by Professor Ron Davis and colleagues at Stanford, measures a unique impedance signature that can differentiate moderate to severe ME/CFS sufferers ($n = 20$) from healthy controls ($n = 20$) [35]. The nanoneedle measures electrical impedance modulations resulting from cellular or molecular interactions in response to an induced high salt stressor. The test was able to differentiate ME/CFS from healthy controls from peripheral blood mononuclear cells (PBMCs) and plasma samples. The origin of the distinct different impedance signature in the ME/CFS group has not yet been identified, but the authors suggest that this may be caused by the Na/K ATPase transmembrane ion pump in ME/CFS cells, or a potential size change in cells as a result of increased osmotic pressure, or a change in the composition of cell membranes in response to the stressor. As yet, this technology has not been shown to distinguish ME/CFS from other related illnesses, and this will take time to resolve.

6. Changes in the Biology of ME/CFS Patients

Emerging molecular technologies have enabled significant insights into the metabolic and physiological abnormalities that sustain ME/CFS. We have applied these technologies in an ongoing preclinical analysis with a group of 10 ME/CFS patients, diagnosed using the CCC criteria, and matched controls for study according to the principles of precision medicine [36] to obtain an integrated 'molecular picture' of the illness. We have collected cytokine (Bio-Plex Human Cytokine 27-plex Assay) [37] and microRNA [38] expression data from patient and control plasma (TaqMan miRNA array), and also genes (RNAseq transcriptome [~13,000 gene transcripts] [38], and SWATH-MSprotein expression data [~1800 proteins], publication in preparation) from peripheral blood mononuclear cells (PBMCs) [38]. Statistically significant changes were identified, despite the small size of the study group with age/gender matched controls. Despite patient heterogeneity in age, gender, and stage of illness, similar patterns of changes in specific processes and pathways were observed. We identified significant dysregulation of immune/inflammatory pathways and oxidative stress linked to metabolic and mitochondrial dysfunction. Immune, inflammatory, cytokine and apoptosis pathways were enhanced, while mitochondrial function, general cellular metabolic and lipid metabolic pathways were suppressed [38]. These findings are consistent with the emerging data from other ME/CFS studies, some with larger cohorts (Table 1) [38–49], and show the utility of the approach utilizing precision medicine to elucidate disease pathology in small patient numbers—a practice used successfully in studies of rare diseases [50].

Table 1. Biological Pathways affected in ME/CFS.

Affected Biological Pathways	References
Immune/inflammation	[37–41,49]
Cytokine regulation	[37,38,42,43,49]
Metabolic dysregulation	[38,44,45,49]
Mitochondrial dysfunction	[38,45,46,49]
Oxidative stress	[38,39,47,49]
Apoptosis	[38,39,47,49]
Circadian rhythm	[48,49]

In particular, our transcriptome study [49] identified the top three upregulated genes in the ME/CFS group, as *IL8*, *NFKBIA* and *TNFAIP3* (see Figure 1), all of which are early-responders to Tumour Necrosis Factor (TNF)-induced Nuclear Factor kappa-light-chain-enhancer of activated B cells (NF-κB) activation [51].

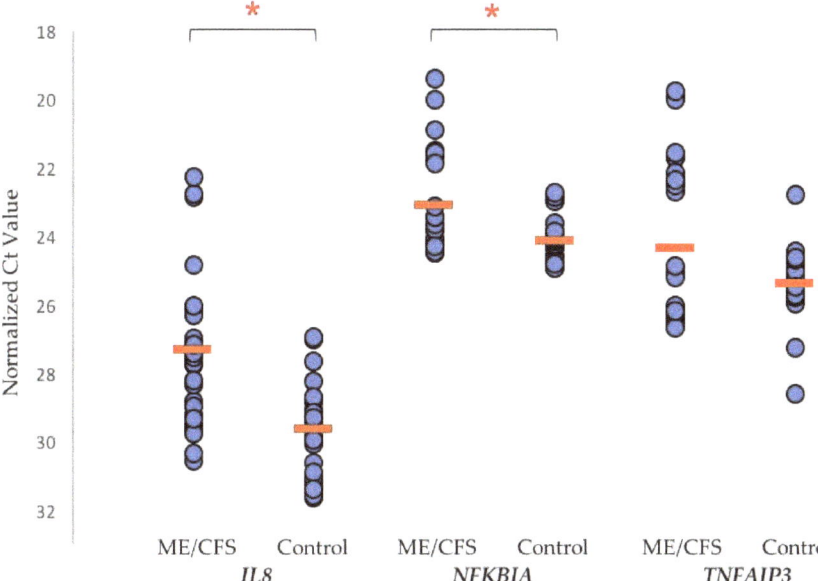

Figure 1. Scatter plot of RT-qPCR assay Ct values (defined below) for *IL8*, *NFKBIA*, and *TNFAIP3*. Each peripheral blood mononuclear cell (PBMC) sample (myalgic encephalomyelitis/chronic fatigue syndrome (ME/CFS) $n = 10$, control $n = 10$) was measured in triplicate, with the mean Ct value for each gene in both ME/CFS and control cohorts shown (orange line). A Ct value is the Reverse Transcription quantitative Polymerase Chain Reaction (RT-qPCR) amplification cycle at which the gene transcript copy number exceeded the individually calculated baseline threshold level for that gene. Figure taken from our own recently published study [49]. Red bars indicate the mean Ct value in each case. Statistical significance ($p < 0.05$) between the two groups is indicated by the *.

Increased *IL8* expression occurs as a result of TNF-induced NF-κB activation, and the proteins A20 (*TNFAIP3*) and Nuclear Factor of Kappa light chain polypeptide gene enhancer in B cells Inhibitor, Alpha (*NFKBIA*) are part of the two main negative feedback loops of NF-κB-driven transcription [51]. Furthermore, TNFα is a potent inducer of IL-8 secretion, through a transcriptional mechanism regulated by NF-κB. Indeed, increases in IL-8 and TNFα have been identified in several ME/CFS cytokine and immune studies. Chronic inflammation is also amplified through the NF-κB signaling pathway. The increase in expression of these three gene transcripts in the ME/CFS group implies that there is an ongoing biological inflammatory response, and a counter-response to the unwanted excess activity of NF-κB and inflammation in ME/CFS, driven by TNFα.

With the same study group, we have investigated the abnormal activation of protein kinase RNA-activated (PKR) as a potential biomarker for ME/CFS. This kinase has been described as a 'universal immunological abnormality' in ME/CFS [52]. ME/CFS often follows an acute viral infection, suggesting that the key role PKR plays in the innate immune response to infection may be significant in ME/CFS symptomology. The efficacy of PKR as a diagnostic biomarker for ME/CFS results from the fact that PKR is phosphorylated when activated. Healthy controls had undetectable phosphorylated PKR in protein extracts of PBMC cells using an in-house affinity purified antibody (two stage purification-positive and negative affinity steps). Phosphorylated PKR (pPKR) was in contrast detected in the protein cell extracts of ME/CFS patients. A ratio of pPKR to inactive unphosphorylated PKR examined between the patients and controls revealed differences between the two groups (see Figure 2).

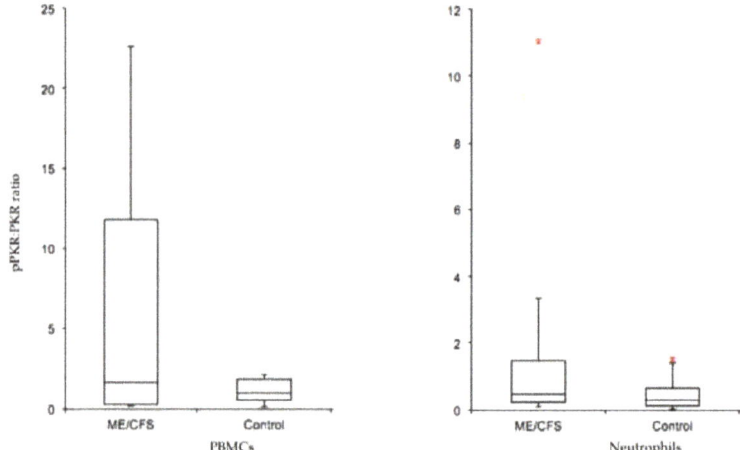

Figure 2. Box-and-whisker plots of ME/CFS and control phosphorylated PKR/protein kinase RNA-activated (pPKR:PKR) ratios in PBMCs and neutrophils. In-house affinity purified antibodies against phosphorylated PKR (active form) and PKR (inactive form) were used to detect the ratio of pPKR:PKR in isolated PBMCs and neutrophils from a matched patient/control ME/CFS study. The median pPKR:PKR ratio is shown, and the interquartile range, maximum and minimum ratio values. Outliers are indicated with a (*). A t-test between ME/CFS and controls gave a P-value of 0.057 in PBMCs (ME/CFS $n = 9$, controls $n = 9$) and 0.142 in Neutrophils (ME/CFS $n = 9$, controls $n = 10$). This figure has been constructed by author ES from data referenced in her PhD thesis, with permission to publish from University of Otago [38].

It should be noted that not all patients scored positive for pPKR, but the study group on average had suffered with their illness for 12 years. It would be important to re-evaluate the pPKR/PKR ratio in larger patient groups undergoing diagnosis at the *early* stage of their illness to determine false negative rates. Then, it will be clear whether PKR has significant promise as a diagnostic tool.

7. Global Research into ME/CFS Biology

7.1. Recent Research Studies Have Focused on Several Key Areas

7.1.1. Microbiome

The chronic nature of ME/CFS suggests that its continuous pathogenesis involves an altered state of body homeostasis. Numerous reports indicate chronic inflammation, characterised by immunological dysfunction, in ME/CFS. Biomarkers of inflammation and leaky gut syndrome [53], possibly as a result of microbiome disturbance and bacterial translocation, have been highlighted [53,54]. Compellingly, most well-studied inflammatory conditions have been linked to microbial imbalance (dysbiosis) of the human microbiome [53]. Impaired mucosal integrity, shown by serum levels of Immunoglobulin A (IgA) and Immunoglobulin M (IgM) against enterobacteria, may explain both inflammation and the hypersensitivity to food in ME/CFS [55]. Recent gut microbiome studies have found lowered microbial diversity in ME/CFS fecal samples [56,57]. Next-generation sequencing of peripheral blood samples identified a 'multifactorial microbial component' that correlated with a disease-severity quality of life measure in ME/CFS patients [58]. Sequencing small ribosomal subunit 16S rRNAs from the collective bacterial population indicated an increase in pro-inflammatory microbiota species and a decrease in anti-inflammatory species [56]. Intracellular pathogens like bacteriophages can drive microbiome dysbiosis by directly interfering with the bacterial molecular biology. Interestingly, a study of monozygotic twins discordant for ME/CFS found an increase in bacteriophages belonging to the tailed double stranded Ribonucleic Acid (dsRNA) *Caudovirales* order [56].

As yet, however, there is no general agreement on changes in specific microbiota phyla/genera among reported ME/CFS studies [53–60].

7.1.2. Metabolome

ME/CFS metabolomics studies have identified a consistent set of disease characteristics, including increased oxidative stress, depleted amino acids, depleted lipids, TCA cycle and purine metabolites, a reduced folate cycle, and increased sugars [44,61]. Recent studies also show a range of plasma metabolites at abnormally low concentrations in ME/CFS, implying that ME/CFS is a 'hypometabolic' syndrome. Naviaux et al. (2016) [44] used broad-spectrum metabolomics to examine metabolites from 63 biochemical pathways and abnormalities were identified in 20 of them. They involved oxidative peroxisomes, mitochondrial metabolism, branch chain amino acids, as well as pathways for sphingolipids, phospholipids and cholesterol. Significantly, despite a diverse heterogeneity of factors leading to the illness of the ME/CFS cohort within the study, the results reflected a lowered cellular metabolic response as a common feature in the patients. It was likened to 'dauer', a protective hibernation-like state [44].

The suggestion that hypometabolic syndrome is a feature of ME/CFS may be underpinned by changes in expression of key genes in the pathways concerned. Changes in the DNA methylation (epigenetic code) across the promoter region of genes for these pathways could be a key factor. DNA methylation is an epigenetic modification process where DNA methyltransferases add a methyl group to the 5' position of the cytosine base of 5'-Cytosine-phosphate-Guanine-3' (CpG) dinucleotides [62], and the extent and pattern of this methylation dictates the rate of gene expression [63]. DNA methylation can also recruit transcriptional co-repressors to inhibit the transcription of certain genes [62]. Epigenetic modifications have been suggested to play important roles in inflammatory and autoimmune diseases that share many similarities with ME/CFS [64]. Multiple DNA methylation studies have now shown both hypo-methylation and hyper-methylation at specific gene promoters in ME/CFS patients, including in our own ongoing unpublished studies. We have found that of the changes observed hyper-methylation was proportionally much higher at promoters than throughout the whole genome. Generally, a loss of methylation accounted for most of the genome-wide changes between the ME/CFS study group and the controls. The addition of methyl groups at promoters may contribute to a hypometabolic state by down-regulating the expression of genes involved in key metabolic pathways. The ME/CFS phenotype is linked to differential methylation in genes associated with immune function and cellular metabolism [48,65,66]. For example, a 2017 study [48] detected 12,608 differentially methylated sites predominantly at cellular metabolism genes, changes that also could be related to patient quality of life health scores. Among these, glucocorticoid sensitivity was associated with differential methylation at 13 loci, implicating this process, along with immune and HPA axis dysfunctions, in ME/CFS [48]. A study focusing on CD4+ T-cells of patients affected by ME/CFS, rheumatoid arthritis and multiple sclerosis found differential methylation around the major Histocompatibility complex, class II, DQ beta 1 gene (HLA-DQB1) [67]. HLA-DQB1 encodes a cell surface receptor essential in immune signaling. Overall, these findings align with recent ME/CFS work pointing towards impairment in cellular energy production and immune dysfunction in the patient population.

7.1.3. Mitochondria

Detailed studies on energy production pathways in ME/CFS implicate dysfunctional mitochondria in the disease pathogenesis. Crucial fatigue symptoms of exercise intolerance and myalgia associated with ME/CFS are shared by patients with primary mitochondrial diseases and known mutations in either nuclear or mitochondrial DNA [68]. A recent study found lower maximal respiration in ME/CFS PBMCs, suggesting a reduced ability to elevate their respiration rate to compensate in times of physiological stress [46], and we have found a similar result in ongoing studies within our patient cohort. Another study showed a reduced abundance of the amino acids that fuel oxidative metabolism via the citric acid cycle in mitochondria. The changed amino acid pattern suggested the functional impairment of a key enzyme, pyruvate dehydrogenase (PDH) [45], supported by the identification of the increased expression of transcripts of kinases that inhibit PDH. Interestingly, myoblasts grown in serum from severe ME/CFS patients showed metabolic adaptations, including increased mitochondrial respiration and lactate secretion [45].

7.1.4. Transient Receptor Potential (TRP) Ion Channels

A recent study has documented extensively the dysfunction of a TRP ion channel and Ca^{2+} mobilisation in ME/CFS [69]. The **T**ransient **R**eceptor **P**otential group **M** (TRPM) subfamily participates in store operated calcium entry (SOCE) in the white matter of the CNS [69]. Previous investigations have proposed that Natural Killer (NK) cells from ME/CFS patients have a significantly reduced expression of TRPM3 and a subsequent reduction in intracellular Ca^{2+} mobilisation [70,71]. Five single nucleotide polymorphisms (SNPs) have now been identified in the TRPM3 gene in ME/CFS patients that may confer susceptibility to the disease [72]. A significant reduction in NK cell cytotoxicity, a Ca^{2+} dependent process, is consistently reported in both severe and moderate ME/CFS [73]. Related to ME/CFS symptomology, TRPM3 ion channels also have a role in the detection of heat and in pain transmission in the CNS [74]. Collectively, these results suggest that disturbed TRPM3 expression or activity may play an important role in the pathophysiology of ME/CFS.

7.1.5. Genetic Susceptibility

Single Nucleotide Polymorphism (SNP) analyses generally have provided weight to a genetic susceptibility for ME/CFS. Associations but not causative mutations have been found between several SNPs and ME/CFS pathology. An evaluation of 116, 204 SNPs found 65 SNPs associated with ME/CFS that included a glutamate receptor, ionotropic kinase 2 (GRIK2) (decreased expression), and neuronal 'Per-Arnt-Sim' (PAS) domain protein 2 (NPAS2) (increased expression) implicating a pathological role for genes involved in glutamatergic neurotransmission and circadian rhythm [75]. Interestingly, transcripts associated with circadian rhythm were identified as significantly changed in our transcriptome study [49]. Most recently, Schlauch et al. evaluated 906, 600 SNPs and found 442 associated with ME/CFS [76].

8. Has Biomedical Research Informed the Clinic, and Assisted Diagnosis and Treatment?

With a myriad of clinical case definitions to choose from, and a lack of understanding of the fundamental pathophysiology of ME/CFS, coupled with a lack of a definitive molecular biomarker, health practitioners have not had a clear direction for the diagnosis and treatment of ME/CFS. In our experience, this has led to frustration both at the feet of the practitioners and the affected patients, and to a long period of debate among the health profession about the true nature of the illness. It has hindered funding for much needed research and has created inertia for researchers to join the research effort. Excitingly, the last 3–4 years have signaled dramatic change. With growing understanding of the disease biology, and with promising diagnostic tools on the horizon, the outlook is much more promising for both practitioners and patients alike. Current biomedical research is on the cusp of providing tools that can be utilised in the clinic, but already the identification of affected pathways like inflammation and disturbed immunity, or changes in energy production and key metabolic pathways, and the identification of potential biomarkers for those changes are starting to inform the clinic today. Therapeutic interventions have been 'trial and error' applications of available drugs but with no universal benefit, and at best very mixed results. We are entering a new phase where the directed design of therapies seems possible. Examples are antioxidants that might target and reduce an energy production insufficiency, and targeted anti-inflammatory drugs to improve impaired central nervous system function. The ultimate goal of the biomedical research is to find the primary cause of the significant downward spiral in health that results in the long-term debilitating illness of ME/CFS.

9. Discussion

Future Directions and Unresolved Questions

While major steps have been made in our understanding of the biological processes involved in ME/CFS, there are important unresolved questions remaining. These include: (i) Is there a genetic susceptibility that causes some individuals, after exposure to a viral or toxic chemical or a traumatic emotional assault, to 'switch' into a life-long ME/CFS 'dauer' state? (ii) What is the key initial physiological trigger causing the dramatic downward spiral in health? (iii) Are the molecular changes and aberrant energy producing pathways observed a consequence of, rather than the cause, of the disease state? (iv) Is there an unidentified 'molecular factor' that facilitates cell alterations, as implied from the effects of ME/CFS serum on healthy cells? (v) Why does the 'switch' triggering a physiological response to the initial assault not return to normal, as for most viral illnesses? and, (vi) Why do characteristic frequent relapses occur in the chronic stage of ME/CFS, implying a hypersensitivity to even minor stress?

ME/CFS was classified originally by the World Health Organization as a neurological disease in 1969 [77], and many symptoms like lack of refreshing sleep and cognitive 'brain fog' must be directly related to a poorly functioning brain. We have proposed a neuro-inflammatory model of ME/CFS, in an attempt to describe its unexplained and diverse characteristics and wide array of symptoms [78]. We believe that a centre within the hypothalamus, a cluster of neurons called the paraventricular nucleus that is key in resolving stress, may be critical to the perpetuation of the disease and the relapse/recovery cycles in ME/CFS [78]. One neuroimaging study with ME/CFS patients [78] provides support for this hypothesis, with the discovery of enhanced activated glial cells (a marker for neuro-inflammation) in the limbic system. The degree of glial activation correlated with the severity of ME/CFS symptoms [79]. To test these ideas, targeted advanced imaging studies are needed which will provide a better understanding of the specific mechanisms in the brain that are affected to cause such a severe phenotype in ME/CFS.

Current global ME/CFS research has focused on identifying changes in physiological and biochemical pathways, with special emphasis on energy metabolism and Ca^{2+} metabolism. More detailed research on the deficiencies coupled with genetic analyses to explain the hypo-metabolism may prove vital in understanding what it is in ME/CFS that sustains the illness and its complex symptoms.

With the powerful new analytical tools available to researchers, rapid advancement is being made in our understanding of the underlying biology of ME/CFS, and several promising potential disease biomarkers have been identified. What is now needed are significant follow-up investigation of these markers, with large patient numbers and across different centres. Most importantly, these biomarkers will need to be validated against diseases that share similar features with ME/CFS.

Author Contributions: Conceptualization: W.T., R.V., E.S.; methodology: E.S., C.E., A.N., A.H.; software: A.N., E.S., A.H., M.R.; validation: R.V., C.E., E.S., M.R., A.M.; formal analysis: E.S., A.N., A.H., A.M.; resources: W.T.; writing—original draft preparation: W.T., E.S.; writing—review and editing: W.T., E.S., M.R.; supervision: W.T., M.R.; project administration: W.T., A.N.; funding acquisition: W.T.

Funding: We thank the National ME/CFS Disease Association-Associated New Zealand ME Society (ANZMES) for their ongoing support to WT. We acknowledge grants from Lottery Health (New Zealand) to WT and to AM, the Healthcare Otago Charitable Trust to WT, the Otago Medical Research Foundation (Otago Community Trust Annual Grant CT376) to WT, and from those generous people who have given private bequests.

Acknowledgments: We gratefully acknowledge Torsten Kleffmann, Protein Chemistry Centre, University of Otago for the Mass Spectrometry proteome analyses. We especially wish to thank the patients and healthy control participants who took part in our study.

Conflicts of Interest: The authors declare no conflict of interest.

References

1. Bansal, A.S.; Bradley, A.S.; Bishop, K.N.; Kiani-Alikhan, S.; Ford, B. Chronic fatigue syndrome, the immune system and viral infection. *Brain Behav. Immun.* **2012**, *26*, 24–31. [CrossRef] [PubMed]
2. Hunt, G. *$3 Million Research Funding for Chronic Fatigue Syndrome*; Media Release; Australian Government Department of Health: Canberra, Australia, 27 March 2019. Available online: https://beta.health.gov.au/ministers/the-hon-greg-hunt-mp/media/3-million-research-funding-for-chronic-fatigue-syndrome (accessed on 10 July 2019).
3. Associated New Zealand ME Society (ANZMES). Available online: http://anzmes.org.nz/ (accessed on 4 April 2019).
4. Simpson, L.O. Myalgic Encephalomyelitis. *J. R. Soc. Med.* **1991**, *84*, 633. [PubMed]
5. Price, J.L. Myalgic encephalomyelitis. *Lancet* **1961**, *1*, 737–738. [CrossRef]
6. IOM (Institute of Medicine). *Beyond Myalgic Encephalomyelitis/Chronic Fatigue Syndrome: Redefining an Illness*; National Academies Press: Washington, DC, USA, 2015.
7. Johnston, S.; Brenu, E.W.; Staines, D.; Marshall-Gradisnik, S. The prevalence of chronic fatigue syndrome/myalgic encephalomyelitis: A meta analysis. *Clin. Epidemiol.* **2013**, *5*, 105–110. [CrossRef] [PubMed]
8. Fukuda, K.; Straus, S.E.; Hickie, I.; Sharpe, M.C.; Dobbins, J.G.; Komaroff, A. The chronic fatigue syndrome: A comprehensive approach to its definition and study. International Chronic Fatigue Syndrome Study Group. *Ann. Intern. Med.* **1994**, *121*, 953–959. [CrossRef] [PubMed]
9. Siegel, S.D.; Antoni, M.H.; Fletcher, M.A.; Maher, K.; Segota, M.C.; Klimas, N. Impaired natural immunity, cognitive dysfunction, and physical symptoms in patients with chronic fatigue syndrome: Preliminary evidence for a subgroup? *J. Psychosom. Res.* **2006**, *60*, 559–566. [CrossRef]
10. Lorusso, L.; Mikhaylova, S.V.; Capelli, E.; Ferrari, D.; Ngonga, G.K.; Ricevuti, G. Immunological aspects of chronic fatigue syndrome. *Autoimmun. Rev.* **2009**, *8*, 287–291. [CrossRef]
11. Devanur, L.D.; Kerr, J.R. Chronic fatigue syndrome. *J. Clin. Virol.* **2006**, *37*, 139–150. [CrossRef]
12. Holgate, S.T.; Komaroff, A.L.; Mangan, D.; Wessely, S. Chronic fatigue syndrome: Understanding a complex illness. *Nat. Rev. Neurosci.* **2011**, *12*, 539–544. [CrossRef]
13. Crawley, E. The epidemiology of chronic fatigue syndrome/myalgic encephalitis in children. *Arch. Dis. Child.* **2014**, *99*, 171–174. [CrossRef]
14. Vallings, R. *Chronic Fatigue Syndrome M.E. Symptoms: Diagnosis & Management*; Calico Publishing Ltd.: Auckland, New Zealand, 2012.
15. Buchwald, D.; Herrell, R.; Ashton, S.; Belcourt, M.; Schmaling, K.; Sullivan, P.; Neale, M.; Goldberg, J. A twin study of chronic fatigue. *Psychosom. Med.* **2001**, *63*, 936–943. [CrossRef] [PubMed]

16. Sabath, D.E.; Barcy, S.; Koelle, D.M.; Zeh, J.; Ashton, S.; Buchwald, D. Cellular immunity in monozygotic twins discordant for chronic fatigue syndrome. *J. Infect. Dis.* **2002**, *185*, 828–832. [CrossRef] [PubMed]
17. Sullivan, P.F.; Evengard, B.; Jacks, A.; Pedersen, N.L. Twin analyses of chronic fatigue in a Swedish national sample. *Psychol. Med.* **2005**, *35*, 1327–1336. [CrossRef] [PubMed]
18. Shepherd, C.; Chaudhuri, A. *ME/CFS/PVFS: An Exploration of the Key Clinical Issues*, 9th ed.; The ME Association: Gawcott, UK, 2017.
19. Agmon-Levin, N.; Zafrir, Y.; Kivity, S.; Balofsky, A.; Amital, H.; Shoenfeld, Y. Chronic fatigue syndrome and fibromyalgia following immunization with the hepatitis B vaccine: Another angle of the 'autoimmune (auto-inflammatory) syndrome induced by adjuvants' ASIA. *Immun. Res.* **2014**, *60*, 376–383. [CrossRef] [PubMed]
20. Carruthers, B.M.; van de Sande, M.I.; De Meirleir, K.L.; Klimas, N.G.; Broderick, G.; Mitchell, T.; Staines, D.; Powles, A.C.; Speight, N.; Vallings, R.; et al. Myalgic encephalomyelitis: International Consensus Criteria. *J. Intern. Med.* **2011**, *270*, 327–338. [CrossRef] [PubMed]
21. Friedberg, F.C.; Bateman, L.; Bested, A.C.; Davenport, T.; Friedman, K.; Gurwitt, A.; Jason, L.A.; Lapp, C.W.; Stevens, S.R.; Underhill, R.A.; et al. *Chronic Fatigue Syndrome/Myalgic Encephalomyelitis: A Primer for Clinical Practitioners*; International Association for Chronic Fatigue Syndrome/Myalgic Encephalomyelitis: Chicago, IL, USA, 2012.
22. Cairns, R.; Hotopf, M. A systematic review describing the prognosis of chronic fatigue syndrome. *Occup. Med.* **2005**, *55*, 20–31. [CrossRef] [PubMed]
23. Brurberg, K.G.; Fonhus, M.S.; Larun, L.; Flottorp, S. Case definitions for chronic fatigue syndrome/myalgic encephalomyelitis (CFS/ME): A systematic review. *BMJ Open* **2014**, *4*, 1–12. [CrossRef]
24. Carruthers, B.M.; Kumar Jain, A.; de Meirleir, K.L.; Peterson, L.; Klimas, N.G.; Lerner, M.; Bested, A.C.; Flor-Henry, P.; Joshi, P.; Powles, P.; et al. Myalgic Encephalomyelitis/Chronic Fatigue Syndrome: Clinical Working Case Definition, Diagnostic and Treatment Guidelines, A Consensus Document. *J. Chronic Fatigue Syndr.* **2003**, *11*, 7–115. [CrossRef]
25. Johnston, S.; Brenu, E.; Staines, D.; Marshall-Gradisnik, S. The role of clinical guidelines for chronic fatigue syndrome/myalgic encephalomyelitis in research settings. *Fatigue* **2014**, *2*, 28–39. [CrossRef]
26. Whiting, P.; Bagnall, A.M.; Sowden, A.J.; Cornell, J.E.; Mulrow, C.D.; Ramírez, G. Interventions for the treatment and management of chronic fatigue syndrome: A systematic review. *JAMA* **2001**, *286*, 1360–1368. [CrossRef]
27. Fluge, O.; Mella, O. Clinical impact of B-cell depletion with the anti-CD20 antibody rituximab in chronic fatigue syndrome: A preliminary case series. *BMC Neurol.* **2009**, *9*, 28–34. [CrossRef] [PubMed]
28. Fluge, O.; Bruland, O.; Risa, K.; Storstein, A.; Kristoffersen, E.K.; Sapkota, D.; Naess, H.; Dahl, O.; Nyland, H.; Mella, O. Benefit from B-lymphocyte depletion using the anti-CD20 antibody rituximab in chronic fatigue syndrome. A double-blind and placebo-controlled study. *PLoS ONE* **2011**, *6*, e26358. [CrossRef] [PubMed]
29. Fluge, O.; Risa, K.; Lunde, S.; Alme, K.; Gurvin Rekeland, I.; Sapkota, D.; Kleboe Kristofferson, E.; Sorland, K.; Bruland, O.; Dahl, O.; et al. B-Lymphocyte depletion in myalgic encephalopathy/chronic fatigue syndrome. an open-label phase II study with rituximab maintenance treatment. *PLoS ONE* **2015**, *10*, 0129898. [CrossRef] [PubMed]
30. Maxmen, A. A reboot for chronic fatigue syndrome research. *Nature* **2018**, *553*, 14–17. [CrossRef] [PubMed]
31. Montoya, J.G.; Anderson, J.N.; Adolphs, D.L.; Bateman, L.; Klimas, N.; Levine, S.M.; Garvert, D.; Kaiser, J.D. KPAX002 as a treatment for myalgic encephalomyelitis/chronic fatigue syndrome (ME/CFS): A prospective, randomized trial. *Int. J. Clin. Exp. Med.* **2018**, *11*, 2890–2900.
32. Sharpe, M.; Goldsmith, K.A.; Johnson, A.L.; Chalder, T.; Walker, J.; White, P.D. Rehabilitative treatments for chronic fatigue syndrome: Long-term follow-up from the PACE trial. *Lancet Psychiatry* **2015**, *2*, 1067–1074. [CrossRef]
33. Coyne, J.C.; Laws, K.R. Results of the PACE follow-up study are uninterpretable. *Lancet Psychiatry* **2016**, *3*, e6–e7. [CrossRef]
34. Marks, D.F. Special issue: The PACE Trial. *J. Health Psychol.* **2017**, *22*, 1103–1216. [CrossRef]
35. Esfandyarpour, R.; Kashi, A.; Nemat-Gorgani, M.; Wilhelmy, J.; Davis, R.W. A nanoelectronics-blood-based diagnostic biomarker for myalgic encephalomyelitis/chronic fatigue syndrome (ME/CFS). *Proc. Natl. Acad. Sci. USA* **2019**, *116*, 10250–10257. [CrossRef]

36. Tate, W.P.; Sweetman, E.C.; Noble, A.J.K.; Edgar, C.; Bateman, G.; Mackay, A.; Ryan, M.; Hodges, L.; Vallings, R. Tackling ME/CFS in New Zealand by the principles of precision medicine. *IiME* **2016**, *10*, 46–55.
37. Noble, A.J.K. Exploring Potential Biomarkers for ME/CFS. Ph.D. Thesis, University of Otago, Dunedin, New Zealand, 2017.
38. Sweetman, E.C. Comprehensive Molecular Analysis of Different Classes of Molecules in a Myalgic Encephalomyelitis/Chronic Fatigue Syndrome Pilot Study Group, and Investigation of RNA-activated Protein Kinase R (PKR) as a Diagnostic Biomarker. Ph.D. Thesis, University of Otago, Dunedin, New Zealand, 2018.
39. Gow, J.W.; Hagan, S.; Herzyk, P.; Cannon, C.; Behan, P.O.; Chaudhuri, A. A gene signature for post-infectious chronic fatigue syndrome. *BMC Med. Genom.* **2009**, *2*, 38–40. [CrossRef] [PubMed]
40. Brenu, E.W.; Ashton, K.J.; Batovska, J.; Staines, D.R.; Marshall-Gradisnik, S.M. High-throughput sequencing of plasma microRNA in chronic fatigue syndrome/myalgic encephalomyelitis. *PLoS ONE* **2014**, *9*, e102783. [CrossRef] [PubMed]
41. Nguyen, C.B.; Alsøe, L.; Lindvall, J.M.; Sulheim, D.; Fagermoen, E.; Winger, A.; Kaarbo, M.; Nilsen, H.; Wyller, V.B. Whole blood gene expression in adolescent chronic fatigue syndrome: An exploratory cross-sectional study suggesting altered B cell differentiation and survival. *J. Transl. Med.* **2017**, *15*, 102–122. [CrossRef] [PubMed]
42. Broderick, G.; Katz, B.Z.; Fernandes, H.; Fletcher, M.A.; Klimas, N.; Smith, F.A.; O'Gorman, M.R.; Vernon, S.D.; Taylor, R. Cytokine expression profiles of immune imbalance in post-mononucleosis chronic fatigue. *J. Transl. Med.* **2012**, *10*, 191–201. [CrossRef] [PubMed]
43. Montoya, J.G.; Holmes, T.H.; Anderson, J.N.; Maecker, H.T.; Rosenberg-Hasson, Y.; Valencia, I.; Chu, L.; Younger, J.W.; Tato, C.M.; Davis, M.M. Cytokine signature associated with disease severity in chronic fatigue syndrome patients. *Proc. Natl. Acad. Sci. USA* **2017**, *114*, E7150–E7158. [CrossRef]
44. Naviaux, R.K.; Naviaux, J.C.; Li, K.; Bright, A.T.; Alaynick, W.A.; Wang, L.; Baxter, A.; Nathan, N.; Anderson, W.; Gordon, E. Metabolic features of chronic fatigue syndrome. *Proc. Natl. Acad. Sci. USA* **2016**, *113*, E5472–E5480. [CrossRef]
45. Fluge, O.; Mella, O.; Bruland, O.; Risa, K.; Drystad, S.E.; Alme, K.; Rekeland, I.G.; Sapkota, D.; Rosland, G.V.; Fossa, A.; et al. Metabolic profiling indicates impaired pyruvate dehydrogenase function in myalgic encephalopathy/chronic fatigue syndrome. *JCI Insight* **2016**, *1*, e89376. [CrossRef]
46. Tomas, C.; Brown, A.; Strassheim, V.; Elson, J.L.; Newton, J.; Manning, P. Cellular bioenergetics is impaired in patients with chronic fatigue syndrome. *PLoS ONE* **2017**, *12*, e0186802. [CrossRef]
47. Armstrong, C.W.; McGregor, N.R.; Lewis, D.P.; Butt, H.L.; Gooley, P.R. The association of fecal microbiota and fecal, blood serum and urine metabolites in myalgic encephalomyelitis/chronic fatigue syndrome. *Metabolomics* **2017**, *13*, 8–20. [CrossRef]
48. de Vega, W.C.; Herrera, S.; Vernon, S.D.; McGowan, P.O. Epigenetic modifications and glucocorticoid sensitivity in myalgic encephalomyelitis/chronic fatigue syndrome. *BMC Med. Genom.* **2017**, *10*, 11–24. [CrossRef]
49. Sweetman, E.C.; Ryan, M.; Edgar, C.; Mackay, A.; Vallings, R.; Tate, W. Changes in the transcriptome of circulating immune cells of a New Zealand cohort with Myalgic encephalomyelitis/chronic fatigue syndrome. *Int. J. Immunopathol. Pharmacol.* **2019**, *33*, 1–8. [CrossRef] [PubMed]
50. Newman, S.K.; Jayanthan, R.K.; Mitchell, G.W.; Carreras Tartak, J.A.; Croglio, M.P.; Suarez, A.; Liu, A.Y.; Razzo, B.M.; Oyeniran, E.; Ruth, J.R.; et al. Taking control of castleman disease: Leveraging precision medicine technologies to accelerate rare disease research. *Yale J. Biol. Med.* **2015**, *88*, 383–388. [PubMed]
51. Lee, R.E.C.; Walker, S.R.; Savery, K.; Frank, D.A.; Gaudet, S. Fold-change of nuclear NF-κB determines TNF-induced transcription in single cells. *Mol. Cell* **2014**, *53*, 867–879. [CrossRef] [PubMed]
52. Meeus, M.; Nijs, J.; McGregor, N.; Meeusen, R.; De Schutter, G.; Truijen, S.; Fremont, M.; Van Hoof, E.; De Meirler, K. Unravelling intracellular immune dysfunctions in chronic fatigue syndrome: Interactions between protein kinase R activity, RNase L cleavage and elastase activity, and their clinical relevance. *In Vivo* **2008**, *22*, 115–122. [PubMed]
53. Shukla, S.K.; Cook, D.; Meyer, J.; Vernon, S.D.; Le, T.; Clevidence, D.; Robertson, C.E.; Schrodi, S.J.; Yale, S.; Frank, D.N. Changes in gut and plasma microbiome following exercise challenge in myalgic encephalomyelitis/chronic fatigue syndrome (ME/CFS). *PLoS ONE* **2015**, *10*, e0145453. [CrossRef]

54. Mandarano, A.H.; Giloteaux, L.; Keller, B.A.; Levine, S.M.; Hanson, M.R. Eukaryotes in the gut microbiota in myalgic encephalomyelitis/chronic fatigue syndrome. *PeerJ* **2018**, *6*, e4282. [CrossRef]
55. Maes, M.; Mihaylova, I.; Leunis, J.C. Increased serum IgA and IgM against LPS of enterobacteria in chronic fatigue syndrome (CFS): Indication for the involvement of gram-negative enterobacteria in the etiology of CFS and for the presence of an increased gut-intestinal permeability. *J. Affect. Disord.* **2007**, *99*, 237–240. [CrossRef]
56. Giloteaux, L.; Hanson, M.R.; Keller, B.A. A pair of identical twins discordant for myalgic encephalomyelitis/chronic fatigue syndrome differ in physiological parameters and gut microbiome composition. *Am. J. Case Rep.* **2016**, *17*, 720–729. [CrossRef]
57. Giloteaux, L.; Goodrich, J.K.; Walters, W.A.; Leine, S.M.; Ley, R.E.; Hanson, M.R. Reduced diversity and altered composition of the gut microbiome in individuals with myalgic encephalomyelitis/chronic fatigue syndrome. *Microbiome* **2016**, *4*, 30–41. [CrossRef]
58. Ellis, J.E.; Missan, D.S.; Shabilla, M.; Martinez, D.; Fry, S.E. Microbial community profiling of peripheral blood in myalgic encephalomyelitis/chronic fatigue syndrome. *Hum. Microbiome J.* **2018**, *9*, 16–21. [CrossRef]
59. Nagy-Szakal, D.; Williams, B.L.; Mishra, N.; Che, X.; Lee, B.; Bateman, L.; Klimas, N.G.; Komaroff, A.L.; Levine, S.; Montoya, J.G.; et al. Fecal metagenomics profiles in subgroups of patients with myalgic encephalomyelitis/chronic fatigue syndrome. *Microbiome* **2017**, *5*, 44–60. [CrossRef] [PubMed]
60. Armstrong, C.W.; McGregor, N.R.; Lewis, D.P.; Butt, H.L.; Gooley, P.R. Metabolic profiling reveals anomalous energy metabolism and oxidative stress pathways in chronic fatigue syndrome patients. *Metabolomics* **2015**, *11*, 1626–1639. [CrossRef]
61. Yamano, E.; Sugimoto, M.; Hirayama, A.; Kume, S.; Yamato, M.; Jin, G.; Tajima, S.; Goda, N.; Iwai, K.; Fukuda, S.; et al. Index markers of chronic fatigue syndrome with dysfunction of TCA and urea cycles. *Sci. Rep.* **2016**, *6*, 34990–34998. [CrossRef] [PubMed]
62. Moore, L.D.; Le, T.; Fan, G. DNA methylation and its basic function. *Neuropsychopharmacology* **2013**, *38*, 23–38. [CrossRef] [PubMed]
63. Laszlo, A.H.; Derrington, I.M.; Brinkerhoff, H.; Lanford, K.W.; Nova, I.C.; Samson, J.M.; Bartlett, J.j.; Pavlenok, M.; Gundlach, J.H. Detection and mapping of 5-methylcytosine and 5-hydroxymethylcytosine with nanopore MspA. *Proc. Natl. Acad. Sci. USA* **2013**, *110*, 18904–18909. [CrossRef] [PubMed]
64. de Vega, W.C.; Erdman, L.; Vernon, S.D.; Goldenberg, A.; McGowan, P.O. Integration of DNA methylation and health scores identifies subtypes in myalgic encephalomyelitis/chronic fatigue syndrome. *Epigenomics* **2018**, *10*, 539–557. [CrossRef] [PubMed]
65. Herrera, S.; de Vega, W.C.; Ashbrook, D.; Vernon, S.D.; McGowan, P.O. Genome-epigenome interactions associated with myalgic encephalomyelitis/chronic fatigue syndrome. *Epigenetics* **2018**, *5*, 1–17. [CrossRef] [PubMed]
66. de Vega, W.C.; Vernon, S.D.; McGowan, P.O. DNA methylation modifications associated with chronic fatigue syndrome. *PLoS ONE* **2014**, *9*, e104757. [CrossRef] [PubMed]
67. Brenu, E.W.; Staines, D.R.; Marshall-Gradisnik, S. Methylation profile of CD4+ T cells in chronic fatigue syndrome/myalgic encephalomyelitis. *J. Clin. Cell Immunol.* **2014**, *5*, 228–241.
68. Gorman, G.S.; Elson, J.L.; Newman, J.; Payne, B.; McFarland, R.; Newton, J.L.; Turnbull, D.M. Perceived fatigue is highly prevalent and debilitating in patients with mitochondrial disease. *Neuromuscul. Disord.* **2015**, *25*, 563–566. [CrossRef] [PubMed]
69. Staines, D.R.; Du Preez, S.; Cabanas, H.; Balinas, C.; Eaton, N.; Passmore, R.; Maksoud, R.; Redmayne, J.; Marshall-Gradisnik, S. Transient receptor potential ion channels in the etiology and pathomechanism of chronic fatigue syndrome/myalgic encephalomyelitis. *Int. J. Clin. Med.* **2018**, *9*, 445–453. [CrossRef]
70. Nguyen, T.; Johnston, S.C.; Clarke, L.; Smith, P.; Marshall-Gradisnik, S. Imparied calcium mobilization in natural killer cells from chronic fatigue syndrome/myalgic encephalomyelitis patients is associated with transient receptor potential melastatin 3 ion channels. *Clin. Exp. Immunol.* **2017**, *187*, 284–293. [CrossRef] [PubMed]
71. Nguyen, T.; Staines, D.R.; Nilius, B.; Smith, P.; Marshall-Gradisnik, S. Novel identification and characterisation of transient receptor potential melastatin 3 ion channels on natural killer cells and b lymphocytes: Effects on cell signalling in chronic fatigue syndrome/myalgic encephalomyelitis. *Biol. Res.* **2016**, *49*, 27–34. [CrossRef] [PubMed]

72. Marshall-Gradisnik, S.; Johnston, S.; Chacko, A.; Nguyen, T.; Smith, P.; Staines, D. Single nucleotide polymorphisms and genotypes of transient receptor potential ion channel and acetylcholine receptor genes from isolated b lymphocytes in myalgic encephalomyelitis/chronic fatigue syndrome patients. *J. Int. Med. Res.* **2016**, *44*, 1381–1394. [CrossRef] [PubMed]
73. Cabanas, H.; Muraki, K.; Eaton, N.; Balinas, C.; Staines, D.; Marshall-Gradisnik, S. Loss of transient receptor potential melastatin 3 ion channel function in natural killer cells from chronic fatigue syndrome/myalgic encephalomyelitis patients. *Mol. Med.* **2018**, *24*, 44–53. [CrossRef]
74. Held, K.; Voets, T.; Vriens, J. TRPM3 in temperature sensing and beyond. *Temperature* **2015**, *2*, 201–213. [CrossRef]
75. Smith, A.K.; Fang, H.; Whistler, T.; Unger, E.R.; Rajeevan, M.S. Convergent genomic studies identify association of GRIK2 and NPAS2 with chronic fatigue syndrome. *Neuropsychobiology* **2011**, *64*, 183–194. [CrossRef]
76. Schlauch, K.A.; Khaiboullina, S.F.; De Meirleir, K.L.; Rawat, S.; Petereit, J.; Rizvanov, A.A.; Blatt, N.; Mijatovic, T.; Kulick, D.; Palotas, A.; et al. Genome-wide association analysis identifies genetic variations in subjects with myalgic encephalomyelitis/chronic fatigue syndrome. *Transl. Psychiatry* **2016**, *6*, e730. [CrossRef]
77. World Health Organization. *International Classification of Diseases, Eighth Revision (ICD-8): I (Code 323): 158*; World Health Organization: Geneva, Switzerland, 1967.
78. Mackay, A.; Tate, W.P. A compromised paraventricular nucleus within a dysfunctional hypothalamus: A novel neuroinflammatory paradigm for ME/CFS. *Int. J. Immunopathol. Pharmacol.* **2018**, *32*, 1–8. [CrossRef]
79. Nakatomi, Y.; Mizuno, K.; Ishii, A.; Wada, Y.; Tanaka, M.; Tazawa, S.; Onoe, K.; Fukuda, S.; Kawabe, J.; Takahashi, K.; et al. Neuroinflammation in patients with chronic fatigue syndrome/Myalgic encephalomyelitis: An 11C-(R)-PK11195 PET study. *J. Nucl. Med.* **2014**, *55*, 945–950. [CrossRef]

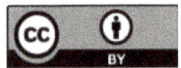

© 2019 by the authors. Licensee MDPI, Basel, Switzerland. This article is an open access article distributed under the terms and conditions of the Creative Commons Attribution (CC BY) license (http://creativecommons.org/licenses/by/4.0/).

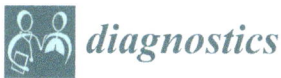

Perspective

Myalgic Encephalomyelitis or What? The International Consensus Criteria

Frank Twisk *

ME-de-Patiënten Foundation, Zonnedauw 15, 1906 HB Limmen, The Netherlands

Received: 13 November 2018; Accepted: 16 December 2018; Published: 20 December 2018

Abstract: Myalgic encephalomyelitis (ME) is a neuromuscular disease with two distinctive types of symptoms (muscle fatigability or prolonged muscle weakness after minor exertion and symptoms related to neurological disturbance, especially of sensory, cognitive, and autonomic functions) and variable involvement of other bodily systems. Chronic fatigue syndrome (CFS), introduced in 1988 and re-specified in 1994, is defined as (unexplained) chronic fatigue accompanied by at least four out of eight listed (ill-defined) symptoms. Although ME and CFS are two distinct clinical entities (with partial overlap), CFS overshadowed ME for decades. In 2011, a panel of experts recommended abandoning the label CFS and its definition and proposed a new definition of ME: the International Consensus Criteria for ME (ME-ICC). In addition to post-exertional neuroimmune exhaustion (PENE), a mandatory feature, a patient must experience at least three symptoms related to neurological impairments; at least three symptoms related to immune, gastro-intestinal, and genitourinary impairments; and at least one symptom related to energy production or transportation impairments to meet the diagnosis of ME-ICC. A comparison between the original definition of ME and the ME-ICC shows that there are some crucial differences between ME and ME-ICC. Muscle fatigability, or long-lasting post-exertional muscle weakness, is the hallmark feature of ME, while this symptom is facultative for the diagnosis under the ME-ICC. PENE, an abstract notion that is very different from post-exertional muscle weakness, is the hallmark feature of the ME-ICC but is not required for the diagnosis of ME. The diagnosis of ME requires only two type of symptoms (post-exertional muscle weakness and neurological dysfunction), but a patient has to experience at least eight symptoms to meet the diagnosis according to the ME-ICC. Autonomic, sensory, and cognitive dysfunction, mandatory for the diagnosis of ME, are not compulsory to meet the ME-ICC subcriteria for 'neurological impairments'. In conclusion, the diagnostic criteria for ME and of the ME-ICC define two different patient groups. Thus, the definitions of ME and ME-ICC are not interchangeable.

Keywords: myalgic encephalomyelitis; chronic fatigue syndrome; diagnosis; symptoms; muscles; neurology

---

1. Introduction

Myalgic encephalomyelitis (ME) is a distinctive neuromuscular disease [1,2], which was described in the medical literature between 1938 and 1993. Due to the introduction of chronic fatigue syndrome (CFS) [3,4] and the misconception that ME and CFS were "similar disorders" [5], ME was rarely considered until 2011, when a group of experts proposed using the International Consensus Criteria to define ME (ME-ICC) in order to separate a distinct patient group from the heterogeneous group of patients with CFS [4]. This article reviews the similarities and differences between the original definition of ME [1,2] and ME-ICC [6].

1.1. ME (1938–1990)

ME has been described in the medical literature since 1938 [7], often due to outbreaks [8–10]. The endemic form of ME has been acknowledged since the 1950s [11,12]. ME, recognized as a clinical entity since 1956 [13], is primarily a neuromuscular disease, which is distinguished by muscle fatigability or prolonged muscle weakness after minor exertion; neurological symptoms indicating cognitive, autonomic, and sensory dysfunction; and a chronic relapsing course [1,2]. ME is often accompanied by various symptoms implicating the involvement of other systems, including the immune system, the gastrointestinal system, and the respiratory system [1,2].

1.2. CFS (1988–2018)

Much of the confusion relating to the diagnosis and the perception of ME originates from the introduction of the label CFS and its definition in 1988 [3]. The most commonly used definition of CFS, the Centers for Disease Control and Prevention (CDC) Fukuda definition, dates back to 1994 [4]. The only mandatory feature of CFS is (unexplained) chronic fatigue, which must be accompanied by at least four out of a list of eight 'minor' symptoms: substantial impairment in short-term memory or concentration; a sore throat; tender lymph nodes; muscle pain; multi-joint pain without swelling or redness; headaches of a new type, pattern, or severity; unrefreshing sleep; and post-exertional malaise (lasting for more than 24 h) [4]. Due to the disease's nature, the case criteria for CFS [4] define a heterogeneous group of patients with chronic fatigue as the principle complaint.

Many researchers and clinicians consider ME and CFS to be "similar disorders" [14]. However, taking the definitions seriously, ME [1,2], a neuromuscular (polio-like) disease, and CFS [4], an ill-defined fatigue syndrome, are two different entities [15] with partial overlap. For this reason, ME [1,2] and CFS [4] simply cannot be replaced by the hybrid diagnosis systemic exertion intolerance disease (SEID) [5,16], as defined by the Institute of Medicine (now the National Academy of Medicine) [14].

1.3. ME-ICC (2011)

To separate a distinct patient group from the diffuse group of patients with CFS [4], a panel of international experts proposed the International Consensus Criteria for ME (ME-ICC) [6]. To meet the diagnosis of ME-ICC [6], a patient must experience post-exertional neuro-immune exhaustion (PENE), defined as "a pathological inability to produce sufficient energy on demand with prominent symptoms primarily in the neuro-immune regions", as well as neurological impairments (at least one symptom from three of four symptom categories), immune, gastro-intestinal, and genitourinary impairments (at least one symptom from three of five symptom categories), and energy production/transportation impairments (at least one of four symptoms).

2. ME vs. ME-ICC: Similarities and Differences

2.1. Similarities

2.1.1. ME Is a Neurological Disease

The original definitions of ME [1,2] emphasize the great importance of neurological abnormalities, especially of symptoms implicating cognitive, sensory, and autonomic dysfunction as distinctive features [17]. The ME-ICC criteria acknowledge the significance of neurological impairments in a separate category (Table 1: symptom category B).

Table 1. The case criteria of myalgic encephalomyelitis (ME) [1,2] and the International Consensus Criteria for ME (ME-ICC) [6].

ME [1,2]	ME-ICC [6,18]
The pathognomonic features (of ME): 1. a complaint of general or local muscular fatigue following minimal exertion with prolonged recovery time [a]; 2. neurological disturbance, especially of cognitive, autonomic, and sensory functions; 3. variable involvement of cardiac and other systems; 4. prolonged relapsing course. "Other characteristics include [...] variation in intensity of symptoms within and between episodes, tending to chronicity." [1]	A. Post-exertional neuro-immune exhaustion (PENE): mandatory. B. Neurological impairments (at least one symptom from three of the four symptom categories): 1. Neurocognitive impairments a. Difficulty processing information: slowed thought, impaired concentration b. Short-term memory loss 2. Pain a. Headaches b. Significant pain in muscles, muscle-tendon junctions, joints, abdomen, or chest 3. Sleep disturbance a. Disturbed sleep patterns b. Unrefreshing sleep 4. Neurosensory, perceptual, and motor disturbances a. Neurosensory and perceptual symptoms b. Motor dysfunction C. Immune, gastro-intestinal, and genitourinary impairments (at least one symptom from three of five symptom categories): 1. Flu-like symptoms (recurrent or chronic, which typically activate or worsen with exertion) 2. Susceptibility to viral infections with prolonged recovery periods 3. Gastro-intestinal symptoms 4. Genitourinary symptoms 5. Sensitivities to food, medications, odors, or chemicals D. Energy production or transportation impairments (at least one of four symptoms): 1. Cardiovascular symptoms 2. Respiratory symptoms 3. Loss of thermostatic stability 4. Intolerance of extremes of temperature

[a] "ME is a multisystem syndrome [...] distinguished by severe muscle fatigue following trivial exertion." [1].

2.1.2. ME Is a Multisystemic Disease

Both the original definition of ME [1,2] and ME-ICC [6] (Table 1) stipulate that ME is a multisystemic disease that can be associated with a wide range of symptoms, e.g., muscle pain, headaches, neurological dysfunction, immunological symptoms, gastro-intestinal complaints, as well as cardiovascular and respiratory symptoms. ME [1,2] and ME-ICC [6] both acknowledge the "variable involvement of cardiac and other systems" [1], alongside neurological dysfunction and musculoskeletal symptoms.

2.1.3. ME Is Not a Psychogenic Disorder

The authors of the original definition [1,2] make it clear that, although biological abnormalities have not yet been demonstrated, ME should not be misinterpreted as a psychogenic illness. The ME-ICC [6] specifically exclude primary psychiatric and somatoform disorders, i.e., "mental disorders which manifest as physical symptoms".

2.1.4. ME Is Assumed to Be Associated with Neuropathology

The original definition of ME [1,2] proposes that ME is associated with inflammation of the brain and the spinal cord, while the ME-ICC [6] presupposes "neuropathology".

Whether or not neuro-inflammation [19] is present in all ME [1,2] and ME-ICC [6] patients, and whether neuro-inflammation is causing all symptoms is yet unclear. However, this discussion of the definition of the disease, whether it be the original definition [1,2] or the ME-ICC [6], is independent of the most appropriate label for the disease.

2.2. Differences

2.2.1. Muscle Fatigability or Prolonged Post-Exertional Muscle Weakness, Mandatory for the Diagnosis of ME, Is an Optional Element for the Diagnosis of ME-ICC

According to the original definition of ME [1,2], "Muscle fatigability is the dominant and most persistent feature of the disease and […] a diagnosis should not be made without it. Restoration of muscle power after exertion can take three to five days or even longer" [20]. Muscle weakness is mentioned as just one of the examples of symptoms related to motor dysfunction (Table 1, symptoms type B4b) in the ICC, and motor weakness is not obligatory for the diagnosis ME-ICC [6]. Thus, muscle weakness, especially prolonged post-exertional muscle weakness, which is mandatory for the diagnosis of ME [1,2], is not required in order to meet the diagnosis of ME-ICC [6]. In more general terms, while the original definition [1,2] depicts ME as a neuromuscular disease, muscular symptoms are not required to meet the diagnosis of ME-ICC [6].

2.2.2. Post-Exertional Neuro-Immune Exhaustion, Mandatory for ME-ICC, Is Not a Mandatory Feature of ME

Although the risks of over-exertion are acknowledged in the original descriptions of ME [1,2,20], the abstract concepts of post-exertional malaise [4] and post-exertional neuro-immune exhaustion [6] were never described as a mandatory symptom of ME [1,2,20]. To meet the original criteria of ME, [1,2,20] only two symptom clusters are mandatory: muscle fatigability or prolonged post-exertional muscle weakness and neurological disturbance, especially of cognitive, autonomic, and sensory functions, in addition to a prolonged relapsing course and variability of the symptoms [17].

2.2.3. The Diagnosis of ME-ICC Requires Many More Symptoms Than the Diagnosis of ME

Although the original definition of ME [1,2] acknowledges the multisystemic nature of the illness, only two features are mandatory—post-exertional muscle weakness and neurological dysfunction. According to this original definition [1,2], cardiac and other bodily systems are variably involved in ME. ME-ICC [6] requires at least eight symptoms. In addition to post-exertional neuro-immune exhaustion, a patient must experience at least three neurological symptoms (Table 1, symptom category B), at least three symptoms related to immune, gastro-intestinal/genitourinary impairments (symptom category C), and one symptom associated with energy production or transportation impairments (symptom category D). Thus, the diagnosis of ME-ICC [6] requires the presence of symptoms that are optional for the diagnosis of ME [1,2].

2.2.4. Autonomic, Sensory, and Cognitive Dysfunction (Mandatory for the Diagnosis of ME) Are Not Compulsory to Meet the ME-ICC Requirements for Neurological Impairments

One could argue that requiring at least three neurological symptoms (Table 1, category B) is sufficient to guarantee a neurological disturbance, mandatory for the diagnosis of ME [1,2]. However, according to the criteria for ME-ICC [6], a patient experiencing headaches (category B2a), unrefreshing sleep (category B3b), and muscle weakness (even without exertion) (category B4b) meets the requirements of symptom category B without experiencing any specific autonomic, sensory, and cognitive symptoms.

3. Summary

The relationship between ME [1,2] and ME-ICC [6] is illustrated in Figure 1.

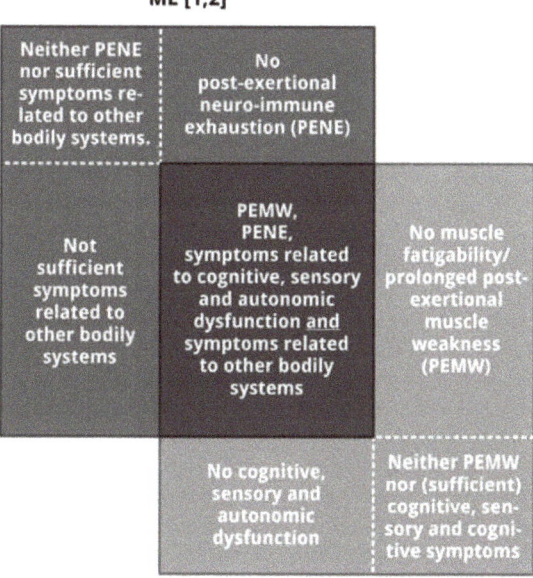

Figure 1. Overlap and differences between the case criteria of ME [1,2] and ME-ICC [6]. Note: Surface size does not reflect proportion. The (relative) number of patients in the seven subpopulations, especially the number of patients meeting the diagnosis of ME [1,2] and ME-ICC [6], and the patient subpopulation in the center are yet unknown. Figure 1 illustrates seven relevant patient subpopulations: patients meeting the diagnostic criteria of both ME and ME-ICC (the darkest grey rectangle in the centre), three ME patients subgroups not meeting the diagnosis ME-ICC (dark grey rectangles), and three groups of patients fulfilling the diagnostic criteria of ME-ICC, but not meeting the diagnosis ME (light grey rectangles).

4. Discussion

ME [1,2] is a neuromuscular disease with distinctive features. The CFS case criteria [4] define a heterogeneous group of patients [21] with chronic fatigue as a common factor. Although a part of the CFS [4] patient group meets the diagnosis of ME [1,2] and a subgroup of patients with ME [1,2] qualifies as having CFS [4], the case criteria of ME [1,2] and CFS [4] define two distinct clinical entities [5]. The ME-ICC [6] criteria are meant to separate a specific patient group from the heterogeneous group of CFS patients [4]. This article reviews similarities and differences between the original definition of ME [1,2] and the ME-ICC [6], in order to determine objectively if the new definition of 'ME' (ME-ICC) [6] is a good alternative for the original definition of ME [1,2].

One could argue that the original definition of ME [1,2] should also be compared with the Canadian Consensus Criteria (CCC) for ME and CFS [22]. However, since the ICC [6] are meant to replace the CCC, as it was stated that "The Canadian Consensus Criteria were used as a starting point, but significant changes were made." [6], a comparison between the original definition of ME [1,2] and ME- and CFS-CCC [22] can be considered irrelevant.

ME [1,2] and CFS [4] are two different clinical entities [15] with partial overlap. For this reason, ME [1,2] and CFS [4] cannot be replaced by the hybrid diagnosis SEID (ME/CFS) [5,16]. Hence, SEID is not a relevant alternative for either ME [1,2] or CFS [4]. This review shows that the case criteria for ME [1,2] and ME-ICC [6] also define two different patient groups. To unravel the etiology and pathophysiology of ME [1,2], ME-ICC [6], and CFS [4] and to develop effective treatments, it is crucial to diagnose patients accurately, using objective tests if possible, [23] and to stratify patients by duration of illness [24], age, and gender [25] in future research.

5. Conclusions

Although the ME-ICC criteria [6] have relevant similarities with the original definition of ME [1,2], there are also several crucial differences. Muscle fatigability or long-lasting post-exertional muscle weakness after exertion, the distinctive feature of ME [1,2], is facultative for the diagnosis ME-ICC [6]. On the other hand, PENE, an abstract notion different from post-exertional muscle weakness, is the hallmark feature of ME-ICC [6] but is not obligatory for the diagnosis of ME [1,2]. While the diagnosis of ME [1,2] requires two types of symptoms (muscle fatigability or post-exertional muscle weakness and neurological dysfunction) [17], a patient has to report at least eight (one mandatory and seven variable) symptoms to meet the diagnosis of ME-ICC [6]. Autonomic, sensory, and cognitive dysfunction, mandatory for the diagnosis of ME [1,2], are not compulsory to meet the ME-ICC [6] requirements for neurological impairments. Although the symptoms required to meet the ICC-criteria for immune, gastro-intestinal, and genitourinary impairments (category C) and energy production and transportation impairments (category D) are often experienced by patients with ME [1], they are not compulsory for the diagnosis of ME according to its original criteria [1,2]. In summary, the diagnostic criteria for ME [1,2] and ME-ICC [6] define different patient groups and are not interchangeable. Future factor analysis studies [26] of the symptoms of patients meeting the discriminative definition of ME [1,2], which only requires two types of symptoms, should clarify to what extent ME [1,2] patients experience the mandatory and other symptoms required by the ME-ICC [6], how they meet the diagnosis of ME-ICC [6], and how many patients meeting the diagnosis of ME-ICC [6] comply with the original definition of ME [1,2].

Funding: This research received no external funding.

Acknowledgments: This article is dedicated to Melvin Ramsay, Elisabeth Dowsett, Donald Acheson, Gordon Parish and other renowned researchers who dedicated their professional career to Myalgic Encephalomyelitis and patients suffering from ME.

Conflicts of Interest: The authors declare no conflict of interest.

References

1. Dowsett, E.G.; Ramsay, A.M.; McCartney, R.A.; Bell, E.J. Myalgic Encephalomyelitis—A persistent enteroviral infection? *Postgrad. Med. J.* **1990**, *66*, 526–530. [CrossRef] [PubMed]
2. Ramsay, A.M.; Dowsett, E.G. Myalgic Encephalomyelitis: Then and now, an epidemiological introduction. In *The Clinical and Scientific Basis of Myalgic Encephalomyelitis/Chronic Fatigue Syndrome*; Hyde, B.M., Goldstein, J., Levine, P., Eds.; Nightingale Research Foundation: Ottawa, ON, Canada, 1992.
3. Holmes, G.P.; Kaplan, J.E.; Gantz, N.M.; Komaroff, A.L.; Schonberger, L.B.; Straus, S.E.; Jones, J.F.; Dubois, A.E.; Cunningham-Rundles, C.; Pahwa, S.; et al. Chronic fatigue syndrome: A working case definition. *Ann. Intern. Med.* **1988**, *108*, 387–389. [CrossRef]
4. Fukuda, K.; Straus, S.E.; Hickie, I.; Sharpe, M.; Dobbins, J.G.; Komaroff, A.L. The chronic fatigue syndrome: A comprehensive approach to its definition and study. *Ann. Intern. Med.* **1994**, *121*, 953–959. [CrossRef] [PubMed]
5. Twisk, F.N.M. Myalgic Encephalomyelitis, chronic fatigue syndrome, and Systemic Exertion Intolerance Disease: Three distinct clinical entities. *Challenges* **2018**, *9*, 19. [CrossRef]
6. Carruthers, B.M.; van de Sande, M.I.; de Meirleir, K.L.; Klimas, N.G.; Broderick, G.; Mitchell, T.; Staines, D.; Powles, A.C.P.; Speight, N.; Vallings, R.; et al. Myalgic encephalomyelitis: International consensus criteria. *J. Intern. Med.* **2011**, *270*, 327–338. [CrossRef]
7. Gilliam, A.G. *Epidemiological study on an epidemic, diagnosed as poliomyelitis, occurring among the personnel of Los Angeles County General Hospital during the summer of 1934*; US Government Printing Office: Washington, DC, USA, 1938; Volume 240, pp. 1–90.

8. The Medical Staff of The Royal Free Hospital. An outbreak of Encephalomyelitis in the Royal Free Hospital Group, London, in 1955. *Br. Med. J.* **1957**, *2*, 895–904. [CrossRef]
9. Sigurdsson, B.; Sigurjonsson, J.; Sigurdsson, J.H.; Thorkelsson, J.; Gudmundsson, K.R. A disease epidemic in Iceland simulating poliomyelitis. *Am. J. Hyg.* **1950**, *52*, 222–238. [CrossRef] [PubMed]
10. Parish, J.G. Early outbreaks of 'epidemic neuromyasthenia'. *Postgrad. Med. J.* **1978**, *54*, 711–717. [CrossRef] [PubMed]
11. Acheson, E.D. The clinical syndrome variously called benign myalgic encephalomyelitis, Iceland disease and epidemic neuromyasthenia. *Am. J. Med.* **1959**, *26*, 569–595. [CrossRef]
12. Ramsay, A.M. Encephalomyelitis in north west London; an endemic infection simulating poliomyelitis and hysteria. *Lancet* **1957**, *270*, 1196–1200. [CrossRef]
13. Acheson, D.E. A new clinical entity? *Lancet* **1956**, *267*, 789–790. [CrossRef]
14. Institute of Medicine. *Beyond Myalgic Encephalomyelitis/Chronic Fatigue Syndrome: Redefining an Illness*; National Academies Press: Washington, DC, USA, 2015.
15. Twisk, F.N.M. The status of and future research into Myalgic Encephalomyelitis and chronic fatigue syndrome: The need of accurate diagnosis, objective assessment, and acknowledging biological and clinical subgroups. *Front. Physiol.* **2014**, *5*, 109. [CrossRef]
16. Twisk, F.N.M. Replacing Myalgic Encephalomyelitis and chronic fatigue syndrome with systemic exercise intolerance disease is not the way forward. *Diagnostics* **2016**, *6*, E10. [CrossRef]
17. Twisk, F.N.M. Myalgic Encephalomyelitis (ME) or what? An operational definition. *Diagnostics* **2018**, *8*, E64. [CrossRef]
18. Carruthers, B.M.; van de Sande, M.I. *Myalgic Encephalomyelitis—Adult & Paediatric: International Consensus Primer for Medical Practioners*; Carruthers and van de Sande: Vancouver/Calgary, BC/AB, Canada, 2012.
19. Nakatomi, Y.; Mizuno, K.; Ishii, A.; Wada, Y.; Tanaka, M.; Tazawa, S.; Onoe, K.; Fukuda, S.; Kawabe, J.; Takahashi, K.; et al. Neuroinflammation in patients with chronic fatigue syndrome/Myalgic Encephalomyelitis: An 11C-(R.)-PK11195 PET study. *J. Nucl. Med.* **2014**, *55*, 945–950. [CrossRef]
20. Ramsay, A.M. *Postviral fatigue syndrome—The saga of Royal Free Disease*, 1st ed.; Gower Medical Publishing: London, UK, 1986.
21. Wilson, A.; Hickie, I.; Hadzi-Pavlovic, D.; Wakefield, D.; Parker, G.; Straus, S.E.; Dale, J.; McCluskey, D.; Hinds, G.; Brickman, A.; et al. What is chronic fatigue syndrome? Heterogeneity within an international multicentre study. *Aust. N. Z. J. Psychiatry* **2001**, *35*, 520–527. [CrossRef]
22. Carruthers, B.M.; Jain, A.K.; de Meirleir, K.; Peterson, D.L.; Klimas, N.G.; Lerner, A.M.; Bested, A.C.; Flor-Henry, P.; Joshi, P.; Peter Powles, A.C.; et al. Myalgic encephalomyelitis/chronic fatigue syndrome: Clinical working case definition, diagnostic and treatment protocols. *J. Chronic Fatigue Syndr.* **2003**, *11*, 7–115. [CrossRef]
23. Twisk FNM. Accurate diagnosis of myalgic encephalomyelitis and chronic fatigue syndrome based upon objective test methods for characteristic symptoms. *World J. Methodol.* **2015**, *5*, 68–87. [CrossRef] [PubMed]
24. Hornig, M.; Montoya, J.G.; Klimas, N.G.; Levine, S.; Felsenstein, D.; Bateman, L.; Peterson, P.L.; Gottschalk, C.G.; Schultz, A.F.; Che, X.; et al. Distinct plasma immune signatures in ME/CFS are present early in the course of illness. *Sci. Adv.* **2015**, *1*, e1400121. [CrossRef]
25. Smylie, A.L.; Broderick, G.; Fernandes, H.; Razdan, S.; Barnes, Z.; Collado, F.; Sol, C.; Fletcher, M.A.; Klimas, N. A comparison of sex-specific immune signatures in Gulf War illness and chronic fatigue syndrome. *BMC Immunol.* **2013**, *14*, 29. [CrossRef] [PubMed]
26. Richardson, A.M.; Lewis, D.P.; Kita, B.; Ludlow, H.; Groome, N.P.; Hedger, M.P.; de Kretser, D.M.; Lidbury, B.A. Weighting of orthostatic intolerance time measurements with standing difficulty score stratifies ME/CFS symptom severity and analyte detection. *J. Transl. Med.* **2018**, *16*, 97. [CrossRef] [PubMed]

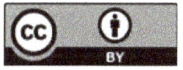

© 2018 by the author. Licensee MDPI, Basel, Switzerland. This article is an open access article distributed under the terms and conditions of the Creative Commons Attribution (CC BY) license (http://creativecommons.org/licenses/by/4.0/).

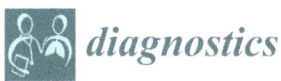

Review

Work Rehabilitation and Medical Retirement for Myalgic Encephalomyelitis/Chronic Fatigue Syndrome Patients. A Review and Appraisal of Diagnostic Strategies

Mark Vink [1,*] and Friso Vink-Niese [2]

1. Family and Insurance Physician, 1096 HZ Amsterdam, The Netherlands
2. Independent Researcher, 49032 Osnabrück, Germany; frisovinkniese@googlemail.com
* Correspondence: markvink.md@outlook.com

Received: 7 June 2019; Accepted: 13 September 2019; Published: 20 September 2019

Abstract: Myalgic Encephalomyelitis/Chronic Fatigue Syndrome leads to severe functional impairment and work disability in a considerable number of patients. The majority of patients who manage to continue or return to work, work part-time instead of full time in a physically less demanding job. The prognosis in terms of returning to work is poor if patients have been on long-term sick leave for more than two to three years. Being older and more ill when falling ill are associated with a worse employment outcome. Cognitive behavioural therapy and graded exercise therapy do not restore the ability to work. Consequently, many patients will eventually be medically retired depending on the requirements of the retirement policy, the progress that has been made since they have fallen ill in combination with the severity of their impairments compared to the sort of work they do or are offered to do. However, there is one thing that occupational health physicians and other doctors can do to try and prevent chronic and severe incapacity in the absence of effective treatments. Patients who are given a period of enforced rest from the onset, have the best prognosis. Moreover, those who work or go back to work should not be forced to do more than they can to try and prevent relapses, long-term sick leave and medical retirement.

Keywords: CFS (Chronic Fatigue Syndrome); ME (Myalgic Encephalomyelitis); medical retirement; prognosis; work rehabilitation

1. Introduction

Myalgic encephalomyelitis (ME) or chronic fatigue syndrome (CFS), often called ME/CFS, is a debilitating disease characterised by post-exertional malaise (PEM) with abnormally prolonged recovery after previously trivial and well tolerated exercise and activities, which differentiates ME/CFS from other fatiguing conditions [1]. Patients experience a substantial loss in quality of life, with severe disruption to occupational, social, and personal activities. It affects more women than men and in the Netherlands it is more common than multiple sclerosis (MS) [2]. There is no diagnostic test, and treatment is based on symptom management. Symptoms occurring in more than 80% of cases are muscle weakness, generalized chronic pain, cognitive dysfunction—for example concentration or short-term memory impairments, difficulty with reading or information processing—hypersensitivity to noise and/or light, new onset headaches or migraines, joint pains, dizziness and episodes of postural orthostatic hypotension [3]. The number of ME literate medical doctors is limited due to the lack of teaching about this disease in medical school and post-graduate training [4]. Most doctors are also not aware of the fact that ME has been classified as a neurological disease by the World Health Organisation [5] since 1969 with CFS as an equivalent. Many still do not believe in the disease. This is partly due to the name, chronic fatigue syndrome, which to many people suggests that patients are just a bit tired. Not many doctors will believe that a disease is serious and very disabling if it can be treated successfully by talking (cognitive behavioural therapy or CBT) and exercise (graded exercise therapy or GET). On top of this, many still think that "most people with CFS recover gradually over a period of 1–3 years" [6] or that there is a "50 to 80 percent recovery after 7 years in protracted chronic fatigue syndrome, when using the Fukuda 1994 diagnostic criteria for patient selection", as stated in the draft report by the Australian Advisory Committee for the Chief Executive Officer of the National Health and Medical Research Council from 2018 [7]. These misconceptions can lead to all sorts of problems for patients including the refusal of benefits or medical retirement.

ME/CFS is not a rare disease [8] and it represents a considerable public health burden with an estimated annual total value of direct and indirect economic costs to society in the US of $17 to $24 billion, including $9.1 billion attributed to lost productivity [9].

The aim of this paper is to answer the following questions by reviewing the current evidence:

1. What is the prognosis of ME/CFS?
2. How does ME/CFS affect a person's ability to work?
3. What can be expected in terms of recovery and return to work?
4. Do CBT and/or GET restore the ability to work in ME/CFS as an influential systematic review by Cairns and Hotopf from 2005 [10] advised to postpone medical retirement until patients had had a course of CBT and GET. Since then, many trials of CBT and/or GET have been published, which will enable us to answer this question.

The answers to these questions are of importance to occupational health physicians, insurance physicians, disability benefit assessors and others who evaluate adults affected by ME/CFS. As such this paper will concentrate on ME/CFS in adults.

A comprehensive search of the literature was undertaken using electronic databases (PubMed, Medline and the Cochrane Database of Clinical Trials and Web of Science) for articles on the natural history of ME/CFS, on work and occupational health in ME/CFS and on the effectiveness of CBT and GET in relation to work in studies that have been published before April 2019. We also searched the reference lists of the articles identified for the review.

2. Overview of ME/CFS

Myalgic Encephalomyelitis got its name after an outbreak in the Royal Free Hospital in London in 1955. The first described outbreak however happened in 1934 when 198 members of the medical and nursing staff of Los Angeles County General Hospital fell ill. The disease was initially known as atypical poliomyelitis. A prominent symptom was muscle fatigue on walking short distances and with the least exertion. The follow up of the Los Angeles cases revealed chronic disability [11].

Over the years, there have been 50 to 60 documented outbreaks, however, lately ME/CFS is mostly sporadic with occasional outbreaks [12]. It usually follows or is triggered by a viral infection, has an unknown aetiology and the onset can be acute or gradual. There are no laboratory diagnostic tests and case definitions (diagnostic criteria) are therefore used to define and diagnose ME/CFS. A group of mainly British psychiatrists came up with the Oxford criteria in 1991 [13], which are primarily used in the UK. Its only requirement is six months or more of unexplained disabling fatigue. The main characteristic of ME/CFS, postexertional malaise [1], however is not required for diagnosis. Consequently, 85% of Oxford-defined cases are healthy subjects with mild fatigue or chronic idiopathic fatigue who are misclassified as ME/CFS according to a large study by Baraniuk [14]. Both the American National Institute of Health (NIH) and the Agency for Healthcare Research and Quality (AHRQ) concluded that the Oxford criteria are flawed and that using the Oxford case definition results in a high risk of including patients who may have an alternate fatiguing illness or whose illness resolves spontaneously with time. Both agencies recommend that the Oxford definition should be retired [15–17].

The most commonly used diagnostic criteria are the Centers for Disease Control and Prevention (CDC) 1994 criteria, better known as the Fukuda criteria [18]. These criteria require 6 months or more of unexplained chronic fatigue and a minimum of 4 out of a list of 8 symptoms as can be seen in Table 1. However, PEM (postexertional malaise) the core symptom of ME/CFS, is only optional and not compulsory for diagnosis, as it is one of the eight additional criteria. Approximately 15% of people labelled by these criteria as having ME/CFS, were in fact healthy people [19]. Newer more restrictive criteria such as the Canadian Consensus Criteria (CCC) [12] and the International Consensus Criteria (ICC) [20] have been created which both require PEM for diagnosis, as can be seen in Table 1. The CCC and ICC select a smaller group of patients than the Fukuda criteria, and those diagnosed with ME are more impaired and less likely to suffer from depression instead of ME/CFS [21].

2.1. Advances in Understanding the Pathophysiology of ME/CFS

For a long time, many doctors have thought that there is nothing wrong in ME/CFS because routine testing does not reveal any abnormalities. However, over the past 35 years, thousands of studies using more advanced tests have documented underlying biological abnormalities involving many organ systems in patients with ME/CFS, as noted by Komaroff in a recent overview [22]. These abnormalities include metabolic changes, immunological abnormalities in lymphocytes—especially in T cells and poorly functioning natural killer cells—and significant elevation of many blood cytokines especially in the first three years of illness which are correlated with the severity of the illness. These studies have also shown widespread neuroinflammation of the brain and cognitive impairments not explained by concomitant psychiatric disorders. Multiple studies demonstrate that during exercise the tissues of patients with ME/CFS have difficulty extracting oxygen leading to impairment of cellular energy production. This impairment is much more prominent during a second exercise tests repeated 24 h after the first [22]. Due to all these abnormalities, the American National Academy of Medicine (NAM), formerly called the Institute of Medicine (IoM), concluded in 2015 that ME/CFS is a chronic and disabling multisystem disease and not a psychiatric or psychosomatic one [23]. The Dutch Health Council came to the same conclusion in 2018 [24].

2.2. Misdiagnosis and under Diagnosing

The lack of a diagnostic test, the lack of standardization of the selection criteria, the lack of teaching about ME/CFS in medical school and the use of the Oxford criteria have resulted in ME/CFS becoming an umbrella term [21]. Consequently, patients with fatigue due to a psychiatric disorder, patients who experience general chronic fatigue but do not meet the other criteria, or experience fatigue as a result of an underlying medical condition, can be misdiagnosed with ME/CFS. This has profound implications, since a false positive diagnosis of ME/CFS may lead to improper interventions, withholding of treatment and a prognosis for a disease they do not have [25,26]. It also leads to the wrong impression about this disease.

It was rare for patients to get an alternative diagnosis in the clinical trials analysed by a systematic review from 2005 [10]. Since then, a number of studies have been published that specifically looked at the subject of misdiagnosis. Nacul et al. found that 24% of GP diagnosed cases did not have ME/CFS [27]. Two studies that analysed GP referrals to tertiary care showed that in 40% [25] and 49% [26] the diagnosis of ME/CFS was incorrect. Johnston et al. [28] found that in a group of 535 Australian patients diagnosed with CFS or ME by a primary care physician, 30.3% met the Fukuda criteria and only a further 32% met both the Fukuda and the ICC. In a tertiary care study by Mariman et al. [29], 228 patients who fulfilled the Fukuda criteria were assessed in a multidisciplinary integrated diagnostic pathway. Subsequently, 35.8% were diagnosed with another illness.

A number of primary-care studies showed the following, 22% of individuals, who believed they had ME/CFS, did not comply with either the Fukuda or Canadian Consensus Criteria [30]. Only 30% of patients who presented to their general practitioners (GPs) with six months or more of unexplained fatigue, had Fukuda defined ME/CFS [31]. But it is not only GPs who get the diagnosis wrong. 21% diagnosed with ME/CFS by one of four specialist physicians in tertiary care got alternative medical (2%) and psychiatric (19%) diagnoses [32].

Table 1. Summary of case definition criteria.

Oxford Criteria (1991) [13]	Fukuda Criteria (1994) [18]	Canadian Consensus Criteria (2003) [12]	International Consensus Criteria (2011) [20]
Chronic disabling fatigue for ≥ 6 months during which it was present for > 50% of the time. No other symptoms required	Chronic fatigue of ≥ 6 months At least 4 of the following symptoms: • Impaired memory/concentration • Sore throat • Tender cervical or axillary lymph nodes • Muscle pain • Multi joint pain • New headaches • Unrefreshing sleep • Post-Exertional malaise	A minimum of 6 months of: • fatigue • post-exertional malaise and/or fatigue • sleep dysfunction • pain Also have two or more neurological/cognitive manifestations and one or more symptoms from two of the categories of autonomic, neuroendocrine, and immune manifestations	A patient will meet the criteria for postexertional neuroimmune exhaustion (A), at least one symptom from three neurological impairment categories (B), at least one symptom from three immune/gastro-intestinal/genitourinary impairment categories (C), and at least one symptom from energy metabolism/transport impairments (D). A. Post exertional neuroimmune exhaustion (PENE): compulsory. Characteristics: • Marked, rapid physical and/or cognitive fatigability in response to exertion, which may be minimal such as activities of daily living or simplemental tasks, can be debilitating and cause a relapse • Postexertional symptom exacerbation • Postexertional exhaustion • Recovery period is prolonged • Low threshold of physical andmental fatigability (lack of stamina) results in a substantial reduction in pre-illness activity level. B. Neurological impairments At least one symptom from three of the following four symptom categories: • Neurocognitive impairments (Difficulty processing information, Short-term memory loss) • Pain (Headaches, significant pain). • Sleep disturbance • Neurosensory, perceptual and motor disturbances C. Immune, gastro-intestinal and genitourinary impairments (symptoms from at least 3 of the following categories): • Flu-like symptoms • Susceptibility to viral infections with prolonged recovery periods • Gastro-intestinal tract symptoms • Genitourinary symptoms • Sensitivities to foods, medications, odors, or chemicals D. Energy production/ion transportation impairments (symptoms from at least 1 of the following categories): • Cardiovascular symptoms • Respiratory symptoms • Loss of thermostatic ability • Intolerance of extremes of temperature Severity: • Mild (an approximate 50% reduction in pre-illness activity level) • Moderate (mostly housebound) • Severe (mostly bedridden) • Very severe (totally bedridden and need help with basic functions).

A number of follow-up studies also reported misdiagnosis. For example, this was 10% in a nine-year follow-up study [33], 23.1% in a three-year follow-up study [34] and 24.5% in a five-year follow-up study [35]. Common alternative medical diagnoses are fatigue associated with a chronic disease, obstructive sleep apnoea, depression or anxiety [25,26,29,34]. These high rates of misdiagnosis underline the importance of evaluating differential diagnoses [35] especially when patients present with new or worsening symptoms.

At the same time, assigning a diagnosis of ME/CFS in the current clinical setting often takes years, as there is no diagnostic test and many physicians are uninformed or misinformed about the disease. Consequently, an estimated 84–91% of patients affected by ME/CFS are not diagnosed with the disease [9].

2.3. Predictors of Outcome

A range of predictors of good and poor outcome have been identified and grouped into a few broad categories [10].

2.3.1. Illness Management in the Initial Stages

The most important prognostic factor is how the illness is managed in its initial stages according to Dr. Ramsay [36], the infectious disease specialist involved in the management of the almost 300 patients, mainly doctors and nurses, who fell ill during the outbreak in the Royal Free Hospital in London in 1955. He also noted that most patients will try to go back to work in the initial stages when they are improving. With many other illnesses that does not pose a problem, yet with ME/CFS it does. Patients who have a period of enforced rest in the initial stages of their illness tend to have the best prognosis [36].

2.3.2. Demographics

Older age was predictive of a worse outcome in a number of studies [37–41] but other studies reported that there was no association between age and outcome [32,42–44]. However, analysis of the outcome of treatments in the National Health Service (NHS) CFS clinics (n = 1643) by Crawley et al. [45] revealed that older age, increased pain and physical function at assessment were associated with poorer physical function at follow-up. Analysis of the data from the UK CFS/ME National Outcomes Database (n = 2170) in 2011 by Collin et al. [46] showed that men and people in older age groups were more likely to have ceased employment due to their fatigue-related symptoms.

2.3.3. Illness Duration

Five studies suggested that illness duration was predictive of a worse outcome [32,38,42,47,48] but this finding was not supported by five other studies that reported no association [34,49–52]. However, the large aforementioned study by Collin et al. [46] from 2011 found that illness duration was predictive of a worse outcome.

2.3.4. Psychiatric Comorbidity

Having a comorbid psychiatric disorder at baseline is associated with a poorer outcome according to a systematic review by Cairns and Hotopf [10].

2.3.5. Illness Severity

Approximately, 25% of ME/CFS patients are severely affected and are homebound or bedbound and dependent on others [53]. Severity is a major factor affecting prognosis [54]. In general, markers of a more severe illness (chronic symptoms, severe disability, more severe fatigue and more physical symptoms) tend to be associated with a poor outcome [30,41,44,47,48,55]. This was confirmed by the above-mentioned evaluation of treatments in the NHS CFS clinics (n = 1643) by Crawley et al. [45]. Leone et al. [56] found that physical functioning at baseline, deterioration of physical functioning between the baseline measurement and 12-month follow-up predicted work disability at 4-year follow-up. Hill et al. [47] who studied the natural history of severe ME, concluded that the prognosis for recovery was extremely poor.

3. ME/CFS and the Occupational Health Physician

3.1. Sickness Absence

Occupational health physicians might have to advise on issues such as sickness absence, fitness for work, work rehabilitation and medical retirement in patients who present with chronic fatigue (CF). Most of them do not suffer from ME/CFS. Postexertional malaise, the main characteristic of ME/CFS, is the single most important factor in discriminating ME/CFS from idiopathic CF or psychiatrically explained CF. Moreover, it is also an important prognostic indicator of poorer outcome at follow-up [57].

From an occupational health point of view, it is important to know that ME/CFS can differ from client to client but also that impairments can fluctuate in nature and severity throughout its course. Symptoms can be such that they can make it difficult for clients to participate in assessments that involve effort and concentration. For this reason, assessments should usually be brief, straightforward and require minimal effort. There may be a need to break longer assessments into smaller segments of 10–20 minutes. For many ME/CFS patients it is difficult to travel. Thus, in-home or phone-based consultations may be viable alternatives [58].

Knowledge of prognostic factors—discussed earlier in this paper—related to occupational outcomes is important because ME/CFS often leads to absenteeism and full work incapacity [56,59]. Since the role of the occupational physicians is to advise on questions relating to work it is important to have some insight into the work-related functions that ME/CFS can affect. It is also important to realise that patients might be worried that they will be unable to perform to an acceptable standard due to the limitations imposed upon them by ME/CFS. At the same time, they might fear that work may have an adverse effect on symptoms and might cause relapses. This might not only interfere with their current capabilities but also with the prospects of eventual improvements, recovery and a return to work. A carefully planned and supervised programme of workplace rehabilitation should therefore also address these fears and problems [60–62]. Such a plan is also important when patients have just fallen ill, because the most important prognostic factor is how the illness is managed in its initial stages as noted before. Patients who have a period of enforced rest in the initial stages of their illness tend to have the best prognosis [36].

ME/CFS can interfere with work-related physical functions like walking, standing, sitting, lifting, pushing, pulling, reaching, carrying, and handling. It can also interfere with mental functions including the ability to understand, remember and carry out simple instructions, the ability to use appropriate judgment, and the ability to respond appropriately to supervision, co-workers, and usual work situations, including changes in a routine work setting [58].

3.2. Employment Status in ME/CFS

A large number of studies into the natural history of ME/CFS—most of them used the Fukuda criteria—also recorded employment status as can be seen in Table 2. However, most of these studies were not set up to for occupational health purposes. Consequently, many studies did not provide employment data at baseline or follow-up which led to heterogeneity in the data in Table 2. Also, a number of studies were fatigue studies containing a proportion of ME/CFS patients. An example of this is the study by Assefi et al. [63]. 37.3% (207/555) of the responders had ME/CFS. There was no follow-up, 61% worked and almost half of them worked less hours. 29% lost their job due to the illness and 30% were in receipt of illness benefits.

Table 2. Work-related outcomes and naturally occurring improvement rate.

Study	Criteria	n	Mean Age in Years	Illness Duration at Baseline	Length of follow-up (FU)	Works Status	Rate of Improvement
Andersen et al. (2007) [33]	Meeting both CDC 1988 and Fukuda	34	46.4 at diagnosis	4 yrs	9 yr	76.5% (26/34) medically retired; 1 worked full time in physically less demanding job, 2 worked part-time, 3 were freelance + on disability payments	As a group patients had not improved; 6% recovered & 10% had received other diagnosis
Assefi et al. (2011) [63]	Fukuda	555 (fatigue study, 207 CFS patients)	38.2	4.4 yr	No FU	Of the CFS patients, 61% worked, 44% worked less hours, 29% lost jobs due to illness, 30% received illness benefits; 23% changed jobs due to illness, 30% took significant pay cut	No FU
Behan et al. (1985) [64]	Unclear	50	37	5 yrs	No FU	4 of the 5 doctors and all 8 nurses were unable to continue work; the medical student withdrew from his course for a yr. No employment data provided for the other 37 patients	The illness was chronic in 37 patients but had a relapsing and remitting course in 13.
Bombardier and Buchwald (1995) [38]	CDC 1988	498 (fatigue study, 226 CFS patients)	38.1	5.2 yrs	1.5 yrs	CFS patients at FU: 40% unable to work at all, 20% unable to work full-time, 22% decreased work performance, 16% increased work performance, 11% resuming full time and 13% part-time work.	2% recovered, 24% had worsened, 12% were unchanged, rest improved slightly to significantly.
Brown et al. (2012) [65]	Bell and Bell 1988	35 (25 CFS + 10 healthy controls HC)	37	25 yrs	25 yr follow-up of patients who fell ill as adolescents; average age at illness onset 12.1 yrs [66]	Full-time employment: 90% HC, 71.4% CFS. CFS: working part time 11.4% and 16.4% on disability	80% remitted yet still showed more impairment on 21 of 23 outcomes compared to healthy controls and on 17 of 23 outcomes there was no difference with those who maintained a CFS diagnosis
Buchwald et al. (1996) [67]	1998 CDC	431 (fatigue clinic patients including 185 CFS) + 99 HC	39	4.7 yrs	No FU	Employed: CFS 46% (part-time and full time) vs. 91% HC	No FU
Castro-Marrero et al. (2017) [3]	Meeting both Fukuda and Canadian criteria	1757	47.7	10 yrs	No FU	62.8% unemployed, 25.6% employed, 11.6% never worked	No FU
Chu et al. (2019) [68]	Fukuda	200, no controls	53.7	Unclear	2 yrs	At baseline, 47% permanently disabled; 15% worked >30 h/week	Response rate: 75% (150/200); 4% improved, 96% no improvement
Ciccone et al. (2010) [44]	Fukuda	94 (women only, no controls)	41.6	5.9 yrs	Biannual telephone surveys over a period of 2.5 yrs	Employed: 50.8% improvers, 29.0% nonimprovers. Disabled: 41.3% improvers, 71.0% nonimprovers	Response rate: 63.5% (94/148); 67% improved but were still far short of recovery
Clark et al. (1995) [37]	1988 CDC	98, no controls; chronic fatigue study, 19 CFS patients	39.9	5.5 yrs	2.5 yrs	Employment status not mentioned	Response rate: 79.6% (78/98), of the CFS patients 7 (37%) recovered and 12 (63%) did not recover
Claypoole et al. (2001) [69]	Fukuda	29 twin pairs (monozygotic twins and their healthy siblings)	41.2	7.2 yrs	No FU	Employed: 43% CFS, 90% HC	24% dropped out.
Collin et al. (2011) [44]	Fukuda	2170	38.6 women, 41.4 men	35 mo currently employed, 48 mo employment discontinued	Single measurement, no FU	40.7% were employed, 50.1% had discontinued work due to CFS	No FU. Employment status recorded for 1991 patients (91.8%).
Garcia-Borreguero et al. (1998) [70]	Fukuda	82 (41 CFS and 41 healthy unrelated neighbours)	37.6 CFS, 38.4 healthy neighbours	5.5 yrs	No FU	Vocational disability: 17.1% partial, 56.1% full CFS, not applicable in healthy neighbours	No FU
Hill et al. (1999) [47]	1988 CDC	23 ("severe" subset of CFS patients)	35	2.4 yrs	3.4 yrs (FU at 1.6 yrs and also at 3.4 yrs)	Employed at baseline: 5 full-time and 1 part time; 2 returned to part-time work at 1st follow-up and 1 of them became disabled again	4% recovered; majority showed no improvement
Huibers et al. (2006) [71] and Leone et al. (2006) [56]	Fukuda	151 fatigued employees (52 with CFS like cases at baseline)	43.9	35.0 mo CFS like cases (at baseline)	4 yrs (FU at 1 yr and 4 yrs)	Work disability CFS like cases: 41% baseline, 20% at 12 month FU, 27% at 4 yr FU. At final follow-up, 59.6% were on sick leave, full or partial work incapacity, unemployed or retired	Response rate: 84% (127/151). 40% went on to meet CFS criteria at follow-up; 16.9% developed a CFS like status during the 4 yrs and 57% still met criteria for severe fatigue.

Table 2. Cont.

Study	Criteria	n	Mean Age in Years	Illness Duration at Baseline	Length of follow-up (FU)	Works Status	Rate of Improvement
Jason et al. (2008) [72] study 1	Fukuda	79 (32 CFS vs. 47 HC)	37	Unclear	No FU	Working full time: 33.3% (CFS) vs. 86.7% (HC); Part-time: 19% vs. 6.7% Unable to work due to illness 42.8% vs. 0%	No FU
Jason et al. (2008) [72] study 2	Fukuda	114 (no control group)	42	Unclear	No FU	Working: 26.4% part-time and 25.3% full-time. 76% had to cut down on their work, 49.4 % were receiving disability or were unemployed due to CFS	No FU
Jason et al. (2011) [41]	Fukuda	213 (study included 32 with CFS and 47 HC)	36.8 CFS 41.4 HC	Unclear	10 yrs	At baseline: on disability 20.8% CFS and 9.1% HC Working part time: 8.3% CFS and 13.6% HC; full-time: 37.5% CFS and 68.2% HC. No employment data provided for follow-up.	86% of CFS patients followed up. Over time the CFS group remained rather ill
Johnston et al. (2016) [28]	CFS diagnosis by their primary physician	535 (30.3% Fukuda cases; a further 32.0% met both Fukuda and ICC; 23.2% CF; 14.6% received other diagnosis)	46.4	14.5 yrs	No FU	Fukuda: 12.4% working full-time, 27.8% part-time; receiving disability 30.3%, unemployed 27.8%, ICC: 9.8% working full-time, 28.0% part-time, 34.7% receiving disability, 25.4% unemployed	No FU
Levine et al. (1992) [73]	Postviral fatigue syndrome defined on the basis of severe persistent fatigue	31 patients following one of four outbreaks in USA	Incline Village + Truckee 40.7; Yerington 31.1; Placerville 41.1	Unclear	3 yrs	No employment data	Response rate: 90.3% (28/31). At 2 years 46.2% (12/26) functioning without limitation, after 2 years almost all study objects were back to pre-illness activity
Lin et al. (2011) [74]	Fukuda	500 (264 chronic fatigue, 112 CFS, 124 HC)	35.8	CFS patients: 53% onset age 25 or later, 15% age 24 or earlier, 32% age unknown	No FU	Working during the last 4 weeks: 71% CFS vs. 95% healthy controls	No FU
Lloyd et al. (1994) [75]	Lloyd 1988	25 (12 male CFS patients, 13 male HC)	33.5	60 mo	No FU	41.7% (5/12) were working on a limited part time basis (CFS) vs. 100% HC (full-time); 58.3% (7/12) had stopped working due to CFS	No FU
Lowry and Pakenham (2008) [76]	Fukuda	139	48.3 yrs	11.2 yrs	No FU	24% in some form of employment, 40% on sick leave or disability benefits, 19% retired, 17% divided equally between the categories of student, unemployed (but able to work), or performing home duties	No FU
Matsuda et al. (2009) [77]	Japanese CFS criteria	155	32.7 yrs	54 mo	22.5 mo	At baseline: 47% were working; 42% unemployed and 11% student. No employment data for follow-up	Response rate: 45% (70/155); 12% recovered, 85% had a poor outcome.
McCrone et al. (2003) [78]	Fukuda	141 (fatigue study, 44 CFS)	40 yrs	Unclear	No FU. Service use assessment.	30% lost employment due to illness	No FU
Naess et al. (2012) [79]	Fukuda	58 (CFS after Giardia enteritis; 38 employees, 20 students)	38.0 females and 31.7 males	2.7 yrs	No FU. Assessment 2.7 yrs after falling ill	34.2% (13/38) Of the employees were working part time, 57.9% (22/38) sick leave, 13.2% (5/38) disability pension, 30% (6/20) of the students studied half time and 70% (14/20) too ill to study.	At the time of assessment 16% (9/58) reported improvement, 28% (16/58) no change, and 57% (33/58) slight or significant worsening.
Natelson et al. (1995) [81]	1988 CDC	113 (41 CFS, 19 MS, 17 major depression, 36 HC)	34.4 CFS, 38.3 MS, 41.9 depression, 34.6 HC	Unclear	No FU	Disabled: 56% CFS, 5% MS, 18% depression, 0% HC. CFS patients who could work were unable to do so without limitations	No FU
Nijs et al. (2005) [8]	Fukuda	54	39	68 mo	No FU	Employment rate 95.0% before CFS; currently 29.4% due to CFS; 50% on disability	No FU
Nisenbaum et al. (2003) [34]	Fukuda	65	46	13.0 yrs	91%, 60% and 37% were followed up for 1, 2 and 3 yrs	Employed: 63.1% at baseline, 61.2% at 1 yr, 55.2% at 2 yr and 55.6% at 3 yr FU. Unemployed due to CFS: 16.9% at baseline, 18.4% at 1 yr, 13.8% at 2 yr and 16.7% at 3 yr FU.	57% had a relapsing remitting course; 23.1% received alternative diagnosis, 10% sustained total remission

Table 2. Cont.

Study	Criteria	n	Mean Age in Years	Illness Duration at Baseline	Length of follow-up (FU)	Works Status	Rate of Improvement
Nyland et al. (2014) [52]	Fukuda	111 (CFS after mononucleosis)	Mean age at onset 23.7	4.7 yrs at baseline and 11.4 yrs at FU	6.5 yrs	At the time of falling ill 47% were employed and 52% were students. At baseline 8% worked full time, 1% part-time, 13.5% were students, 75% received full sickness benefits. At follow-up 27% worked full time, 28% part-time and 68.5% (63/92) received full or partial disability benefits.	Response rate: 83% (92/111). About half of younger patients experienced marked improvement.
Pendergrast et al. (2016) [53]	Unclear	557 (4 groups of CFS patients: from US 216, UK 103 and two from Norway (N1, 175 + N2, 63)); nearly 25% too ill to leave their homes	US 52.0 UK 45.6 N1 43.4 N2 34.9	Unclear	No FU	On disability: 56.7% US, 30.2% UK, 84.0% N1, 76.2% N2. Working full or part-time: 13.5% US, 37.5% UK, 9.7% N1, 19% N2	No FU
Ray et al. (1993) [62]	Oxford	48 (24 CFS, 24 HC)	38.3 CFS, 40 HC	46.6 mo	No FU	Working full-time: 13% (3/24) CFS, 71% (17/24) HC	No FU
Roche et al. (2005) [83]	Fukuda	47	46.9	10.7 yrs	No FU	Working full-time 14.9%, part-time 14.9%, unemployed 70.2%	No FU
Rowe et al. (2019) [84]	Fukuda (PEM, unrefreshing sleep and cognitive symptoms were also required)	784 (40% started after EBV)	22.5 yrs (mean age 14.8 at diagnosis)	Illness duration prior to diagnosis: 13.6 mo	8 yrs (FU on up to 6 occasions, 2 to 16 yrs after diagnosis)	At baseline, 5% not working or studying; 8% less then part time; 24% more than part-time; 63% full-time. In comparison: similarly aged healthy people: 85% worked/studied full-time. 6% able to work but unemployed	Response rate 81.8% (641/784). Reporting recovery: 38% at 5 yrs and 68% at 10 yrs; 58% reported continuous pattern of illness with fluctuating severity; 5% remained very unwell and 20% significantly unwell.
Russo et al. (1998) [85]	1988 CDC	98 (fatigue study, 27% CFS, increased to 42% at follow-up)	39.9	5.5 yrs	2.5 yrs	Number of subjects not working at enrolment not given; 29.5% returned to work. Unclear how many of these had CFS	Response rate 80% (78/98); unclear how many had CFS; 3% (2/78) fully recovered and 26% of the sample worse
Saltzstein et al. (1998) [86]	Fukuda	15 female patients	41.2	Unclear; 46.7% (7/15) were ill for less than 2 yrs	2 yrs	All were in full-time employment before CFS, at assessment 40% (6/15) worked full-time, 33% (5/15) part-time and 26.7% (4/15) were unemployed	20% were worse or the same; 80% were improved of which 20% (3/15) reported recovery
Schmaling et al. (1998) [87]	1988 CDC	37 (15 CFS, 11 depression, 11 HC); all participants were female	39.4 CFS, 43.1 depression, 45.6 HC	Unclear	No FU	Working: 13% CFS, 64% of depression, 91% HC	No FU
Schweitzer et al. (1995) [88]	Lloyd 1988	77 (47 CFS, 30 HC)	38 CFS, 29 HC	5.0 yrs	No FU	CFS unemployed: currently 49%, before CFS 13%; 47% (22/47) retired from employment as a result of CFS. No employment figures for HC	No FU
Sharpe et al. (1992) [43]	Minimum of six weeks of fatigue	177 (fatigue study, 66% had Oxford defined CFS)	34 yrs	25 mo	1 yr	38% had left or changed their job because of their illness. 73% had days during the past month when they had been entirely unable to work. No baseline data available for comparison	Response rate: 81% (144/177). 13% recovered, 65% were functionally impaired at follow-up and could not walk 100 yards (90 m).
Stoothoff et al. (2017) [89]	Unclear	541	46.3	Unclear	No FU	62.5% on disability, 17.5% worked full or part-time. 14% of those constantly getting worse were still working	59.7% described their illness as fluctuating, 15.9% as constantly getting worse, 14.1% persisting, 8.5% relapsing and remitting; and 1.9% as constantly getting better.
Strickland et al. (2001) [40]	1988 CDC	259 (fatigue study after outbreak, 41% had CFS)	47 CFS	10 yrs	10 years after outbreak	No employment data provided	Response rate 47.5% (123/259), 15% of responding CFS patients had recovered

Table 2. Cont.

Study	Criteria	n	Mean Age in Years	Illness Duration at Baseline	Length of follow-up (FU)	Works Status	Rate of Improvement
Thomas and Smith (2019) [41]	Fukuda	226	41.7	62.1 mo	3 yrs	At baseline 34% in employment, 49% unemployed, 16% on sick leave, 24% retired or home-makers.	Response rate: 57.5% (130/226); 29% reported some improvement at 18 mo and 3 yrs FU. Recovery: 2% at 6 mo, 6% at 18 mo and at 3 yrs.
Tiersky et al. (2001) [48]	Fulfilling both the 1988 CDC + Fukuda criteria	47	35.5	25.9 mo	41.9 mo	Employment status did not change; 68% were unable to work due to CFS at baseline and FU; those who worked were only able to perform light duty desk work for 3 to 4 hours a day but even this amount of work required rest periods	Response rate: 74.5% (35/47). 57% improved, 43% did not. The majority remained functionally impaired overtime. Overall the prognosis appears to be poor.
Tirelli et al. (1994) [62]	1988 CDC	265	35	3 yrs	24 mo	38.5% (102/265) stopped working activities for a period ranging from 3 months to 2 years No other employment data provided.	Response rate: 100%, 3% recovered, 8% substantial decrease in symptoms, in 89% symptoms persisted
Tritt et al. (2004) [63]	Fukuda	429	41.7	Unclear	No FU	37.1% had taken sick leave for more than four weeks in the last 12 months and 56.6% less than 4 weeks; 18.9% (81/429) were on long-term sick leave	No FU
Van der Werf et al. (2002) [44]	Fukuda	79	34.8	1.4 yrs (minimum illness duration 6 mo, maximum 24 mo)	1 yr	75% were in paid employment before illness onset vs. 29% at baseline. No employment data available from follow-up.	Response rate: 98.7% (78/79). At FU: 8% no complaints, 38% less complaints, 37% similar, 17% had deteriorated. Spontaneous recovery was rare and only occurred in patients with an illness duration < 1.5 years
Vercoulen et al. (1996) [49]	Oxford	298 CFS patients (comparison data from 53 HC)	39	8.4 yrs (51 patients with illness duration of ≤2 yrs)	18 mo	Employment status at baseline (BL) and at FU: 12% were unemployed; 28% (BL)and 29% (FU) worked; 43% (BL) and 42% (FU) were on sick leave/medically retired and 17% were housewife, retired or at school.	Response rate: 83% (246/298); 3% recovered; 17% improved, 60% remained unchanged and 20% had become worse
Vercoulen et al. (1997) [65]	Oxford	51 CFS, 50 MS and 53 HC	36.3 CFS	5 yrs CFS	No FU	Working: 27% CFS, 28% MS and 47% HC. Invalidity benefits: 43% CFS, 32% MS and 2% HC. Total hours working: 10.4 CFS, 13.3 MS, 35.7 HC	No FU
Vincent et al. (2012) [46]	Fukuda	151 (76 CFS, 75 IF)	38.2 CFS (at fatigue onset)	3.9 yrs CFS	No FU	CFS affected daily activities and work in 95% of cases	No FU
Wilson et al. (1994) [32]	Lloyd 1988	139	42.2	9.2 yrs	3.2 yrs	30% (31/103) patients unable to perform any work at FU and 25% (26/103) were receiving disability benefits because of CFS. No baseline data available for comparison.	Response rate: 74% (103/139); 37% did not improve, 20% could not perform any significant physical activity and 40% no social activity. Only 5.8% (6/103) had completely recovered
Zdunek et al. (2015) [67]	Fukuda	2 groups of CFS patients: USA 162, UK 83	USA 52.0 UK 45.9	Unclear	No FU	Working full or part-time: 11.2% USA, 35.2% UK. On disability: 55.3% US, 35.4% UK.	UK more gradual onset, USA more sudden onset

BL: baseline; CF: chronic fatigue; EBV: Epstein-Barr virus; FU: follow-up; HC: healthy controls; ICF: idiopathic chronic fatigue; IF: idiopathic fatigue; mo: months; MS: multiple sclerosis; yr: year; yrs: years.

ME/CFS studies that did report on employment data at baseline and follow-up showed the following. Employment status did not change in a study with 42 months follow-up [40]. In two studies with 18 months and three-year follow-up respectively, employment status decreased from 31% to 24% [49] and from 63% to 55% [34]. In a study with a follow-up of 3.8 years, 36.5% (19/52) of CFS like cases returned to work [56]. In a nine-year follow-up by Anderson et al. [33], as a group, patients had not improved.

Many studies contained a limited number of patients. However, the following two tertiary care studies contained a large number of patients. In a review by Castro-Marrero et al. [3] (n = 1757), 26% were employed and 63% were unable to work due to ME/CFS. In the aforementioned study by Collin et al. [46] of the NHS database (n = 2170), this was 41% and 50%, respectively.

Finally, studies which were done by ME Associations from Norway, The Netherlands, Australia, Britain and America [98–102], are described in Table 3. They confirm the findings from the long-term follow-up studies that many patients are unable to work due to their illness. Of particular interest is the study by the Dutch ME Association (n = 629) [100], which found that the percentage of patients who were able to work more than 40 h per week decreased from 14.8% to 0.8%. The percentage able to work 24 to 40 h decreased from 43% to 4% and the percentage of patients who were able to work 0 to 8 h increased from 1.4% to 28%. These are similar to the findings by TNO (The Netherlands Organisation for Applied Scientific Research) [2], a renowned independent Dutch research institute. In their evaluation study of 924 patients, 7% had never been on long-term sick leave. However, 2/3 of the 7% had to reduce their hours and 1/3 of them had to change their work due to ME/CFS. 23% who had been on long-term sick leave had gone back to work so that a total of 30% of patients were working. Approximately 77% of these 23%, however, needed adjustments to work. Many had to reduce their hours, were now doing sedentary and less physical work, often involving work behind a computer. Also, less people were able to work in management positions.

Table 3. Work status according to patient charities and independent research Institutes.

Study	n	Works Status
25% ME Group (2004) [103]	437 severely affected patients	In receipt of state illness benefits 98% and disability living allowance 86%
Bringsli (2014) [98]	1096	50% received temporary disability benefits, 25% were medically retired 5% worked full time, 10% part-time
Chu (2013) (FDA Survey) [99]	623	Disabled and unemployed due to CFS 53.4% and 21.9%; working part-time 7.0% and full-time 5.7%
De Kimpe (2016) [100]	629	71.38% worked > 8 h a week before falling ill with CFS. Due to CFS only 45.79% are able to work. Also, those who are able to work: > 40 h decreased from 14.8% to 0.8%; 32 to 40 h decreased from 29.7% to 1.6%; 24 to 32 h decreased from 13.67% to 2.34%; 0 to 8 h increased from 1.43% to 27.98%.
Emerge Australia (2018) [101]	610	74% had to stop working due to CFS, this usually occurred around one yr after the onset of symptoms.
ME Association (UK) (2015) [102]	1428	Net increase in disability benefits of 10% after CBT, 13% GET and 1% after pacing
Nivel (2008) [104]	412	71.0% are (partially) medically retired due to CFS. 20.7% worked, mean 20 h/week; 15% worked > 32 h/week.
TNO (2005) [2]	924	30% were working; 7% had never been on long-term sick leave and 23% had been able to go back to work after long-term sick leave but they were working less hours. They were also less often involved in management and more often did sedentary work behind a computer. 34% were fully and 22% were partially medically retired

Note: Nivel and TNO are two independent Dutch research institutes.

A study by Vercoulen et al. (1997) [95] that used the Oxford criteria, found similar employment rates for CFS (27%) as for MS (28%). It also found that 43% of CFS patients were on invalidity benefits/sick leave compared to 32% of MS patients. However, a study by Natelson et al. [80] used the much stricter 1988 CDC criteria [105], when they compared ME/CFS with MS, major depression and healthy controls. The percentages of patients that were unable to work due to illness were the following: 56% (ME/CFS), 5% (MS), 18% (depression) and 0% (healthy controls). A study by Sharpe et al. [43] showed that despite using the Oxford criteria, 65% were functionally impaired. At one-year follow-up it was found that most patients had been unable to work for prolonged periods. They were also unable to walk 90 m and 38% had abandoned employment due to their illness altogether.

A number of studies also reported on improvements over time. In a three-year follow-up study by Nisenbaum et al. [34], 57% had a relapsing remitting course. A large study by Stoothoff et al. (n = 541) [89] found that 17.3% worked full or part-time; 15.9% were constantly getting worse yet 14% of those constantly getting worse, were still working; 8.5% were relapsing and remitting while only 1.9% were constantly getting better. 59.7% had a fluctuating course which is similar to the 57% found by Nisenbaum et al. [34]. A study by Clarke et al. [37] with a 2.5 year follow-up, found that 3% recovered, 38% improved and 59% got significantly worse or there was no change.

3.3. Work Rehabilitation

Work rehabilitation will usually need to start with a workload and number of hours of work that are dramatically reduced [60] using an individualised return to work plan taking the symptoms and specifics of the disease and the way it is affecting the individual employee into account. In particular, care should be taken to match the proposed duties in employment to the subject's capabilities. Strenuous physical work, long working hours, rapidly changing shift patterns, work requiring sustained high levels of attention and concentration are likely to place sustained high pressure on the employee and are inadvisable or at least require careful monitoring until it is clear that the employee is able to sustain this level of work. Care must be taken not to set definite deadlines in anticipating recovery and future employability to avoid causing relapses [12].

In the UK, most employees with ME/CFS fall under the Disability Discrimination Act 1995 [61]. Most other western countries will likely have a similar Act in place. This Act requires that an employer should make 'reasonable adjustments' to the workplace and to working practices, so that a disabled or chronically ill employee is not at a disadvantage compared to abled bodied employees and is able to work despite his or her disability. Workplace adjustments that fall under this disability act, could include: changing location of work, working from home, limiting working hours, reducing workload and limiting or reducing physical tasks [60–62]. Small modifications to the working environment can make a big difference for ME/CFS patients. Examples of such modifications might be creating a quiet area to rest without being disturbed or the use of an allocated parking space near the entrance of the building [61,62].

People with ME/CFS often feel under pressure to continue working when they first become ill or when their symptoms worsen. Unfortunately, trying to push through this illness is counterproductive, potentially causing longer sickness absences and slower recovery. Returning to work after a period of illness with ME/CFS requires a much more gradual approach than most other phased returns and can require a year or more instead of weeks or months. A return to previous hours within eight weeks, as happens with some other illnesses, is likely to be counter-productive. A slow and gradual return tailored to the individual and his symptoms is more likely to be sustainable without leading to relapses which can cause long term sick leave. It is important that (time to) travel to/from work, is incorporated and taken into account in the work rehabilitation programme [61]. It can be difficult for employees with ME/CFS to maintain a consistent level of working, because of the fluctuating nature of the illness, whereby symptoms can also vary from day-to-day. This can be frustrating and challenging for all parties involved including the employee with ME/CFS. In some cases, flexible working hours might be the solution to that [61,62].

NIVEL, the Netherlands Institute for Health Services Research, published a report (n = 412) about ME/CFS [104]. They found that 20.7% were working a mean of 20 hours per week, 6.1% were going to school or studying and 71.0% were partially or fully medically retired from work due to ME/CFS. According to research by TNO [2] (n = 924), another independent Dutch research institute, 34% were fully and 22% were partially medically retired. The most important problems interfering with work were severe and disabling chronic fatigue, concentration problems/cognitive dysfunction and/or muscle pain (for more information about this TNO report, see earlier). According to the findings by NIVEL, only 22.5% of those who were working, were working more than 24 h per week. The report found that there are a number of important things according to the respondents who were working, which had enabled them to (return to) work. The most important thing for 92% was support in finding the right balance between work and spare time and support and cooperation from the employer to enable patients to continue to work (84%). Other things that respondents found important were the following: supplying information about ME/CFS to colleagues and superiors (62%), changing tasks (61%) and reducing the number of hours they had to work (61%); more rest periods during working times (60%) and the availability of a special rest place at work (45%); working from home (52%), individual support and coaching in general (51%) and by an occupational health physician in particular (44%); adjustments to working conditions (furniture, physical aids) (38%) and a regulation or provision for commuting to work (36%).

3.4. Medical Retirement

In cases when incapacity is prolonged, work rehabilitation is impossible or unsuccessful and prognosis appears to be poor, then medical retirement might be the only option. The occupational physician may then be asked to advise on this if the employee is covered by a company pension scheme which makes this provision. Qualifying criteria inevitably vary, although permanent inability to undertake normal duties for reasons of ill health is a common requirement [60–62].

4. CBT and GET and Work Outcome

A systematic review by Whiting et al. [106] concluded that many studies of behavioural therapies in ME/CFS do not use outcomes that are relevant to patients. Examples of outcomes that would be relevant to them, according to Whiting et al., but also according to a systematic review by Smith et al. [107], would be quality of life, objective outcome measures—like the actometer or the six-minute walk test—and employment and disability status. CBT and GET studies that reported on work outcomes are presented in Table 4.

Akagi 2001 et al. [108], concluded that CBT was effective and that those who worked had increased from 15 to 27 ($n = 94$). However, 10 of those 27 were actually on sick leave, 5 of those 27 were unemployed and 77% of those working changed occupation due to their illness. Also, the dropout rate was 46% (43/94). Moreover, it was a non-randomised study without a control group and patients were selected if they satisfied the Oxford criteria or criteria for neurasthenia yet all of them were classified as having ME/CFS.

Table 4. Cognitive behavioural therapy (CBT) and/or graded exercise therapy (GET) studies reporting on work status.

Study	Intervention	n	Criteria	Length of FU	Control Group	Work Outcome	Dropouts/Missing Data
Akagi et al. (2001) [106]	CBT; non-randomised noncontrolled study	94	Oxford or neurasthenia criteria, all labelled as ME/CFS	20 mo	No control group	Employment status increased from 15 to 27 patients. However, of those 27, 10 were on sick leave and 5 were unemployed. Also, 77% of those working changed occupation due to their illness	46% (43/94) dropped out
Bazelmans et al. (2005) [109]	Group CBT (GCBT), non-randomised trial	67 (patients with CFS or ICF)	Fukuda	6 mo	Waiting list (WL)	No statistically significant difference in hours worked per week at follow-up: 6.4 (GCBT) vs. 6.7 (WL; $p = 0.958$)	3% (2/67) dropped out from GCBT; 0% from WL
Burgess et al. (2012) [103]	Face-to-face CBT versus telephone CBT	80 (35 CBT, 45 telephone CBT)	Fulfilling both Fukuda and Oxford criteria	12 mo	No control group	Job to return to at baseline: 45.5% CBT and 21.9% telephone CBT. No employment data provided at follow-up.	34.3% (12/35 CBT) and 55.6% (25/45 telephone CBT) dropped out
Collin and Crawley (2017) [101]	Evaluation of CBT and GET in 11 NHS CFS clinics	952	NICE criteria	1 yr	No control group; evaluation of NHS treatment	After NHS treatment: 47.2% no change in employment situation; 18.0% returned to work or increased hours; 30.0% stopped working or reduced hours due to CFS and 4.8% for other reasons. 78.8% no change in education; 4.6% returned to or increased hours of education whilst 12.9% ceased or reduced these hours.	Response rate: 46.2% (440/952)
Cox (1999 and 2002) [112,113]	Inpatient Occupational Therapy Programme (IOTP) consisting of CBT and GET; non-randomised study	97 (61 inpatients + comparison group of 36 patients recruited from the pending inpatient admission list)	Fukuda	6 months post-discharge	No treatment control group (waiting-list)	At baseline not working: 92% IOTP; 97% WL, student 25% IOTP; 11% WL, housewife 0% IOTP; 3% WL, unemployed 5% IOTP; 8% WL. No employment data provided at follow-up.	Response rate: 70.5% (43/61) IOTP and 54% (19/36) WL
Deale et al. (2001) [114]	CBT	60	Oxford	5 yrs	Relaxation, poorly matched	No differences between groups in employment status at 5 year FU (p=0.28)	Dropouts: 16.7% (5/30) CBT, 6.7% (2/30) Relax
Dyck et al. (1996) [115]	Rehabilitation programme which included CBT and GET	2	Fukuda	3 mo	No control group	1 made a career change, the other one tried modified work	No drop outs
Friedberg et al. (2016) [104]	Fatigue self-management programme (CBT delivered by booklet and audio CDs) in severe CFS with web diaries and actigraphs; second group with less expensive paper diaries	137 patients with severe CFS	Fukuda	12 mo	Usual care control	At baseline 15.3% (21/137) worked full time, 21.2% (29/137) part-time or half time, 15.3% (21/137) were unemployed and 54.7% (75/137) disabled (participants were able to select multiple employment status categories). No employment data provided at follow-up. Actigraphy, step counter and six minute walk test showed no significant objective change.	5.1% (7/137) dropout rate
Fulcher and White (1997) [77]	GET	66	Oxford	12 mo	Flexibility exercises and relaxation therapy. Poorly matched groups; concerns if this was in fact a trial for ME/CFS patients	At baseline 39% (26/66) were working or studying at least part time, compared with 47% (31/66) after treatment	21% (14/66) dropped out
Hlavaty et al. (2011) [108]	CBT with graded activity, homework compliance	82 (divided over 4 treatment groups)	Fukuda	12 mo	3 other treatment groups: cognitive coping skills, relaxation or anaerobic exercises	At baseline 57.3% were retired, unemployed or on disability; 37.9% worked full-time or part-time; 1.2% working and on disability. No employment data provided at follow-up.	Unclear
Huibers et al. (2004) [102]	CBT delivered by GPs	151 fatigued employees on sick leave (66 met CFS criteria)	Fukuda	12 mo	No treatment	At 4 mo 50% (CBT) and 61% (NT) and at 12 mo 59% (CBT) and 65% (NT) resumed work	Did not complete: 33% (25/76) CBT, 9.3% (7/75) no treatment

94

Table 4. *Cont.*

Study	Intervention	n	Criteria	Length of FU	Control Group	Work Outcome	Dropouts/Missing Data
Janse et al. (2017) [120]	Evaluation of four studies: 2 of CBT, 1 of group CBT and 1 of stepped care CBT *	583 (participants from four trials grouped together)	Fukuda	5 yrs, minimum of 18 mo	No control groups (2 non-randomised noncontrolled studies, one randomised study had no control group and control group from 4th study was not used for this evaluation)	At long-term FU, 54% (264/490) had paid work and 27% (114/430) received a disability pension. Baseline employment data was not provided.	Response rate was 84.0% (490/583, paid work) and 73.8% (430/583, disability pension) respectively. The authors themselves noted that non-responders scored significantly lower on physical functioning at short-term follow-up than responders.
Janse et al. (2018) [121]	Protocol iCBT vs. on demand iCBT **	240	Fukuda	6 mo	Waiting-list (WL)	Paid job at baseline: 65% Protocol iCBT, 71% on demand iCBT and 68% WL. No employment data provided at follow-up.	Dropped out: 6.3% (5/80) Protocol iCBT, 8.8% (7/80) on demand iCBT, 5% (4/80) WL
Jason et al. (2007) [122]	CBT vs. cognitive therapy vs. anaerobic activity	114	Fukuda	12 mo	Relaxation	At baseline, 19.3% were working full time, 20.2% part time, 24.6% on disability, 23.7% unemployed, 6.1% retired, 4.4% part-time students, 0.9% full time students and 0.9% working part time and on disability. No significant interaction effects were found for employment at FU.	25% dropped out; no differences between groups
Koolhaas et al. (2009) [123]	CBT; patient survey by University	100	98% diagnosed by a doctor, 2% by a psychologist	Patient survey		41% worked before, 31% after CBT; patients who were able to work, worked five hours per week less after CBT	Not applicable
Lopez et al. (2011) [124]	Cognitive behavioral stress management (CBSM)	69 (44 CBSM, 25 control group)	Fukuda	12 weeks (end of treatment)	Psycho educational (PE) seminar	At baseline: 13.2% worked full time, 18.8% part time, 15.9% unemployed 4.3% retired, 2.9% student and 44.9% on disability. No employment data provided at follow-up.	13.6% (6/44) CBSM and 20% (5/25) PE lost to FU
Marlin et al. (1998) [125]	Multidisciplinary intervention (MDI) that include CBT; 50% also treated with full dose antidepressants	71 (51 MDI, 20 control) nonrandomised study with patients from a private clinic	Fukuda	33 mo	No treatment control group (many of them had declined MDI)	Average duration of work disability at baseline: 23 mo MDI, 39 mo NT; at FU: 25 mo MDI, 27 mo NT.	69% (49/71) were lost to follow up.
Masuda et al. (2002) [126]	Multidisciplinary treatment *** for both treatment groups	38 (9 postinfectious (PI) and 9 non-infectious (NI) CFS; 20 HC) non-randomised study	CDC 1988	2 yr	No treatment	Illness duration: 8.2 mo PI and 38.2 mo NI (badly matched). Postinfectious group: 3 returned to work, 5 others changed occupation or workplace; non-infectious group: 3 returned to work. No employment date for HC.	No drop outs
McBride et al. (2017) [127]	Online cognitive remediation training programme including CBT+GET (OCRTP) **** vs. CBT+GET alone (CGA). Non-randomised trial	72 (36 in each group)	Fukuda	12 wks	No control group	Baseline characteristics: currently employed 33% CGA, 22% OCRTP; disability pension 14% CGA, 8% OCRTP; hours of employment/week 6 CGA, 19 OCRTP; currently studying 27% CGA, 25% OCRTP; hours of study/week 6 CGA, 11 OCRTP. No employment data provided at follow-up.	Unclear
McDermott et al. (2004) [128]	Lifestyle management programme based on CBT+GET with pacing as the core strategy	98, nonrandomised trial	Fukuda	18 mo	No control group	Of those who attended 4 or more sessions of therapy, 8.5% (5/59) returned to work full time and 10.2% (6/59) part-time	24.5% (24/98) lost to follow up; 79.7% (59/74) completed at least four sessions of treatment
Moss-Morris et al. (2005) [129]	GET	49 self referred patients from a CFS private practice (25 GET, 24 controls)	Fukuda	6 mo	No treatment, poorly matched control group	22.4% were unemployed and unable to work due to disability at baseline. No employment data provided at follow-up. Fitness (VO2peak) deteriorated by 15% after GET	Lost to FU: 36% (9/25) GET, 29.2% (7/24) no treatment
O'Dowd et al. (2006) [130]	Group CBT incorporating graded activity vs. education and support group	153	Fukuda	12 mo	No treatment (SMC)	The authors concluded that group CBT did not significantly improve employment status.	Missing cognitive test data: 28.9% CBT, 13.7% NT
Prins et al. (2001) [131]	CBT versus guided support	278	Oxford	14 mo	No treatment (natural course).	No statistically significant difference in number of hours worked at 8 ($p = 0.3362$) and 14 mo ($p = 0.1134$) between CBT and natural course	40.9% (55/93) CBT and 23.1% (70/91) no treatment (dropouts)

Table 4. Cont.

Study	Intervention	n	Criteria	Length of FU	Control Group	Work Outcome	Dropouts/Missing Data
Powell et al. (2001) and (2004) [132,133]	GET vs. telephone intervention with GET vs. minimum intervention with GET	148	Oxford	2 yrs	No treatment (NT; labelled as SMC; participants received an information booklet that encouraged graded activity and positive thinking)	At baseline: working: 39.5% (15/38) GET, 35.1% (13/37) minimum, 28.2% (11/39) telephone, 32.4% (11/34) NT. Disability benefit: 42.1% (16/38) GET, 17/37 minimum, 16/39 telephone, 15/34 NT. No employment data provided at follow-up.	Response rate: 77.0% (114/148)
Ridsdale et al. (2001) [134]	CBT versus counseling	160 (fatigue study, 28% (45) had CFS)	Fukuda	6 mo	Counselling	At baseline 3.1% (counselling) and 10.9% (CBT) were off sick. Days off work improved by 4.3% (15/350, counselling) vs. deteriorated by 6.6% (55/829, CBT) [135]	36% (29/80) counselling and 31% (25/80) CBT dropped out
Ridsdale et al. (2004) [136]	CBT vs. GET	123 (fatigue study, 29% (36 patients) fulfilled Fukuda criteria (n = 15 CBT, n = 21 GET)	Fukuda	8 mo	Post hoc added non-randomised prospective no treatment control group; badly matched. Patients were given a booklet on self-management of fatigue	Employed at base line: 60% CBT, 73% GET vs. 65% control group. No employment data provided at follow-up. Step test results not published.	29% (18/63) CBT and 40% (24/60) GET did not complete 6 sessions of therapy; 22.5% (9/40) did not provide follow-up data (control group)
Sandler et al. (2016) [137]	Integrated programme of CBT, GET and pacing. Non-randomised noncontrolled trial	264 (245 CFS and 19 post-cancer fatigue (PCF) patients)	Fukuda (for CFS)	24 weeks	No control group	At baseline 39% (104/264) in receipt of sickness benefits or medical pension. Unclear how many of those had CFS. No other employment data provided. Also, no employment data provided at follow-up.	36% (96/264) missing data
Saxty et al. (2005) [138]	Group CBT, non-randomised nonnoncontrolled trial	6	Fukuda	3 mo	No control group	At baseline 1 was working full time, 3 part-time and 2 were on sick leave. At follow-up, the 2 part-time workers had increased their hours. No other employment changes	No drop outs; therapy attendance rate 86.7%
Scheeres et al. (2008) [139]	CBT; non-randomised noncontrolled study	125 (13 did not fulfil the Fukuda criteria)	Fukuda	8 mo	No control group	At baseline 62% had a paid job. Fewer patients had a paid job after treatment than before (percentage not give). The number of contract hours after CBT decreased from 16.2 to 14.9 but the number of hours worked increased from 9.4 to 11.4 per week.	35.7% (40/112) dropped out; the last observation was used in case of missing data
Schreurs et al. (2011) [140]	CBT combined with GET (inpatient rehabilitation programme); non-randomised noncontrolled study	160	Fukuda	6 mo	No control group	At intake 52% (83/160) on disability benefits, 31.2% (50/160) were working mostly part-time, 2.5% (4/160) had own business, 8.8% (14/160) were school going. No employment data provided at follow-up.	27% (44/160) no FU measurements
Stordeur et al. (2008) [141]	Evaluation of CBT and GET in Belgium CFS knowledge centres	655	Fukuda	Treatment evaluation	No control group (treatment evaluation)	Employment status decreased from 18.3% to 14.9%; sickness allowance status increased from 54% to 57%	28% dropped out
Vos-Vromans et al. (2016 and 2017) [142,43]	Multidisciplinary rehabilitation treatment (MRT) which contained an element of CBT versus CBT	122	Fukuda	12 mo	No control group	At baseline 68% (39/57) MRT and 52% (27/52) CBT had paid work and were working 26.1 (MRT) and 29.8 (CBT) hours per week. No employment data provided at follow-up. Objective improvement: 5.8% MRT and 6.5% CBT (activity monitor)	20% (12/60) CBT and 10% (6/62) MRT (dropped out)
Wearden et al. (1998) [144]	2 treatment groups: exercise and 20 mg fluoxetine versus appointments only and 20 mg fluoxetine	136	Oxford	6 mo	2 control groups: exercise and placebo drug; appointments and placebo drug	At baseline 84% had changed occupation. No employment data provided at follow-up.	37% (25/67, exercise) vs. 22% (15/69, non-exercise) (dropouts); drop-outs were significantly more likely than trial completers to have changed or given up their occupation as a result of their illness (95% vs. 79%); 34% (23/67) complied fully with GET, 78% (54/69) complied fully with exercise placebo

Table 4. Cont.

Study	Intervention	n	Criteria	Length of FU	Control Group	Work Outcome	Dropouts/Missing Data
Wearden et al. (2010, 2012 and 2013) [45–47]	Pragmatic rehabilitation (CBT, GET and explanation about CFS to patients) vs. supportive listening	296	Oxford	70 wks	No treatment (GP treatment as usual)	At baseline 65% (187/296) in receipt of benefits. No other employment data provided at baseline or follow-up. Step test showed no objective improvement	13% (39/296) dropped out
White et al. (2011) [48]	CBT vs. GET vs. APT (all 3 also contained SMC)	641	Oxford	52 wks (with long-term follow-up (LTFU) at 31 months [49]).	SMC (no treatment)	Lost employment: remained 84% (CBT); increased from 83% at baseline to 86% (GET) at FU. Income benefits increased from 10% to 13% (CBT) and from 14% to 20% (GET); illness/disability benefits increased from 32% to 38% (CBT) and from 31% to 36% (GET); payments from income protection schemes or private pensions increased from 6% to 12% (CBT) and from 8% to 16% (GET) [56]. No employment data provided at LTFU.	Dropouts: 10.5% (17/161) CBT, 6.3% (10/160) GET. Missing step test data: 33.8% (54/160) GET and 29.8% (48/161) CBT [51]
Witkowski et al. (2004) [152]	Group CBT; non-randomised noncontrolled trial	6	Fukuda	3 mo	No control group	1 returned to full-time employment and 1 worked part-time on a phased return	33% (2/6) dropped out
Worm-Smeitink et al. (2016) [153]	Comparison of efficacy of CBT in two leading international centres (UK and Netherlands)	NL: 293, UK: 163	NL: Fukuda, UK: Oxford	Unclear	Outcomes after CBT in the other country	At baseline employed: 67.6% NL, 55.2% UK; number of hours worked: 9.88 NL, 13.80 UK; on sick leave: 51.5% NL, 20% UK. No employment data provided at follow-up.	Dropped out: NL 7.8% (23/293), UK: 6.7% (11/163)
Worm-Smeitink et al. (2019) [154]	Prescheduled or on-demand internet-based CBT (iCBT) followed by face-to-face (f2f) CBT when necessary versus f2f CBT *****	363	Fukuda (7 patients had <4 of the required 4 or more additional symptoms)	Unclear	No control group	Paid job at baseline: 68.9% prescheduled iCBT, 65.8% on-demand iCBT, 64.7% f2f CBT. No employment data provided at follow-up.	Dropped out plus <4 CDC criteria: 5% (6/121) prescheduled iCBT, 11.6% (14/121) on-demand iCBT, 31.4% (38/121) f2f CBT; of those who met step-up criteria 55.4% (51/92) prescheduled iCBT and 41.9% (39/93) on-demand iCBT declined f2f CBT

APT: adaptive pacing therapy; FU: follow-up; HC: healthy controls; ICF: idiopathic chronic fatigue; NT: no treatment; SMC: specialist medical care; vs.: versus; WL: waiting list. * Janse et al. (2017) [120] reviewed the efficacy of different forms of CBT of the following four trials at long-term follow-up (5 years with a minimum of 18 months). Heins et al. [155] (n = 232) and Knoop et al. [156] (n = 112) were 2 non-randomised noncontrolled trials of CBT. Tummers et al. [157] (n = 171) was a randomised trial without a control group. They compared guided self-instruction, followed by CBT with CBT alone. Wiborg et al. [158] (n = 204) was a waiting-list controlled trial of group CBT. This wait-list group (n = 68) was not assessed by Janse et al. Consequently, all 4 studies in the review by Janse et al. (2017) were noncontrolled. ** Janse et al. (2018) [121] [126]: Protocol iCBT: Internet-based CBT with protocol-driven therapist feedback; on demand iCBT: Internet-based CBT with therapist feedback on demand. *** Masuda et al. (2002) [126]: Multidisciplinary treatment consisting of three-stage treatment programs was carried out for all patients. Each stage of treatment required 3 weeks. The 1st stage consisted of drug therapy, rehabilitation, and counseling. The second stage consisted of cognitive behavioral therapy and family therapy, and the third stage consisted of exercise therapy. **** McBride et al. (2017) [127]: online cognitive remediation training programme (OCKTP; cognitive exercise therapy; CET) in addition to CBT+GET compared to CBT+GET alone (CGA). ***** Worm-Smeitink et al. (2019) [154] was a three-arm, parallel, randomized, noninferiority trial. In 2 arms, the patients received stepped care (SC) consisting of I-CBT, either with protocol-driven feedback (SC-protocol-driven feedback) or with feedback on demand (SC-feedback-on-demand), followed by face-to-face (f2f) CBT when necessary, that is, still severely fatigued (CIS fatigue severity >35) or disabled (SIP >700) after I-CBT. The third arm was f2f CBT after a variable waiting period.

Dyck et al. [115] was a case study (n = 2) of a multidisciplinary programme including 30 min of fitness twice a week. Such a workload would exclude most patients with ME/CFS. Fulcher and White (n = 66) [117] created a study that used the Oxford criteria. 39% were working or studying at least part time at trial entry, compared with 47% after treatment. However, as found by the reanalysis of the Cochrane exercise review for ME/CFS [159], there were a number of issues with this study. Participants in the exercise group had sessions of five to fifteen minutes, increasing to a maximum of thirty minutes, at least five days a week. Such a workload would exclude most patients with ME/CFS. Moreover, the normal fitness scores (VO2max) at baseline in the GET group (31.8) cast further doubts about the diagnosis as this score is well above the score for mildly impaired ME/CFS patients (22.1) according to VanNess et al. [160]. It is also well above the threshold of impairment (25) according to the American Medical Association [161]. Moreover, patients with a common symptom of ME/CFS (sleep disturbances) were excluded yet patients on full dose antidepressants were not. All this together raises serious concerns about whether this was in fact a trial for patients with ME/CFS. Finally, there was an important difference of the fitness of the GET group at baseline compared to the control group (VO2max score 31.8 versus 28.2).

In a non-randomised non-controlled trial by McDermott et al. [128], 9.2% (9/98) returned to work full time and 6.1% (6/98) part-time after a lifestyle management programme. This programme used the principles of CBT and graded activity for ME/CFS within a biopsychosocial framework [113] with pacing as the core strategy [128]. Pacing is an illness management strategy to stay within one's energy envelope which has been practiced by patients for a long time as a strategy to try and prevent relapses and optimise the things they can do [162].

A non-randomised non-controlled trial of six patients that tested the efficacy of group CBT by Saxty et al. [138], found that the two people who had been working part time had increased their hours and the one patient who was working full time continued to do so. Wittkowski et al. [152] conducted a non-randomised non-controlled trial of group CBT that also only included six patients. Two of them dropped out, one patient returned to full time employment while another worked part time on a phased return. Scheeres et al. [139] was another non-randomised non-controlled study in which "relatively many patients (62%) had a paid job" at baseline according to the authors. The number of contract hours after CBT decreased from 16.2 to 14.9 but the number of hours worked increased from 9.4 to 11.4 per week.

Marlin et al. (1998) [125] was a non-randomised study in a privately funded clinic of a multidisciplinary intervention consisting of medical treatment if needed, pharmacological treatment of comorbid defective or anxiety disorders and CBT for ME/CFS. 50% of the participants in the treatment group were treated with full-dose antidepressant, which suggests that they were suffering from depression. There was 25.5% (13/51) and 21.6% (11/51) in the treatment group and 0% and 5% in the no treatment control group had resumed work at the end of treatment and follow-up, respectively. Many in the no treatment group had refused to take part in a behavioural intervention programme. Also, 69% (49/71) were lost to follow up.

Friedberg et al. [116] was set up to assess the efficacy of behavioural self-management (CBT delivered by a booklet and audio CDs) in severe ME/CFS. The authors concluded that there was significantly reduced fatigue at three months but not at twelve-month follow-up compared to the no treatment control group (usual care). Also, that it appeared to be less effective in comparison to findings reported for higher functioning groups by other trials. The trial found that behavioural self-management did not lead to objective improvement (actigraphy, step counter and six-minute walk test). At baseline, 15.3% (21/137) worked full time and 21.2% (29/137) part-time or halftime. No employment data is available from follow up. The high rate of participants working at baseline together with the distance walked during the six-minute walk test (336 m), raises serious concerns about whether this was in fact a trial for patients with severe ME/CFS.

Other trials of behavioural interventions that provided employment data at baseline but not at follow-up, were conducted by for example Hlavaty et al., Lopez et al., Schreurs et al., Vos-Vromans et al. and Wearden et al. [118,124,140,142,145].

Trials by Bazelmans et al., Jason et al., O'Dowd et al. and Prins et al. [109,122,130,131], with follow-up ranging from 6 to 14 months, found no statistically significant difference in employment status between the treatment and control group at follow-up. This was also found by Deale et al. [114] at 5-year follow-up.

More patients had resumed work at 4- and 12-months follow-up in the no treatment control group compared to the group that was treated with CBT delivered by GPs in a trial by Huibers et al. [119].

An evaluation of the efficacy of CBT in the Netherlands by Koolhaas et al. [123] found that after CBT, patients worked five hours per week less and the percentage of patients who were able to work, had decreased from 41% to 31%.

In the PACE trial ($n = 641$) by White et al. [148], lost employment remained the same (84%) after CBT and increased from 83% to 86% after GET. The number of participants on income benefits increased from 10% to 13% (CBT) and from 14 to 20% (GET); disability benefits increased from 32% to 38% (CBT) and from 31% to 36% (GET); payments from income protection schemes or private pensions increased from 6% to 12% (CBT) and from 8% to 16% (GET) [150]. Evaluation of the efficacy of CBT and GET in the Belgian CFS knowledge centres ($n = 655$) showed that employment status decreased from 18.3% to 14.9% and sickness allowance status increased from 54% to 57% [141].

Collin and Crawley [111] analysed the efficacy of treatments provided by 11 CFS/ME specialist services in the UK ($n = 952$). These services treated patients with CBT, GET, a combination of both or activity management which was more effective in fatigue reduction at 12 months follow-up than CBT and GET. Also, there was no change in employment situation after treatment in the NHS clinics in 47.2 % cases. 18.0% were able to return to work or increase their hours and 30.0% stopped working or reduced their hours because of ME/CFS. Therefore, the net effect was that 12% stopped working or reduced their hours after NHS treatment.

5. Discussion

A large supplier of nationwide occupational health services had questions about medical retirement for ME/CFS, how ME/CFS affects a person's ability to work and what can be expected in terms of recovery. Yet they were unable to find an article in the medical literature addressing these questions. We were also unable to find such an article. Therefore, we reviewed the literature to see if we could answer these questions.

The name, chronic fatigue syndrome, has had a huge impact on the medical, scientific and patient communities—how it is viewed and how patients are treated by the medical profession [163]. That together with the fact that most ME/CFS patients look well and have no outward signs of illness, combined with the lack of training in medical school and during post graduate education, means that many doctors are not aware of the severity of ME/CFS [164] or that 25% are too ill to leave their homes [53]. Nor are they aware of the fact that the quality of life in ME/CFS is worse than in other severe illnesses like MS, lung cancer, chronic renal failure or stroke [165].

Most cases tend to start as an unremarkable viral infection. However, instead of recovering, patients begin to experience profound muscular (and cognitive) fatigue—for example heavy legs—following activities which were previously completed without difficulty. Also typical is an abnormally prolonged delay in the restoration of muscle (and brain) power [166]. Consequently, people with ME/CFS are often unable to engage in economically productive work and typically request sick leave as a solution to their health crisis [167]. Prior to developing ME/CFS, most patients were healthy, sporty and active [4]. There is no diagnostic test, therefore diagnostic criteria are used to diagnose ME/CFS. Over the last 35 years and especially in the last 5 to 10 years, many different biological abnormalities have been found in patients with ME/CFS distinguishing them from healthy controls [22]. Due to these, the Institute of Medicine—now called the American National Academy of Medicine—concluded in 2015 that ME/CFS is a severely debilitating chronic multisystem disease [23]. A great deal more is known today about the underlying biology of ME/CFS but unfortunately, we do not have a diagnostic test yet. However, a recently published small study of 20 cases and 20 controls, reported that a test they had developed involving a nanoelectric chip, which is capable of measuring minuscule energy changes in cells in the blood to gauge their health when exposed to stress. In this case salt, was able to distinguish between cases and controls with 100% certainty [168]. A much larger study is now needed to confirm the accuracy of this test. Not only to distinguish cases from healthy controls but also to distinguish them from other fatiguing illnesses.

Growing awareness of the underlying biological underpinnings has created increased international awareness and interest in the illness. This will accelerate research and the finding of a diagnostic test and effective pharmacological treatment [22]. However, we will have to continue to rely on diagnostic criteria to diagnose the illness as has been the case so far until such a test becomes available.

Just like with most other illnesses, illness severity can vary between patients. Mildly affected patients have a substantial activity reduction according to the Fukuda criteria [18], and at least a 50% activity reduction in comparison to before they fell ill according to the 1988 CDC criteria [105] and the 2011 International Consensus Criteria [20]. Unfortunately, postexertional malaise (PEM), the main characteristic of the disease, is not a requirement for diagnosis according to the Oxford criteria [13] which are primarily used in the UK. Moreover, it is only an optional requirement according to the Fukuda criteria [18], the most commonly used criteria to diagnose ME/CFS. PEM is compulsory for diagnosis according to newer diagnostic criteria—the Canadian Consensus Criteria and its revised version, the International Consensus Criteria [12,20] as can be seen in Table 1. The consequence of using criteria that do not require the main characteristic of the disease to be present is that in a substantial number of cases, as discussed earlier, patients do not suffer from ME/CFS but they have a self-limiting illness [15,16] or a disease which in many cases would be treatable if patients had gotten the right diagnosis. The combination of a lack of a diagnostic test, using different diagnostic criteria and the lack of adequate training about this illness in medical school has led to 2 problems. First of all, up to 50% of patients diagnosed with ME/CFS have an alternative explanation for their symptoms [25,26]. Many of the alternative diagnoses are currently treatable which would mean that many patients could go back to work if they would get the right diagnosis and treatment. The diagnosis of ME/CFS should be reconsidered if none of the following key features are present:: post-exertional fatigue or malaise, cognitive difficulties, sleep disturbance (unrefreshing sleep or reversal of sleep pattern) and chronic pain [8]. The diagnosis should also be reconsidered if patients deteriorate or get new symptoms. Secondly, according to estimates, around 90% of patients affected by ME/CFS are not diagnosed with the disease. Improving diagnosis and optimizing management can have significant economic and public health consequences [9]. In particular because shorter illness duration is a significant predictor of sustained remission, and thus early detection of ME/CFS is of utmost importance [34].

A meta-analysis by Franklin et al. [169] of 32 studies found that ME/CFS patients have a substantially reduced VO2peak compared to healthy sedentary controls. If occupational health physicians have doubts about the legitimacy or the severity of the disease in a specific case then this physiological abnormality, together with postexertional malaise, can be detected by two-day cardiopulmonary exercise testing (CPET) using the protocol of the Workwell Foundation [170]. The downside of CPET in ME/CFS however is that it is expensive, it can lead to relapses and severely affected patients are too ill and disabled to do it. Alternatively, in such a case, it could be worthwhile considering a second opinion by a ME/CFS literate medical doctor.

5.1. What Can Be Expected If a Patient Is Diagnosed with ME/CFS?

A comprehensive review of the literature on the natural course of ME/CFS in adults showed that the illness runs a chronic course. A progression or worsening of symptoms is seen in 10 to 20% of cases and overall the prognosis in terms of return to work is poor. Also, only 5% will recover [10]. In clinical trials of ME/CFS, the term recovery often reflects less than full restoration of health. A more appropriate and accurate label for this would be clinically significant improvement [164]. However, it's not only clinical trials that suffer from this problem. Brown et al. [65] found that adults who labelled themselves as recovered from ME/CFS, showed significant impairments on 21 out of 23 outcomes compared to healthy controls. Moreover, on 17 of those 23 outcomes, the impairments were the same as for those who were still ill with ME/CFS, which suggests that patients adapt to their impairments instead of recover from them. A working group, reporting to the Chief Medical Officer (CMO) for England [55], concluded that most of those who feel recovered stabilise at a lower level of functioning than that before their illness. Consequently, even a recovery percentage as low as 5, might well be too optimistic.

Contrary to typical patterns of chronic disease, where the most severe cases present to medical professionals, severe cases of ME/CFS are less likely to do that [28] due to being bedridden and too ill to attend. Several studies have shown that the prognosis for patients with severe ME/CFS, including young patients with severe ME/CFS, is worse than for ME/CFS in general. Early management of the illness appeared the most important determinant of severity [54]. Dr Melvin Ramsay [36], the infectious disease specialist who witnessed and documented the outbreak of ME in the Royal Free Hospital in London in 1955, wrote the following about that: "The degree of physical incapacity varies greatly, but the dominant clinical feature of profound fatigue is directly related to the length of time the patient persists in physical effort after its onset; put in another way, those patients who are given a period of enforced rest from the onset have the best prognosis." In the absence of effective treatment, this is the only thing that occupational health physicians and other doctors can do in the beginning of the illness, to try and prevent chronic and severe physical incapacity, long-term sick leave and medical retirement later on in the course of the disease.

5.2. Factors Predictive of a Worse Outcome

Illness severity is strongly implicated in a poor prognosis for ME/CFS [54]. Those who are more fatigued experience a greater number of somatic symptoms and an increase in functional limitations. These factors make it more difficult to recover from ME/CFS [41]. A systematic review by Cairns and Hotopf [10] found that having a comorbid psychiatric disorder at baseline was associated with poorer outcome and Vercoulen et al. [49] found the same for cognitive factors. Psychosocial factors show little relationship to recovery [171]. Smoking and personality are not risk factors [172]. Neurotic traits are more frequent among the less severely ill. Conscientiousness is not related to severity [54]. Patients with ME/CFS and Fibromyalgia (FM)—FM is a comorbidity in 50% to 60% of cases—are three times more likely to become non-improvers than those without FM [44]. Patients who are more ill and have comorbidities are less likely to be able to work than those with milder ME/CFS without comorbidities [3]. While there is good reason to suggest that a positive attitude will help in the prognosis of any disease, including ME/CFS, there is little empirical evidence to support the assertion that attitudes, behaviour or underlying personality have a major role in determining outcomes [54]. Men, people in older age groups, and people who have been ill for longer are more likely to have ceased employment due to their illness. These factors are predictive of a worse outcome [45,46]. Poorer outcome is also predicted by increased pain and worse physical functioning at onset [45]. Disability was the main independent predictor of discontinuation of employment in a study of employees on long-term sick leave due to fatigue [56]. The NHS database findings suggest that people with ME/CFS continue in employment despite the primary (fatigue and pain) and secondary effects (depression and anxiety) of ME/CFS. Instead, loss of physical capacity is the ultimate arbiter of inability to continue working [46]. The prognosis is better if patients developed ME/CFS during an outbreak [173], after glandular fever/mononucleosis [52] or after Giardia enteritis [35,79].

5.3. Employment Status

The inability to work due to ME/CFS is high [59]. Between 27% and 65% of CFS patients are reported not to be working, and less than a third of patients are estimated to resume employment within three years after diagnosis, as found by a systematic review [10]. Many who improve, experience the majority of their improvement relatively quickly [55]. Van der Werf et al. [94] found that after a follow-up period of 12-months, spontaneous recovery was rare and only occurred in patients with an illness duration of less than 1.5 years. A prospective study by Vercoulen et al. [49] followed up

298 patients with a relatively long duration of complaints—median 4.5 years—for 18 months. They found no improvement in employment and benefit status. This despite the fact that the study included 51 patients with an illness duration of less than two years, who according to the same study are more likely to improve. Nine-year follow-up of a Danish group of CFS patients, showed that recovery and substantial improvement are uncommon and that patients as a group neither improved nor deteriorated since diagnosis [33].

Studies that reported on employment status found large differences between ME/CFS patients and healthy controls (see Table 2) but also between ME/CFS, MS, depression and healthy sedentary controls [80]. These data are often from small(er) studies, larger studies show the following. Castro-Marrero et al. [3] (n = 1757) found that 62.8% were unemployed due to ME/CFS and 25.6% were employed. The rest had never worked. Collin et al. [46] who analysed the NHS database (n = 2170) found that 41% were employed and 50% had discontinued work due to ME/CFS which is similar to the 54% found by a systematic review by Ross et al. [59]. TNO, an independent Dutch research institute [2] (n = 924) found that 30% were working; 7% had never been on long-term sick leave and 23% had been able to go back to work after long-term sick leave but they were working less hours. They were also less often involved in management and more often did sedentary work behind a computer. Nivel, another independent Dutch research institute [104] (n = 412), found similarly high rates of patients unable to work due to their ME/CFS. It also found that only 1/4 of patients who worked, were able to work more than 24 hours a week. Reports by ME Associations from around the world [98–102] also highlight the large number of patients who are unable to work due to ME/CFS (see Table 3).

5.4. Medical Retirement

In cases where incapacity is prolonged, work rehabilitation is impossible or unsuccessful and prognosis appears to be poor, then the occupational health physician may be asked to advice on the possibility of retirement on the grounds of ill health if an employee with ME/CFS is covered by a company pension scheme which makes this provision. Qualifying criteria inevitably vary, although permanent inability to undertake normal duties for reasons of ill health is a common requirement [60]. Important aspects of a work capability and functional capacity assessment are the influence of symptoms such as pain, fatigue and cognitive problems on the ability to work, bearing in mind that cognitive problems, together with physical problems are often the reason why patients stopped working [46]. It is estimated that between 74% and 95% of ME/CFS patients have some type of cognitive deficit [174,175] which are cited as some of the most disruptive and functionally disabling symptoms of ME/CFS [114]. Studies of objective neuropsychological functioning in ME/CFS consistently document impairment in information-processing speed, auditory attention and memory [176]. In addition, Chu et al. [68] found that cognitive symptoms present at the beginning of the illness tend to persist, declining by only 4–10%.

Although many patients are eventually retired, such action should be a last resort. On the other hand, the prognosis for recovery and substantial improvement that enables a return to work is poor if patients have been off work for 2 to 3 years. This was confirmed by the Inspectorate Work and Pay of the Dutch Ministry of Work and Social Affairs [177]. This Inspectorate concluded that if patients have been on long-term sick leave for two years or more and treatment with CBT did not make a difference, then the prognosis for a return to work is poor.

If employees are mildly affected yet unable to work and the occupational health physician is reluctant to award medical retirement than it seems reasonable to award retirement benefits for a limited time followed by a case review in six months to a year. Long-term compensation to secure the socioeconomic position does not inhibit return to work, but may be an essential contributor to becoming employed later on [52]. The reason for this might be that it prevents patients from going over their limits if they would be forced to do work which they are unable to do which might seriously disrupt the naturally occurring recovery or improvement process in persons with ME/CFS.

5.5. Strengths and Limitations of This Review

Limitations of this review are caused by the use of different selection criteria by the studies in the review, so that patients might have been included who do not have ME/CFS. Also, by the variability in follow-up periods. Furthermore, some studies are prospective whilst others are retrospective. In some studies patients were seen by physicians to check the diagnosis, other studies relied on questionnaires only. Studies did not consistently report about work status at both baseline and follow-up. Nor did they consistently describe employment status as full-time or part-time, previous or new work, or duration before returning to work. Studies also only measured outcomes at baseline and one follow-up moment but not more frequently. Therefore, in those studies it was impossible to see whether self-rated improvement or recovery and return to work was maintained or temporary.

Despite these limitations, one conclusion supported by all studies is that ME/CFS patients who fulfil strict diagnostic criteria, have worse prognosis compared to patients fulfilling lenient criteria and that the prognosis in general is poor. Reports by two independent Dutch research institutes, the large Spanish study by Castro-Marrero et al., the evaluation reports of the Belgian CFS clinics, the British NHS CFS clinics and the NHS database [2,3,45,46,104,111,141] provide detailed analyses about employment status in CFS adding to the strength of the evidence gathered by this review. Another strength of this review is that 38 CBT and/or GET studies that reported on work status were reviewed. Previously, a systematic review by Ross et al. (2004) [59] reviewed 4 CBT and/or GET studies that did so. Systematic reviews by Cairns and Hotopf (2005), Castro-Marrero et al. (2017), Chambers et al. (2006), Malouff et al. (2007), Smith et al. (2015) and Whiting et al. (2001) [10,106,107,178–180], a systematic review and meta-analysis by Marques et al. (2015) [181] and a meta-analysis by Castell et al. (2011) [182] did not review this.

5.6. Do CBT and GET Restore the Ability to Work in ME/CFS?

An influential systematic review by Cairns and Hotopf [10] concluded in 2005 that because there is increasing evidence for the effectiveness of CBT and GET, that "Medical retirement should be postponed until a trial of such treatment has been given." Consequently, many patients in The Netherlands have been forced to undergo these treatments and illness benefits and medical retirement were often not awarded if patients refused to do so. The Dutch Health Council concluded in March 2018 that ME/CFS is a serious and chronic multisystem disease and that CBT and GET are not adequate medical treatments for ME/CFS [24]. It also concluded that patients should not be forced to undergo these treatments. However, the chairman of the Dutch Association of Insurance Physicians said in a recent interview in a Dutch medical journal [183] that he did not agree with this. He was also urging insurance physicians to question patients' recovery behaviour if they refused to be treated with CBT and GET and to force patients to undergo these treatments. In the Netherlands the more than 700 insurance physicians of the UWV (Uitvoeringsinstituut Werknemersverzekeringen or Employee Insurance Agency) [177] decide if employees will be granted (temporary) medical retirement.

This raises the question if these treatments restore the ability to work. To answer this question, we analysed studies that tested the efficacy of CBT and/or GET and reported on employment outcomes (see Table 4). One of these studies was a study by Prins et al. (2001) [131], the largest CBT trial from the Netherlands (n = 278) which found that CBT does not improve employment status compared to doing nothing. Another important study was the PACE trial (n = 641) [148], the largest CBT and GET trial ever conducted. The efficacy of these treatment has also been assessed in real life outside of clinical trials, in the Belgium CFS knowledge centres (n = 655) and the NHS CFS clinics (n = 952) [111,141]. These evaluations, just like the PACE trial itself, showed that CBT and GET do not improve employment and illness benefit status. As a matter of fact, both deteriorated. After treatment, more patients were unable to work and more were receiving illness benefits. Also, a systematic review by Ross et al. [59] concluded in 2004 that CBT and GET did not prove effective in restoring the ability to work. Chambers et al. and Castro-Marrero et al. [178,179] documented this conclusion by Ross et al. in their systematic reviews in 2006 and 2017, respectively. Consequently, being treated with CBT and GET should not be a requirement to be eligible for medical retirement. Moreover, there is also no point in questioning patients' recovery behaviour or forcing them to undergo these treatments.

6. Conclusions

Myalgic Encephalomyelitis/Chronic Fatigue Syndrome leads to severe functional impairment and work disability in a considerable number of patients. The majority of patients who manage to continue or return to work, work part-time instead of full time in a physically less demanding job. The prognosis in terms of returning to work is poor if patients have been on long-term sick leave for more than two to three years. Being older and more ill when falling ill are associated with a worse employment outcome. Cognitive behavioural therapy and graded exercise therapy do not restore the ability to work. Consequently, many patients will eventually be medically retired depending on the requirements of the retirement policy, the progress that has been made since they have fallen ill in combination with the severity of their impairments compared to the sort of work they do or are offered to do. However, there is one thing that occupational health physicians and other doctors can do to try and prevent chronic and severe incapacity in the absence of effective treatments. Patients who are given a period of enforced rest from the onset, have the best prognosis. Moreover, those who work or go back to work should not be forced to do more than they can to try and prevent relapses, long-term sick leave and medical retirement.

Funding: This research received no external funding. The article publication charges were paid for by Emerge Australia. An Australia-wide organisation for information, support services, research and news about ME/CFS. Emerge Australia was not involved in the review or writing of the article.

Acknowledgments: The authors would like to thank M.V.'s parents for typing out his speech memos and Kasia for her help in improving the article. Finally, we would like to thank Emerge Australia for paying the article publication charges and the peer reviewers for their help in improving the article.

Conflicts of Interest: The authors declare no conflicts of interest.

References

1. Brurberg, K.G.; Fønhus, M.S.; Larun, L.; Flottorp, S.; Malterud, K. Case definitions for chronic fatigue syndrome/myalgic encephalomyelitis (CFS/ME): A systematic review. *BMJ Open* **2014**, *4*, e003973. [CrossRef] [PubMed]
2. Blatter, B.M.; van den Berg, R.; van Putten, D.J. Werk, Uitval en Reïntegratie bij Patiënten met ME/CVS *TBV* 13, nr. 7 (juli 2005). Available online: https://huisartsvink.files.wordpress.com/2019/05/blatter-werk-uitval2005-werk.pdf (accessed on 30 May 2019).
3. Castro-Marrero, J.; Faro, M.; Aliste, L.; Sáez-Francàs, N.; Calvo, N.; Martínez-Martínez, A.; de Sevilla, T.F.; Alegre, J. Comorbidity in Chronic Fatigue Syndrome/Myalgic Encephalomyelitis: A Nationwide Population-Based Cohort Study. *Psychosomatics* **2017**, *58*, 533–543. [CrossRef] [PubMed]
4. Bested, A.C.; Marshall, L.M. Review of Myalgic Encephalomyelitis/Chronic Fatigue Syndrome: An evidence-based approach to diagnosis and management by clinicians. *Revs. Environ. Health* **2015**, *30*, 223–249. [CrossRef] [PubMed]
5. WHO (World Health Organization). Volume 1: Tabular List. In *International Statistical Classification of Diseases and Health Related Problems (the) ICD-10*, 2nd ed.; WHO: Geneva, Switzerland, 2010.
6. Campbell Murdoch, J. Chronic fatigue syndrome The patient centred clinical method—A guide for the perplexed. *Aust. Fam. Physician* **2003**, *32*, 883–887.
7. Australian Myalgic Encephalomyelitis/Chronic Fatigue Syndrome Advisory Committee Report to the NHMRC Chief Executive Officer Draft for Public Consultation. December 2018. Available online: https://huisartsvink.files.wordpress.com/2019/05/australian-publicconsultationdraftceoreportME/CFS.pdf (accessed on 30 May 2019).
8. NICE Guidelines ME/CFS Criteria Chronic Fatigue Syndrome/Myalgic Encephalomyelitis (or Encephalopathy): Diagnosis and Management Clinical Guideline [CG53]. Published date: August 2007. Available online: https://www.nice.org.uk/guidance/cg53/resources/chronic-fatigue-syndromemyalgic-encephalomyelitisor-encephalopathy-diagnosis-and-management-pdf-975505810885 (accessed on 28 May 2019).

9. Valdez, A.R.; Hancock, E.E.; Adebayo, S.; Kiernicki, D.J.; Proskauer, D.; Attewell, J.R.; Bateman, L.; DeMaria, A., Jr.; Lapp, C.W.; Rowe, P.C.; et al. Estimating Prevalence, Demographics, and Costs of ME/CFS Using Large Scale Medical Claims Data and Machine Learning. *Front. Pediatr.* **2019**, *6*, 412. [CrossRef] [PubMed]
10. Cairns, R.; Hotopf, M.A. systematic review describing the prognosis of chronic fatigue syndrome. *Occup. Med. (Lond.)* **2005**, *55*, 20–31. [CrossRef] [PubMed]
11. Parish, J.G. Early outbreaks of 'epidemic neuromyasthenia'. *Postgrad. Med. J.* **1978**, *54*, 711–717. [CrossRef]
12. Carruthers, B.M.; Jain, A.K.; De Meirleir, K.L.; Peterson, D.L.; Klimas, N.G.; Lerner, A.M.; Bested, A.C.; Flor-Henry, P.; Joshi, P.; Powles, A.C.P.; et al. Myalgic encephalomyelitis/chronic fatigue syndrome: Clinical working case definition, diagnostic and treatment protocols. *J. Chronic Fatigue Syndr.* **2003**, *11*, 7–115. [CrossRef]
13. Sharpe, M.C.; Archard, L.C.; Banatvala, J.E.; Borysiewicz, L.K.; Clare, A.W.; David, A.; Edwards, R.H.; Hawton, K.E.; Lambert, H.P.; Lane, R.J.; et al. A report—Chronic fatigue syndrome: Guidelines for research. *J. R. Soc. Med.* **1991**, *84*, 118–121. [CrossRef]
14. Baraniuk, J. Chronic fatigue syndrome prevalence is grossly overestimated using Oxford criteria compared to Centers for Disease Control (Fukuda) criteria in a U.S. population study. *Fatigue Biomed. Health Behavs.* **2017**, *5*, 215–230. [CrossRef]
15. Green, C.R.; Cowan, P.; Elk, R.; O'Neil, K.M.; Rasmussen, A.L. Draft Executive Summary: National Institutes of Health-Pathways to Prevention Workshop: Advancing the Research on Myalgic Encephalomyelitis/Chronic Fatigue Syndrome. 2014. Available online: https://huisartsvink.files.wordpress.com/2018/08/green-draftreport-odp-mecfs-1.pdf (accessed on 16 September 2019).
16. Green, C.R.; Cowan, P.; Elk, R.; O'Neil, K.M.; Rasmussen, A.L. Final Report: National Institutes of Health-Pathways to Prevention Workshop: Advancing the Research on Myalgic Encephalomyelitis/Chronic Fatigue Syndrome, Executive Summary. 2014. Available online: https://huisartsvink.files.wordpress.com/2018/08/green-odp-finalreport-p2p-mecfs.pdf (accessed on 16 September 2019).
17. Smith, M.E.B.; Nelson, H.D.; Haney, E.; Pappas, M.; Daeges, M.; Wasson, N.; McDonagh, M. Diagnosis and Treatment of Myalgic Encephalomyelitis/Chronic Fatigue Syndrome. Evidence Reports/Technology Assessments, No. 219. (Prepared by the Pacific Northwest Evidence-based Practice Center under Contract No. 290-2012-00014-I.) AHRQ Publication No. 15-E001-EF. Rockville, MD: Agency for Healthcare Research and Quality; December 2014. Addendum July 2016. Available online: https://huisartsvink.files.wordpress.com/2018/08/ahrq-smith-et-al-2016-chronic-fatigue_research.pdf (accessed on 30 May 2019).
18. Fukuda, K.; Straus, S.E.; Hickie, I.; Sharpe, M.C.; Dobbins, J.G.; Komaroff, A. The chronic fatigue syndrome: A comprehensive approach to its definition and study. *Ann. Intern. Med.* **1994**, *121*, 953–959. [CrossRef] [PubMed]
19. Friedberg, F.; Dechene, L.; McKenzie, M.J., 2nd; Fontanetta, R. Symptom patterns in long-duration chronic fatigue syndrome. *J. Psychosom. Res.* **2000**, *48*, 59–68. [CrossRef]
20. Carruthers, B.M.; van de Sande, M.I.; De Meirleir, K.L.; Klimas, N.G.; Broderick, G.; Mitchell, T.; Staines, D.; Powles, A.C.P.; Speight, N.; Vallings, R.; et al. Myalgic encephalomyelitis: International consensus criteria. *J. Intern. Med.* **2011**, *270*, 327–338. [CrossRef] [PubMed]
21. Jason, L.A.; McManimen, S.; Sunnquist, M.; Brown, A.; Furst, J.; Newton, J.L.; Strand, E.B. Case definitions integrating empiric and consensus perspectives. *Fatigue* **2016**, *4*, 1–23. [CrossRef] [PubMed]
22. Komaroff, A.L. Advances in Understanding the Pathophysiology of Chronic Fatigue Syndrome. *JAMA* **2019**, *322*, 499–500. [CrossRef] [PubMed]
23. Institute of Medicine (IOM); Committee on the Diagnostic Criteria for Myalgic Encephalomyelitis/Chronic Fatigue Syndrome; Board on the Health of Select Populations. *Beyond Myalgic Encephalomyelitis/Chronic Fatigue Syndrome: Redefining an Illness*; National Academies Press: Washington, DC, USA, 2015.
24. Dutch Health Council. Aan: De Voorzitter van de Tweede Kamer der Staten-Generaal Nr. 2018, Den Haag 19 maart 2018 Gezondheidsraad|Nr. 2018/07. 2018. Available online: https://www.gezondheidsraad.nl/sites/default/files/grpublication/kernadvies_me_cvs_1.pdf (accessed on 30 May 2019).
25. Newton, J.L.; Mabillard, H.; Scott, A.; Hoad, A.; Spickett, G. The Newcastle NHS Chronic Fatigue Syndrome Service: Not all fatigue is the same. *J. R. Coll. Physicians Edinb.* **2010**, *40*, 304–307. [CrossRef] [PubMed]
26. Devasahayam, A.; Lawn, T.; Murphy, M.; White, P.D. Alternative diagnoses to chronic fatigue syndrome in referrals to a specialist service: Service evaluation survey. *JRSM Short Rep.* **2012**, *3*, 4. [CrossRef] [PubMed]

27. Nacul, L.C.; Lacerda, E.M.; Pheby, D.; Campion, P.; Molokhia, M.; Fayyaz, S.; Drachler, M.L. Prevalence of myalgic encephalomyelitis/chronic fatigue syndrome (ME/CFS) in three regions of England: A repeated cross-sectional study in primary care. *BMC Med.* **2011**, *9*, 91. [CrossRef] [PubMed]
28. Johnston, S.C.; Staines, D.R.; Marshall-Gradisnik, S.M. Epidemiological characteristics of chronic fatigue syndrome/myalgic encephalomyelitis in Australian patients. *Clin. Epidemiol.* **2016**, *8*, 97–107. [CrossRef] [PubMed]
29. Mariman, A.; Delesie, L.; Tobback, E.; Hanoulle, I.; Sermijn, E.; Vermeir, P.; Pevernagie, D.; Vogelaers, D. Undiagnosed and comorbid disorders in patients with presumed chronic fatigue syndrome. *J. Psychosom. Res.* **2013**, *75*, 491–496. [CrossRef] [PubMed]
30. Strassheim, V.S.J.; Sunnquist, M.; Jason, L.A.; Newton, J.L. Defining the prevalence and symptom burden of those with self-reported severe chronic fatigue syndrome/myalgic encephalomyelitis (CFS/ME): A two-phase community pilot study in the North East of England. *BMJ Open* **2018**, *8*, e020775. [CrossRef] [PubMed]
31. Darbishire, L.; Ridsdale, L.; Seed, P.T. Distinguishing patients with chronic fatigue from those with chronic fatigue syndrome: A diagnostic study in UK primary care. *Br. J. Gen. Pract.* **2003**, *53*, 441–445. [PubMed]
32. Wilson, A.; Hickie, I.; Lloyd, A.; Hadzi-Pavlovic, D.; Boughton, C.; Dwyer, J.; Wakefield, D. Longitudinal study of outcome of chronic fatigue syndrome. *BMJ* **1994**, *308*, 756–759. [CrossRef] [PubMed]
33. Andersen, M.M.; Permin, H.; Albrecht, F. Nine-year follow-up of Danish chronic fatigue syndrome (CFS) patients' impact on health, social, vocational, and personal lives. *J. Chron. Fatigue Syndr.* **2007**, *14*, 7–23. [CrossRef]
34. Nisenbaum, R.; Jones, J.F.; Unger, E.R.; Reyes, M.; Reeves, W.C. A population-based study of the clinical course of chronic fatigue syndrome. *Health Qual. Life Outcomes* **2003**, *1*, 49. [CrossRef] [PubMed]
35. Mørch, K.; Hanevik, K.; Rivenes, A.C.; Bødtker, J.E.; Næss, H.; Stubhaug, B.; Wensaas, K.A.; Rortveit, G.; Eide, G.E.; Hausken, T.; et al. Chronic fatigue syndrome 5 years after giardiasis: Differential diagnoses, characteristics and natural course. *BMC Gastroenterol.* **2013**, *13*, 28. [CrossRef] [PubMed]
36. Ramsay, M. *Myalgic Encephalomyelitis: A Baffling Syndrome with a Tragic Aftermath*; ME Association: Gawcott, UK, 1986.
37. Clark, M.R.; Katon, W.; Russo, J.; Kith, P.; Sintay, M.; Buchwald, D. Chronic fatigue: Risk factors for symptom persistence in a 2 1/2-year follow-up study. *Am. J. Med.* **1995**, *98*, 187–195. [CrossRef]
38. Bombardier, C.H.; Buchwald, D. Outcome and prognosis of patients with chronic fatigue vs chronic fatigue syndrome. *Arch. Intern. Med.* **1995**, *155*, 2105–2110. [CrossRef]
39. Hinds, G.M.E.; McCluskey, D.R. A retrospective study of chronic fatigue syndrome. *Proc. R. Coll. Physicians Edinb.* **1993**, *23*, 10–14.
40. Tiersky, L.A.; DeLuca, J.; Hill, N.; Dhar, S.K.; Johnson, S.K.; Lange, G.; Rappolt, G.; Natelson, B.H. Longitudinal assessment of neuropsychological functioning, psychiatric status, functional disability and employment status in chronic fatigue syndrome. *Appl. Neuropsychol.* **2001**, *8*, 41–50. [CrossRef]
41. Jason, L.A.; Porter, N.; Hunnell, J.; Brown, A.; Rademaker, A.; Richman, J.A. A natural history study of chronic fatigue syndrome. *Rehabil. Psychol.* **2011**, *56*, 32–42. [CrossRef] [PubMed]
42. Pheley, A.M.; Melby, D.; Schenck, C.; Mandel, J.; Peterson, J.K. Can we predict recovery in chronic fatigue syndrome? *Minn. Med.* **1999**, *82*, 52–56. [PubMed]
43. Sharpe, M.; Hawton, K.; Seagroatt, V.S.; Pasvol, G. Follow-up of patients presenting with fatigue to an infectious diseases clinic. *Br. Med. J.* **1992**, *305*, 147–152. [CrossRef] [PubMed]
44. Ciccone, D.S.; Chandler, H.K.; Natelson, B.H. Illness trajectories in the chronic fatigue syndrome: A longitudinal study of improvers versus non-improvers. *J. Nerv. Ment. Dis.* **2010**, *198*, 486–493. [CrossRef] [PubMed]
45. Crawley, E.; Collin, S.M.; White, P.D.; Rimes, K.; Sterne, J.A.; May, M.T.; UK CFS/ME National Outcomes Database. Treatment outcome in adults with chronic fatigue syndrome: A prospective study in England based on the CFS/ME National Outcomes Database. *QJM* **2013**, *106*, 555–565. [CrossRef] [PubMed]
46. Collin, S.M.; Crawley, E.; May, M.T.; Sterne, J.A.; Hollingworth, W.; UK CFS/ME National Outcomes Database. The impact of CFS/ME on employment and productivity in the UK: A cross-sectional study based on the CFS/ME national outcomes database. *BMC Health Servs. Res.* **2011**, *11*, 217. [CrossRef] [PubMed]
47. Hill, N.; Tiersky, L.; Scavalla, V.S.; Natelson, B. The fluctuation and outcome of chronic fatigue syndrome (CFS) over time. *J. Chronic Fatigue Syndr.* **1999**, *5*, 93–94.
48. Andersen, M.M.; Permin, H.; Albrecht, F. Illness and disability in Danish Chronic Fatigue Syndrome patients at diagnosis and 5-year follow-up. *J. Psychosom. Res.* **2004**, *56*, 217–229. [CrossRef]

49. Vercoulen, J.H.M.N.; Swanink, C.M.A.; Fennis, J.F.M.; Galama, J.M.D.; Van der Meer, J.W.M.; Bleijenberg, G. Prognosis in chronic fatigue syndrome: A prospective study on the natural course. *J. Neurol. Neurosurg. Psychiatry Bombard.* **1996**, *60*, 489–494. [CrossRef]
50. Ray, C.; Jeffries, S.; Weir, W.R.C. Coping and other predictors of outcome in chronic fatigue syndrome: A 1-year follow-up. *J. Psychosom. Res.* **1997**, *43*, 405–415. [CrossRef]
51. Reyes, M.; Dobbin, J.G.; Nisenbaum, R.; Subedar, N.; Randall, B.; Reeves, W.C. Chronic fatigue syndrome progression and self-defined recovery: Evidence from CDC surveillance system. *J. Chronic Fatigue Syndr.* **1999**, *5*, 17–27. [CrossRef]
52. Nyland, M.; Naess, H.; Birkeland, J.S.; Nyland, H. Longitudinal follow-up of employment status in patients with chronic fatigue syndrome after mononucleosis. *BMJ Open* **2014**, *4*, e005798. [CrossRef] [PubMed]
53. Pendergrast, T.; Brown, A.; Sunnquist, M.; Jantke, R.; Newton, J.L.; Strand, E.B.; Jason, L.A. Housebound versus nonhousebound patients with myalgic encephalomyelitis and chronic fatigue syndrome. *Chronic Illn* **2016**, *12*, 292–307 20. [CrossRef] [PubMed]
54. Pheby, D.; Saffron, L. Risk factors for severe ME/CFS. *Biol. Med.* **2009**, *1*, 50–74.
55. Independent Working Group. *A Report of the CFS/ME Working Group*; Report to the Chief Medical Officer of an Independent Working Group; Department of Health: London, UK, 2002; Available online: https://huisartsvink.files.wordpress.com/2019/05/cmo-report-2002.pdf (accessed on 30 May 2019).
56. Leone, S.S.; Huibers, M.J.; Kant, I.; Van Schayck, C.P.; Bleijenberg, G.; André Knottnerus, J. Long-term predictors of outcome in fatigued employees on sick leave: A 4-year follow-up study. *Psychol. Med.* **2006**, *36*, 1293–1300. [CrossRef] [PubMed]
57. Jason, L.J.; Taylor, R.R. Applying cluster analysis to define a typology of chronic fatigue syndrome in a medically-evaluated, random community sample. *Psychol. Health* **2002**, *17*, 323–337. [CrossRef]
58. Taylor, R.R.; Kielhofner, G.W. An Occupational Therapy Approach to Persons with Chronic Fatigue Syndrome: Part Two, Assessment and Intervention. *Occup. Ther. Health Care* **2003**, *17*, 63–87. [CrossRef] [PubMed]
59. Ross, S.D.; Estok, R.P.; Frame, D.; Stone, L.R.; Ludensky, V.S.; Levine, C.B. Disability and chronic fatigue syndrome: A focus on function. *Arch. Intern. Med.* **2004**, *164*, 1098–1107. [CrossRef] [PubMed]
60. Mounstephen, A.; Sharpe, M. Chronic fatigue syndrome and occupational health. *Occup. Med. (Lond.)* **1997**, *47*, 217–227. [CrossRef]
61. Action for ME, M.E. and Work. 2013. Available online: https://huisartsvink.files.wordpress.com/2019/05/actionforme-returnwork.pdf (accessed on 30 May 2019).
62. NHS Plus Evidence Based Guideline Project. Occupational Aspects of the Management of Chronic Fatigue Syndrome: A National Guideline Workplace Management of Chronic Fatigue Syndrome. October 2006. Available online: https://huisartsvink.files.wordpress.com/2019/05/nhs-occupational-aspects-cfs_full_guideline.pdf (accessed on 30 May 2019).
63. Assefi, N.P.; Coy, T.V.S.; Uslan, D.; Smith, W.R.; Buchwald, D. Financial, occupational, and personal consequences of disability in patients with chronic fatigue syndrome and fibromyalgia compared to other fatiguing conditions. *J. Rheumatol.* **2003**, *30*, 804–808.
64. Behan, P.O.; Behan, W.M.; Bell, E.J. The postviral fatigue syndrome—An analysis of the findings in 50 cases. *J. Infect.* **1985**, *10*, 211–222. [CrossRef]
65. Brown, M.M.; Bell, D.S.; Jason, L.A.; Christos, C.; Bell, D.E. Understanding long-term outcomes of chronic fatigue syndrome. *J. Clin. Psychol.* **2012**, *68*, 1028–1035. [CrossRef] [PubMed]
66. Bell, D.S.; Jordan, K.; Robinson, M. Thirteen-year follow-up of children and adolescents with chronic fatigue syndrome. *Pediatrics* **2001**, *107*, 994–998. [PubMed]
67. Buchwald, D.; Pearlman, T.; Umali, J.; Schmaling, K.; Katon, W. Functional status in patients with chronic fatigue syndrome, other fatiguing illnesses, and healthy individuals. *Am. J. Med.* **1996**, *101*, 364–370. [CrossRef]
68. Chu, L.; Valencia, I.J.; Garvert, D.W.; Montoya, J.G. Onset Patterns and Course of Myalgic Encephalomyelitis/Chronic Fatigue Syndrome. *Front. Pediatr.* **2019**, *7*, 12. [CrossRef] [PubMed]
69. Claypoole, K.; Mahurin, R.; Fischer, M.E.; Goldberg, J.; Schmaling, K.B.; Schoene, R.B.; Ashton, S.; Buchwald, D. Cognitive compromise following exercise in monozygotic twins discordant for chronic fatigue syndrome: Fact or artifact? *Appl. Neuropsychol.* **2001**, *8*, 31–40. [CrossRef]
70. García-Borreguero, D.; Dale, J.K.; Rosenthal, N.E.; Chiara, A.; O'Fallon, A.; Bartko, J.J.; Straus, S.E. Lack of seasonal variation of symptoms in patients with chronic fatigue syndrome. *Psychiatry Res.* **1998**, *77*, 71–77. [CrossRef]

71. Huibers, M.J.; Leone, S.S.; Kant, I.J.; Knottnerus, J.A. Chronic fatigue syndrome-like caseness as a predictor of work status in fatigued employees on sick leave: Four year follow up study. *Occup. Environ. Med.* **2006**, *63*, 570–572. [CrossRef]
72. Jason, L.A.; Benton, M.C.; Valentine, L.; Johnson, A.; Torres-Harding, S. The economic impact of ME/CFS: Individual and societal costs. *Dyn. Med.* **2008**, *7*, 6. [CrossRef]
73. Levine, P.H.; Jacobson, S.; Pocinki, A.G.; Cheney, P.; Peterson, D.; Connelly, R.R.; Weil, R.; Robinson, S.M.; Ablashi, D.V.S.; Salahuddin, S.Z.; et al. Clinical, epidemiologic, and virologic studies in four clusters of the chronic fatigue syndrome. *Arch. Intern. Med.* **1992**, *152*, 1611–1616. [CrossRef]
74. Lin, J.S.; Resch, S.C.; Brimmer, D.J.; Johnson, A.; Kennedy, S.; Burstein, N.; Simon, C.J. The economic impact of chronic fatigue syndrome in Georgia: Direct and indirect costs. *Cost Eff. Resour. Alloc.* **2011**, *9*, 1. [CrossRef] [PubMed]
75. Lloyd, A.; Gandevia, S.; Brockman, A.; Hales, J.; Wakefield, D. Cytokine production and fatigue in patients with chronic fatigue syndrome and healthy control subjects in response to exercise. *Clin. Infect. Dis.* **1994**, *18* (Suppl. 1), S142–S146. [CrossRef] [PubMed]
76. Lowry, T.J.; Pakenham, K.I. Health-related quality of life in chronic fatigue syndrome: Predictors of physical functioning and psychological distress. *Psychol. Health Med.* **2008**, *13*, 222–238. [CrossRef] [PubMed]
77. Matsuda, Y.; Matsui, T.; Kataoka, K.; Fukada, R.; Fukuda, S.; Kuratsune, H.; Tajima, S.; Yamaguti, K.; Kato, Y.H.; Kiriike, N. A two-year follow-up study of chronic fatigue syndrome comorbid with psychiatric disorders. *Psychiatry Clin. Neurosci.* **2009**, *63*, 365–373. [CrossRef] [PubMed]
78. McCrone, P.; Darbishire, L.; Ridsdale, L.; Seed, P. The economic cost of chronic fatigue and chronic fatigue syndrome in UK primary care. *Psychol. Med.* **2003**, *33*, 253–261. [CrossRef] [PubMed]
79. Naess, H.; Nyland, M.; Hausken, T.; Follestad, I.; Nyland, H.I. Chronic fatigue syndrome after Giardia enteritis: Clinical characteristics, disability and long-term sickness absence. *BMC Gastroenterol.* **2012**, *12*, 13. [CrossRef] [PubMed]
80. Natelson, B.H.; Johnson, S.K.; DeLuca, J.; Sisto, S.; Ellis, S.P.; Hill, N.; Bergen, M.T. Reducing heterogeneity in chronic fatigue syndrome: A comparison with depression and multiple sclerosis. *Clin. Infect. Dis.* **1995**, *21*, 1204–1210. [CrossRef] [PubMed]
81. Nijs, J.; Van de Putte, K.; Louckx, F.; De Meirleir, K. Employment status in chronic fatigue syndrome. A cross-sectional study examining the value of exercise testing and self-reported measures for the assessment of employment status. *Clin. Rehabil.* **2005**, *19*, 895–899. [CrossRef] [PubMed]
82. Ray, C.; Phillips, L.; Weir, W.R. Quality of attention in chronic fatigue syndrome: Subjective reports of everyday attention and cognitive difficulty, and performance on tasks of focused attention. *Br. J. Clin. Psychol.* **1993**, *32 Pt 3*, 357–364. [CrossRef]
83. Roche, R.; Taylor, R.R. Coping and Occupational Participation in Chronic Fatigue Syndrome. *OTJR Occup. Particip. Health* **2005**. [CrossRef]
84. Rowe, K.S. Long Term Follow up of Young People with Chronic Fatigue Syndrome Attending a Pediatric Outpatient Service. *Front. Pediatr.* **2019**, *7*, 21. [CrossRef] [PubMed]
85. Russo, J.; Katon, W.; Clark, M.; Kith, P.; Sintay, M.; Buchwald, D. Longitudinal changes associated with improvement in chronic fatigue patients. *J. Psychosom. Res.* **1998**, *45*, 67–76. [CrossRef]
86. Saltzstein, B.J.; Wyshak, G.; Hubbuch, J.T.; Perry, J.C. A naturalistic study of the chronic fatigue syndrome among women in primary care. *Gen. Hosp. Psychiatry* **1998**, *20*, 307–316. [CrossRef]
87. Schmaling, K.B.; Hamilos, D.L.; Diclementi, J.D.; Jones, J.F. Pain Perception in Chronic Fatigue Syndrome. *J. Chronic Fatigue Syndr.* **1998**, *4*, 13–22. [CrossRef]
88. Schweitzer, R.; Kelly, B.; Foran, A.; Terry, D.; Whiting, J. Quality of life in chronic fatigue syndrome. *Soc. Sci. Med.* **1995**, *41*, 1367–1372. [CrossRef]
89. Stoothoff, J.; Gleason, K.; McManimen, S.; Thorpe, T.; Jason, L.A. Subtyping Patients with Myalgic Encephalomyelitis (ME) and Chronic Fatigue Syndrome (CFS) By Course of Illness. *J. Biosens. Biomark. Diagn.* **2017**, *2*. [CrossRef]
90. Strickland, P.S.; Levine, P.H.; Peterson, D.L.; O'Brien, K.; Fears, T. Neuromyasthenia and chronic fatigue syndrome (CFS) in Northern Nevada/California: A ten-year follow-up of an outbreak. *J. Chronic Fatigue Syndr.* **2001**, *9*, 3–14. [CrossRef]

91. Thomas, M.; Smith, A.P. Can the Improvements Reported by Individuals with Chronic Fatigue Syndrome Following Multi-Convergent Therapy Be Sustained in the Longer-Term: A Three-Year Follow-Up Study. *J. Health Med. Sci.* **2019**, *2*, 122–130. [CrossRef]
92. Tirelli, U.; Marotta, G.; Improta, S.; Pinto, A. Immunological abnormalities in patients with chronic fatigue syndrome. *Scand. J. Immunol.* **1994**, *40*, 601–608. [CrossRef]
93. Tritt, K.; Nickel, M.; Mitterlehner, F.; Nickel, C.; Forthuber, P.; Leiberich, P.; Rother, W.; Loew, T. Chronic fatigue and indicators of long-term employment disability in psychosomatic inpatients. *Wiener Klinische Wochenschrift* **2004**, *116*, 182–189. [CrossRef]
94. Van der Werf, S.P.; de Vree, B.; Alberts, M.; van der Meer, J.W.M.; Beijenberg, G. Natural course and predicting self-reported improvement in patients with chronic fatigue syndrome with a relatively short illness duration. *J. Psychosom. Res.* **2002**, *53*, 749–753. [CrossRef]
95. Vercoulen, J.H.; Bazelmans, E.; Swanink, C.M.; Fennis, J.F.; Galama, J.M.; Jongen, P.J.; Hommes, O.; Van der Meer, J.W.; Bleijenberg, G. Physical activity in chronic fatigue syndrome: Assessment and its role in fatigue. *J. Psychiatr. Res.* **1997**, *31*, 661–673. [CrossRef]
96. Vincent, A.; Brimmer, D.J.; Whipple, M.O.; Jones, J.F.; Boneva, R.; Lahr, B.D.; Maloney, E.; St Sauver, J.L.; Reeves, W.C. Prevalence, incidence, and classification of chronic fatigue syndrome in Olmsted County, Minnesota, as estimated using the Rochester Epidemiology Project. *Mayo Clin. Proc.* **2012**, *87*, 1145–1152. [CrossRef]
97. Zdunek, M.; Jason, L.A.; Evans, M.; Jantke, R.; Newton, J.L. A Cross Cultural Comparison of Disability and Symptomatology Associated with CFS. *Int. J. Psychol. Behavs. Sci.* **2015**, *5*, 98–107.
98. Bringsli, G.J.; Gilje, A. *Getz Wold, B.K. The Norwegian ME Association National Survey Abridged English Version*; Norwegian ME-Association: Oslo, Norway, 2014; Available online: https://huisartsvink.files.wordpress.com/2018/08/bringsli-2014-me-nat-norwegian-survey-abr-eng-ver-2.pdf (accessed on 30 May 2019).
99. Chu, L. Patient Survey Results for FDA Drug Development Meeting for ME and CFS. 25–26 April 2013. Available online: https://huisartsvink.files.wordpress.com/2019/09/chu-fda_survey_results_july2013.pdf (accessed on 16 September 2019).
100. De Kimpe, A.; Crijnen, B.; Kuijper, J.; Verhulst, I.I.; van der Ploeg, Y. Care for ME Survey of ME Patients about their Experiences with Health Care in The Netherlands. 2016. Available online: https://huisartsvink.files.wordpress.com/2018/07/de-kimpe-2016-rapport-2.pdf (accessed on 30 May 2019).
101. Emerge Australia. Health and Wellbeing Survey of Australians with ME/CFS Report of Key Findings. September 2018. Available online: https://huisartsvink.files.wordpress.com/2019/09/emerge-australia-health-and-wellbeing-survey-of-australians-with-mecfs-2018.pdf (accessed on 16 September 2019).
102. ME Association. *ME/CFS Illness Management Survey Results: No Decisions about ME without ME. Patient Survey*; ME Association: Gawcott, UK, 2015; Available online: http://www.meassociation.org.uk/wp-content/uploads/2015-ME-Association-Illness-Management-Report-No-decisions-about-me-without-me-30.05.15.pdf (accessed on 30 May 2019).
103. 25% ME Group. Severely Affected ME (Myalgic Encephalomyelitis) Analysis Report on Questionnaire Issued January 2004. Troon, Scotland. 1 March 2014. Available online: https://huisartsvink.files.wordpress.com/2018/09/severely-affected-me.pdf (accessed on 30 May 2019).
104. De Veer, A.J.E.; Francke, A.L. Zorg Voor ME/CVS-Patiënten: Ervaringen van de Achterban van Patiënten Organisaties met de Gezondheidszorg. Utrecht: NIVEL. 2008. Available online: https://www.nivel.nl/sites/default/files/bestanden/Rapport-draagvlakmeting-CVS-ME-2008.pdf (accessed on 30 May 2019).
105. Holmes, G.P.; Kaplan, J.E.; Gantz, N.M.; Komaroff, A.L.; Schonberger, L.B.; Straus, S.E.; Jones, J.F.; Dubois, R.E.; Cunningham-Rundles, C.; Pahwa, S.; et al. Chronic fatigue syndrome: A working case definition. *Ann. Intern. Med.* **1988**, *108*, 387–389. [CrossRef]
106. Whiting, P.; Bagnall, A.M.; Sowden, A.J.; Cornell, J.E.; Mulrow, C.D.; Ramírez, G. Interventions for the Treatment and Management of Chronic Fatigue Syndrome—A Systematic Review. *JAMA* **2001**, *286*, 1360–1368. [CrossRef]
107. Smith, M.E.; Haney, E.; McDonagh, M.; Pappas, M.; Daeges, M.; Wasson, N.; Fu, R.; Nelson, H.D. Treatment of Myalgic Encephalomyelitis/Chronic Fatigue Syndrome: A Systematic Review for a National Institutes of Health Pathways to Prevention Workshop. *Ann. Intern. Med.* **2015**, *162*, 841–850. [CrossRef]
108. Akagi, H.; Klimes, I.; Bass, C. Cognitive behavioral therapy for chronic fatigue syndrome in a general hospital—Feasible and effective. *Gen. Hosp. Psychiatry* **2001**, *23*, 254–260. [CrossRef]

109. Bazelmans, E.; Prins, J.B.; Lulofs, R.; van der Meer, J.W.; Bleijenberg, G. Netherlands Fatigue Research Group Nijmegen. Cognitive behaviour group therapy for chronic fatigue syndrome: A non-randomised waiting list controlled study. *Psychother. Psychosom.* **2005**, *74*, 218–224. [CrossRef]
110. Burgess, M.; Andiappan, M.; Chalder, T. Cognitive behaviour therapy for chronic fatigue syndrome in adults: Face to face versus telephone treatment: A randomized controlled trial. *Behavs. Cogn. Psychother.* **2012**, *40*, 175–191. [CrossRef]
111. Collin, S.M.; Crawley, E. Specialist treatment of chronic fatigue syndrome/ME: A cohort study among adult patients in England. *BMC Health Servs. Res.* **2017**, *17*, 488. [CrossRef]
112. Cox, D.L. Chronic fatigue syndrome: An occupational therapy programme. *Occup. Ther. Int.* **1999**, *6*, 52–56. [CrossRef]
113. Cox, D.L. Chronic Fatigue Syndrome: An evaluation of an Occupational Therapy Inpatient Intervention. *Br. J. Occup. Ther.* **2002**, *65*, 461–468. [CrossRef]
114. Deale, A.; Hussain, K.; Chalder, T.; Wessely, S. Long-term outcome of cognitive behavior therapy for chronic fatigue syndrome: A 5-year follow-up study. *Am. J. Psychiatry* **2001**, *158*, 2038–2042. [CrossRef]
115. Dyck, D.; Allen, S.; Barron, J.; Marchi, J.; Price, B.A.; Spavor, L.; Tateishi, S. Management of chronic fatigue syndrome: Case study. *AAOHN. J.* **1996**, *44*, 85–92. [CrossRef]
116. Friedberg, F.; Adamowicz, J.; Caikauskaite, I.; Seva, V.S.; Napoli, A. Efficacy of two delivery modes of behavioral self-management in severe chronic fatigue syndrome. *Fatigue Biomed. Health Behavs.* **2016**, *4*, 158–174. [CrossRef]
117. Fulcher, K.Y.; White, P.D. Randomised controlled trial of graded exercise in patients with chronic fatigue syndrome. *BMJ* **1997**, *314*, 1647–1652. [CrossRef]
118. Hlavaty, L.E.; Brown, M.M.; Jason, L.A. The effect of homework compliance on treatment outcomes for participants with myalgic encephalomyelitis/chronic fatigue syndrome. *Rehabil. Psychol.* **2011**, *56*, 212–218. [CrossRef]
119. Huibers, M.J.; Beurskens, A.J.; Van Schayck, C.P.; Bazelmans, E.; Metsemakers, J.F.; Knottnerus, J.A.; Bleijenberg, G. Efficacy of cognitive behavioural therapy by general practitioners for unexplained fatigue among employees: Randomised controlled trial. *Br. J. Psychiatry* **2004**, *184*, 240–246. [CrossRef]
120. Janse, A.; Nikolaus, S.; Wiborg, J.F.; Heins, M.; van der Meer, J.W.M.; Bleijenberg, G.; Tummers, M.; Twisk, J.; Knoop, H. Long-term follow-up after cognitive behaviour therapy for chronic fatigue syndrome. *J. Psychosom. Res.* **2017**, *97*, 45–51. [CrossRef]
121. Janse, A.; Worm-Smeitink, M.; Bleijenberg, G.; Donders, R.; Knoop, H. Efficacy of web-based cognitive-behavioural therapy for chronic fatigue syndrome: Randomised controlled trial. *Br. J. Psychiatry* **2018**, *212*, 112–118. [CrossRef]
122. Jason, L.; Torres-Harding, S.; Friedberg, F.; Corradi, K.; Njoku, M.G.; Donalek, J.; Reynolds, N.; Brown, M.; Weitner, B.B.; Rademaker, A.; et al. Non-pharmacologic interventions for CFS: A randomized trial. *J. Clin. Psychol. Med. Settings* **2007**, *172*, 485–490. [CrossRef]
123. Koolhaas, M.P.; de Boorder, H.; van Hoof, E. Cognitieve Gedragstherapie bij het Chronische Vermoeidheidssyndroom ME/CVS Vanuit het Perspectief van de Patiënt Februari. 2008. Available online: https://ccgt.nl/pics_cs/csmrt2009.pdf (accessed on 30 May 2019).
124. Lopez, C.; Antoni, M.; Penedo, F.; Weiss, D.; Cruess, S.; Segotas, M.C.; Helder, L.; Siegel, S.; Klimas, N.; Fletcher, M.A. A pilot study of cognitive behavioral stress management effects on stress, quality of life, and symptoms in persons with chronic fatigue syndrome. *J. Psychosom. Res.* **2011**, *70*, 328–334. [CrossRef]
125. Marlin, R.G.; Anchel, H.; Gibson, J.C.; Goldberg, W.M.; Swinton, M. An evaluation of multidisciplinary intervention for chronic fatigue syndrome with long-term follow-up, and a comparison with untreated controls. *Am. J. Med.* **1998**, *105*, 110S–114S. [CrossRef]
126. Masuda, A.; Nakayama, T.; Yamanaka, T.; Koga, Y.; Tei, C. The prognosis after multidisciplinary treatment for patients with postinfectious chronic fatigue syndrome and noninfectious chronic fatigue syndrome. *J. Behavs. Med.* **2002**, *25*, 487–497. [CrossRef]
127. McBride, R.L.; Horsfield, S.; Sandler, C.X.; Cassar, J.; Casson, S.; Cvejic, E.; Vollmer-Conna, U.; Lloyd, A.R. Cognitive remediation training improves performance in patients with chronic fatigue syndrome. *Psychiatry Res.* **2017**, *257*, 400–405. [CrossRef]

128. McDermott, C.; Richards, S.C.M.; Ankers, S.; Selby, M.; Harmer, J.; Moran, C.J. An Evaluation of a Chronic Fatigue Lifestyle Management Programme Focusing on the Outcome of Return to Work or Training. *Br. J. Occup. Ther.* **2004**, *67*. [CrossRef]
129. Moss-Morris, R.; Sharon, C.; Tobin, R.; Baldi, J.C. A randomized controlled graded exercise trial for chronic fatigue syndrome: Outcomes and mechanisms of change. *J. Health Psychol.* **2005**, *10*, 245–259. [CrossRef]
130. O'Dowd, H.; Gladwell, P.; Rogers, C.; Hollinghurst, S.; Gregory, A. Cognitive behavioural therapy in chronic fatigue syndrome: A randomised controlled trial of an outpatient group programme. *Health Technol. Assess.* **2006**, *10*, 1–121. [CrossRef]
131. Prins, J.B.; Bleijenberg, G.; Bazelmans, E.; Elving, L.D.; de Boo, T.M.; Severens, J.L.; van der Wilt, G.J.; Spinhoven, P.; van der Meer, J.W. Cognitive behaviour therapy for chronic fatigue syndrome: A multicentre randomised controlled trial. *Lancet* **2001**, *357*, 841–847. [CrossRef]
132. Powell, P.; Bentall, R.P.; Nye, F.J.; Edwards, R.H. Randomised controlled trial of patient education to encourage graded exercise in chronic fatigue syndrome. *BMJ* **2001**, *322*, 387–390. [CrossRef]
133. Powell, P.; Bentall, R.P.; Nye, F.J.; Edwards, R.H. Patient education to encourage graded exercise in chronic fatigue syndrome. 2-year follow-up of randomised controlled trial. *Br. J. Psychiatry* **2004**, *184*, 142–146. [CrossRef]
134. Ridsdale, L.; Godfrey, E.; Chalder, T.; Seed, P.; King, M.; Wallace, P.; Wessely, S. Fatigue Trialists' Group. Chronic fatigue in general practice: Is counselling as good as cognitive behaviour therapy? A UK randomised trial. *Br. J. Gen. Pract.* **2001**, *51*, 19–24.
135. Chisholm, D.; Godfrey, E.; Ridsdale, L.; Chalder, T.; King, M.; Seed, P.; Wallace, P.; Wessely, S.; Fatigue Trialists' Group. Chronic fatigue in general practice: Economic evaluation of counselling versus cognitive behaviour therapy. *Br. J. Gen. Pract.* **2001**, *51*, 15–18.
136. Ridsdale, L.; Darbishire, L.; Seed, P.T. Is graded exercise better than cognitive behaviour therapy for fatigue? A UK randomized trial in primary care. *Psychol. Med.* **2004**, *34*, 37–49. [CrossRef]
137. Sandler, C.X.; Hamilton, B.A.; Horsfield, S.L.; Bennett, B.K.; Vollmer-Conna, U.; Tzarimas, C.; Lloyd, A.R. Outcomes and predictors of response from an optimised, multidisciplinary intervention for chronic fatigue states. *Intern. Med. J.* **2016**, *46*, 1421–1429. [CrossRef]
138. Saxty, M.; Hansen, Z. Group Cognitive Behavioural Therapy for Chronic Fatigue Syndrome: A Pilot Study. *Behavs. Cogn. Psychother.* **2005**, *33*, 311–318. [CrossRef]
139. Scheeres, K.; Wensing, M.; Bleijenberg, G.; Severens, J.L. Implementing cognitive behavior therapy for chronic fatigue syndrome in mental health care: A costs and outcomes analysis. *BMC Health Servs. Res.* **2008**, *8*, 175. [CrossRef]
140. Schreurs, K.M.; Veehof, M.M.; Passade, L.; Vollenbroek-Hutten, M.M. Cognitive behavioural treatment for chronic fatigue syndrome in a rehabilitation setting: Effectiveness and predictors of outcome. *Behavs. Res. Ther.* **2011**, *49*, 908–913. [CrossRef]
141. Stordeur, S.; Thiry, N.; Eyssen, M. *Chronisch Vermoeidheidssyndroom: Diagnose, Behandeling en Zorgorganisatie [Fatigue Syndrome: Diagnosis, Treatment and Organisation of Care]*; KCE Technical Report 88A; Belgian Healthcare Knowledge Center: Brussels, Belgium, 2008; (In Dutch). Available online: https://kce.fgovs.be/sites/default/files/page_documents/d20081027358.pdf (accessed on 30 May 2019).
142. Vos-Vromans, D.; Smeets, R.J.; Huijnen, I.P.; Köke, A.J.; Hitters, W.M.; Rijnders, L.J.; Pont, M.; Winkens, B.; Knottnerus, J.A. Multidisciplinary rehabilitation treatment versus cognitive behavioural therapy for patients with chronic fatigue syndrome: a randomized controlled trial. *J. Intern. Med.* **2016**, *279*, 268–282. [CrossRef]
143. Vos-Vromans, D.; Evers, S.; Huijnen, I.; Köke, A.; Hitters, M.; Rijnders, N.; Pont, M.; Knottnerus, A.; Smeets, R. Economic evaluation of multidisciplinary rehabilitation treatment versus cognitive behavioural therapy for patients with chronic fatigue syndrome: A randomized controlled trial. *PLoS ONE* **2017**, *12*, e0177260. [CrossRef]
144. Wearden, A.J.; Morriss, R.K.; Mullis, R.; Stricland, P.L.; Pearson, D.J.; Appleby, L.; Campbell, I.T.; Morris, J.A. Randomised, double-blind, placebo controlled treatment trial of fluoxetine and graded exercise for chronic fatigue syndrome. *Br. J. Psychiatry* **1998**, *178*, 485–492. [CrossRef]
145. Wearden, A.J.; Dowrick, C.; Chew-Graham, C.; Bentall, R.P.; Morriss, R.K.; Peters, S.; Riste, L.; Richardson, G.; Lovell, K.; Dunn, G.; et al. Fatigue Intervention by Nurses Evaluation (FINE) trial writing group and the FINE trial group. Nurse led, home based self help treatment for patients in primary care with chronic fatigue syndrome: Randomised controlled trial. *BMJ* **2010**, *340*, c1777. [CrossRef]

146. Wearden, A.J.; Dunn, G.; Dowrick, C.; Morriss, R.K. Depressive symptoms and pragmatic rehabilitation for chronic fatigue syndrome. *Br. J. Psychiatry* **2012**, *201*, 227–232. [CrossRef]
147. Wearden, A.J.; Emsley, R. Mediators of the effects on fatigue of pragmatic rehabilitation for chronic fatigue syndrome. *J. Consult. Clin. Psychol.* **2013**, *81*, 831–838. [CrossRef]
148. White, P.D.; Goldsmith, K.A.; Johnson, A.L.; Potts, L.; Walwyn, R.; DeCesare, J.C.; Baber, H.L.; Burgess, M.; Clark, L.V.S.; Cox, D.L.; et al. Comparison of adaptive pacing therapy, cognitive behaviour therapy, graded exercise therapy, and specialist medical care for chronic fatigue syndrome (PACE): A randomised trial. *Lancet* **2011**, *377*, 823–836. [CrossRef]
149. Sharpe, M.; Goldsmith, K.A.; Johnson, A.L.; Chalder, T.; Walker, J.; White, P.D. Rehabilitative treatments for chronic fatigue syndrome: Long-term follow-up from the PACE trial. *Lancet Psychiatry* **2015**, *2*, 1067–1074. [CrossRef]
150. McCrone, P.; Sharpe, M.; Chalder, T.; Knapp, M.; Johnson, A.L.; Goldsmith, K.A.; White, P.D. Adaptive pacing, cognitive behaviour therapy, graded exercise, and specialist medical care for chronic fatigue syndrome: A cost-effectiveness analysis. *PLoS ONE* **2012**, *7*, e40808. [CrossRef]
151. Supplement to: Chalder, T.; Goldsmith, K.A.; White, P.D.; Sharpe, M.; Pickles, A.R. Rehabilitative therapies for chronic fatigue syndrome: A secondary mediation analysis of the PACE trial. *Lancet Psychiatry* **2015**, *2*, 141–152. [CrossRef]
152. Wittkowski, A.; Toye, K.; Richards, H.L. A cognitive behaviour therapy group for patients with chronic fatigue syndrome: A preliminary investigation. *Behavs. Cogn. Psychother.* **2004**, *32*, 107–112. [CrossRef]
153. Worm-Smeitink, M.; Nikolaus, S.; Goldsmith, K.; Wiborg, J.; Ali, S.; Knoop, H.; Chalder, T. Cognitive behaviour therapy for chronic fatigue syndrome: Differences in treatment outcome between a tertiary treatment centre in the United Kingdom and the Netherlands. *J. Psychosom. Res.* **2016**, *87*, 43–49. [CrossRef]
154. Worm-Smeitink, M.; Janse, A.; van Dam, A.; Evers, A.; van der Vaart, R.; Wensing, M.; Knoop, H. Internet-Based Cognitive Behavioral Therapy in Stepped Care for Chronic Fatigue Syndrome: Randomized Noninferiority Trial. *J. Med. Internet Res.* **2019**, *21*, e11276. [CrossRef]
155. Heins, M.J.; Knoop, H.; Burk, W.J.; Bleijenberg, G. The process of cognitive behaviour therapy for chronic fatigue syndrome: Which changes in perpetuating cognitions and behaviour are related to a reduction in fatigue? *J. Psychosom. Res.* **2013**, *75*, 235–241. [CrossRef]
156. Knoop, H.; Bleijenberg, G.; Gielissen, M.F.; van der Meer, J.W.; White, P.D. Is a full recovery possible after cognitive behavioural therapy for chronic fatigue syndrome? *Psychother. Psychosom.* **2007**, *76*, 171–176. [CrossRef]
157. Tummers, M.; Knoop, H.; Bleijenberg, G. Effectiveness of stepped care for chronic fatigue syndrome: A randomized noninferiority trial. *J. Consult. Clin. Psychol.* **2010**, *78*, 724–731. [CrossRef]
158. Wiborg, J.F.; van Bussel, J.; van Dijk, A.; Bleijenberg, G.; Knoop, H. Randomised controlled trial of cognitive behaviour therapy delivered in groups of patients with chronic fatigue syndrome. *Psychother. Psychosom.* **2015**, *84*, 368–376. [CrossRef]
159. Vink, M.; Vink-Niese, A. Graded exercise therapy for myalgic encephalomyelitis/chronic fatigue syndrome is not effective and unsafe. Re-analysis of a Cochrane review. *Health Psychol. Open* **2018**, *5*. [CrossRef]
160. Vanness, J.M.; Snell, C.R.; Strayer, D.R.; Dempsey, L., 4th; Stevens, S.R. Subclassifying chronic fatigue syndrome through exercise testing. *Med. Sci. Sports Exerc.* **2003**, *35*, 908–913. [CrossRef]
161. Gunnar, A.B.; Occhiarella, L. *Guide to the Evaluation of Permanent Impairment*, 3rd ed.; American Medical Association: Chicago, IL, USA, 2000; pp. 27–28.
162. Jason, L.A.; Brown, M.; Brown, A.; Evans, M.; Flores, S.; Grant-Holler, E.; Sunnquist, M. Energy Conservation/Envelope Theory Interventions to Help Patients with Myalgic Encephalomyelitis/Chronic Fatigue Syndrome. *Fatigue* **2013**, *1*, 27–42.
163. Jason, L.A.; Richman, J.A. How science can stigmatize: The case of chronic fatigue syndrome. *J. Chronic Fatigue Syndr.* **2008**, *14*, 85–103. [CrossRef]
164. Devendorf, A.R.; Jackson, C.T.; Sunnquist, M.; Jason, L.A. Defining and measuring recovery from myalgic encephalomyelitis and chronic fatigue syndrome: The physician perspective. *Disabil. Rehabil.* **2019**, *41*, 158–165. [CrossRef] [PubMed]
165. Falk Hvidberg, M.; Brinth, L.S.; Olesen, A.V.S.; Petersen, K.D.; Ehlers, L. The Health-Related Quality of Life for Patients with Myalgic Encephalomyelitis/Chronic Fatigue Syndrome (ME/CFS). *PLoS ONE* **2015**, *10*, e0132421. [CrossRef]

166. Howes, S.; Goudsmit, E.M. Progressive Myalgic Encephalomyelitis (ME) or A New Disease? A Case Report. *Phys. Med. Rehabil. Int.* **2015**, *2*, 1052.
167. Fennell, P.A. The Four Progressive Stages of the CFS Experience. *J. Chronic Fatigue Syndr.* **1995**, *1*, 69–79. [CrossRef]
168. Esfandyarpour, R.; Kashi, A.; Nemat-Gorgani, M.; Wilhelmy, J.; Davis, R.W. A nanoelectronics-blood-based diagnostic biomarker for myalgic encephalomyelitis/chronic fatigue syndrome (ME/CFS). *Proc. Natl. Acad. Sci. USA* **2019**, *116*, 10250–10257. [CrossRef] [PubMed]
169. Franklin, J.D.; Atkinson, G.; Atkinson, J.M.; Batterham, A.M. Peak Oxygen Uptake in Chronic Fatigue Syndrome/Myalgic Encephalomyelitis: A Meta-Analysis. *Int. J. Sports Med.* **2019**, *40*, 77–87. [CrossRef] [PubMed]
170. Stevens, S.; Snell, C.; Stevens, J.; Keller, B.; VanNess, J.M. Cardiopulmonary Exercise Test Methodology for Assessing Exertion Intolerance in Myalgic Encephalomyelitis/Chronic Fatigue Syndrome. *Front. Pediatr.* **2018**, *6*, 242. [CrossRef]
171. Camacho, J.; Jason, L.A. Psychosocial factors show little relationship to chronic fatigue syndrome recovery. *J. Psychol. Behavs. Sci.* **1998**, *12*, 60–70.
172. Le Bon, O.; Cappeliez, B.; Neu, D.; Stulens, L.; Hoffmann, G.; Hansenne, M.; Lambrecht, L.; Ansseau, M.; Linkowski, P. Personality Profile of Patients with Chronic Fatigue Syndrome. *J. Chronic Fatigue Syndr.* **2007**, *14*, 55–68. [CrossRef]
173. Levine, P.H. Epidemiologic advances in chronic fatigue syndrome. *J Psychiatr. Res.* **1997**, *31*, 7–18. [CrossRef]
174. Komaroff, A.L.; Buchwald, D. Symptoms and signs in chronic fatigue syndrome. *Revs. Infect. Dis.* **1991**, *13*, S8–S11. [CrossRef] [PubMed]
175. Vercoulen, J.H.M.M.; Bazelmans, E.; Swanink, C.M.A.; Galama, J.M.D.; Fennis, J.F.M.; Van der Meer, J.W.M.; Bleijenberg, G. Evaluating neuropsychological impairment in chronic fatigue syndrome. *J. Clin. Exp. Neuropsychol.* **1998**, *20*, 144–156. [CrossRef] [PubMed]
176. Tiersky, L.A.; Johnson, S.K.; Lange, G.; Natelson, B.H.; DeLuca, J. Neuropsychology of chronic fatigue syndrome: A critical review. *J. Clin. Exp. Neuropsychol.* **1997**, *19*, 560–586. [CrossRef] [PubMed]
177. Inspectorate Work and Pay, Now the Inspectorate SZW of the Dutch Ministry of Work and Social Affairs Het Chronisch Vermoeidheidssyndroom De Beoordeling Door Verzekeringsartsen. Programma Inkomenszekerheid Nummer R 10/08, November 2010. Available online: https://huisartsvink.files.wordpress.com/2019/05/inspectie-2010_cvs-verzekeringsartsen.pdf (accessed on 30 May 2019).
178. Castro-Marrero, J.; Sáez-Francàs, N.; Santillo, D.; Alegre, J. Treatment and management of chronic fatigue syndrome/myalgic encephalomyelitis: All roads lead to Rome. *Br. J. Pharm.* **2017**, *174*, 345–369. [CrossRef] [PubMed]
179. Chambers, D.; Bagnall, A.M.; Hempel, S.; Forbes, C. Interventions for the treatment, management and rehabilitation of patients with chronic fatigue syndrome/myalgic encephalomyelitis: An updated systematic review. *J. R. Soc. Med.* **2006**, *819*, 506–520.
180. Malouff, J.M.; Thorsteinsson, E.B.; Rooke, S.E.; Bhullar, N.; Schutte, N.S. Efficacy of cognitive behavioral therapy for chronic fatigue syndrome: A meta-analysis. *Clin. Psychol. Revs.* **2008**, *28*, 736–745. [CrossRef] [PubMed]
181. Marques, M.M.; De Gucht, V.S.; Gouveia, M.J.; Leal, I.; Maes, S. Differential effects of behavioral interventions with a graded physical activity component in patients suffering from Chronic Fatigue (Syndrome): An updated systematic review and meta-analysis. *Clin. Psychol. Revs.* **2015**, *40*, 123–137. [CrossRef] [PubMed]
182. Castell, B.D.; Kazantzis, N.; Moss-Morris, R.E. Cognitive behavioral therapy and graded exercise for chronic fatigue syndrome: A meta-analysis. *Clin. Psychol.* **2011**, *18*, 311–324. [CrossRef]
183. Maassen, H. Interview Verzekeringsarts Rob Kok: 'Wij mogen patiënten aanspreken op hun herstelgedrag' Medisch Contact 16–17|18 April 2019. Available online: https://www.medischcontact.nl/nieuws/laatste-nieuws/artikel/verzekeringsarts-rob-kok-wij-mogen-patienten-aanspreken-op-hun-herstelgedrag.htm (accessed on 30 May 2019).

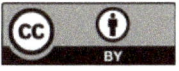

© 2019 by the authors. Licensee MDPI, Basel, Switzerland. This article is an open access article distributed under the terms and conditions of the Creative Commons Attribution (CC BY) license (http://creativecommons.org/licenses/by/4.0/).

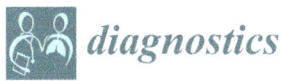

Article

Assessment of Post-Exertional Malaise (PEM) in Patients with Myalgic Encephalomyelitis (ME) and Chronic Fatigue Syndrome (CFS): A Patient-Driven Survey

Carly S. Holtzman, Shaun Bhatia, Joseph Cotler and Leonard A. Jason *

Center for Community Research, Department of Psychology, DePaul University, Chicago, IL 60604, USA; choltzm1@depaul.edu (C.S.H.); sbhatia3@depaul.edu (S.B.); jcotler@depaul.edu (J.C.)
* Correspondence: ljason@depaul.edu; Tel.: +1-773-325-2018

Received: 1 February 2019; Accepted: 26 February 2019; Published: 2 March 2019

Abstract: Considerable controversy has existed with efforts to assess post-exertional malaise (PEM), which is one of the defining features of myalgic encephalomyelitis (ME) and chronic fatigue syndrome (CFS). While a number of self-report questionnaires have been developed to assess this symptom, none have been comprehensive, and a recent federal government report has recommended the development of a new PEM measure. The current study involved a community-based participatory research process in an effort to develop a comprehensive PEM instrument, with critical patient input shaping the item selection and overall design of the tool. A survey was ultimately developed and was subsequently completed by 1534 members of the patient community. The findings of this survey suggest that there are key domains of this symptom, including triggers, symptom onset, and duration, which have often not been comprehensively assessed in a previous PEM instrument. This study indicates that there are unique benefits that can be derived from patients collaborating with researchers in the measurement of key symptoms defining ME and CFS.

Keywords: myalgic encephalomyelitis; chronic fatigue syndrome; post-exertional malaise; assessment; patient-driven questionnaire; participatory research

1. Introduction

Among patients with myalgic encephalomyelitis (ME) and chronic fatigue syndrome (CFS), post-exertional malaise (PEM) has long been considered a hallmark symptom [1]. However, in a field which includes more than twenty case definitions for ME and CFS, there has not been agreement regarding defining PEM [2]. For example, discrepancies occur with two of the most frequently used ME and CFS case definitions, the Fukuda [3] and Canadian Consensus Criteria (CCC; [4]). The Fukuda et al. criteria do not define the term beyond requiring that it last for more than 24 h nor does it make PEM a requirement for diagnosis. In contrast, the CCC case definition requires the presence of PEM for diagnosis and goes further to describe the symptomatic experience as similar to flu-like distress, with a potential delayed onset [4].

Several activity and self-report measurements that assess the extent of activity and how such activity might result in exacerbation of symptoms have been proposed to measure PEM. These include actigraphy, exercise challenges, time logs, and self-reports [5]. For example, following an exercise task, Mateo et al. [6] reported a broad spectrum of PEM-related symptoms including fatigue, muscle/joint pain, cognitive dysfunction, decrease in function, headaches, sleep disturbances, pain, weakness, cardiopulmonary symptoms, lightheadedness, and flu-like symptoms. Others have found using self-report measures that PEM comprises two distinct constructs: muscle-specific fatigue and generalized fatigue [7].

Factors which elicit PEM include physical and cognitive exertion. For some patients, even basic activities of daily living such as toileting, bathing, dressing, communicating, and reading can trigger PEM. However, many patients feel that potential triggers should extend beyond these types of stressors and include infections [8], exposure to chemicals or certain foods [9], or exposure to certain metals [10]. Additionally, many efforts to assess PEM have not included a characteristic delay in the onset of PEM. Chu et al. [11] maintain that this delay is rarely found in other fatiguing illnesses. Another issue that has often not been included in the assessment of PEM is that many patients with ME and CFS take considerably longer to recover from a trigger [12], reporting a substantial increase in symptoms immediately after an exercise test, the next day, and even a week later [13].

In an effort to address these PEM-related discrepancies, the National Institutes of Health/Center for Disease Control and Prevention (NIH/CDC) Common Data Element (CDE) committee's PEM working group attempted to define PEM [14] as "an abnormal response to minimal amounts of physical or cognitive exertion that is characterized by: (1) Exacerbation of some or all of an individual study participant's ME/CFS symptoms. (2) Loss of stamina and/or functional capacity. (3) An onset that can be immediate or delayed after the exertional stimulus by hours, days, or even longer. (4) A prolonged, unpredictable recovery period that may last days, weeks, or even months. (5) Severity and duration of symptoms that is often out-of-proportion to the type, intensity, frequency, and/or duration of the exertion." Yet, there was no set of items with anchor points associated with these 5 descriptors of PEM offered by the NIH/CDC CDE PEM working group. While the general guidance of the committee was helpful, these types of general descriptions need to be operationalized if investigators are to reliably use them to assess PEM. The NIH/CDC CDE's PEM working group also recommended the use of 5 items from the DePaul Symptom Questionnaire (DSQ, [12]) to measure PEM (e.g., physically drained or sick after mild activity). However, the DSQ was not developed as a comprehensive measure of PEM but rather as a measure of ME and CFS symptomatology as a whole. Following the release of the NIH/CDC CDE's PEM recommendations, patients were extremely concerned with the recommendations that had been made [15].

This latest NIH/CDC CDE's recommendations regarding the measurement of PEM needs to be understood in the context of a long history where patients have felt left out of key policy decisions imposed on them, including how to name, define, and treat ME and CFS. As one example, when the Institute of Medicine (IOM; [16]) recommended a new name and case definition, this created considerable controversy, as many feel that both were decisions imposed on the patient community, without first seeking their input and approval.

The recent recommendations made by this NIH/CDC CDE's PEM working group, and the vociferous reactions to it by the patient community, provided an opportunity to engage in community-based participatory research, which equitably involves all partners in the research process [17]. Given the importance of PEM, and the patient community's resentment regarding once again not being active participants in the development of this latest PEM recommendation, the current authors decided to try to develop a comprehensive measure with active collaboration of the patient community. We hypothesized that a valid PEM instrument could be created with the help of the patient community.

2. Materials and Methods

2.1. Methods and Participants

The study began with dialogue between Leonard Jason and a number of leading patient activists who were unhappy with the NIH/CDC CDE's PEM recommendations. A patient poll had indicated that the patient community preferred the NIH/CDC general description of PEM rather than the 5 DSQ items [15], but those general PEM descriptors had not been operationalized in any systematic way. Jason and several patient activists reworked those descriptors into a usable questionnaire, and this was posted on Facebook, Twitter, and LinkedIn social media pages and were widely shared with patient groups internationally. Hundreds of emails were received during the next three months, and Jason and

Holtzman posted nine revisions of the survey for patients to provide comments. The comments and items received helped shape each new revision of the questionnaire. For example, when one participant commented "I also experience different types of PEM. I have the immediate PEM, where I do too much ... But if I stop [exerting myself], these [PEM symptoms] go away fairly quickly ... But if I am not able to stop during this immediate PEM stage and have to push on while experiencing these symptoms, then I get the "Post-PEM" usually two or more days later," we used this input to introduce survey items that asked about both the immediate and delayed onset of PEM and its relationship to potential triggers.

After several months, when we were receiving few additional patient comments regarding our survey that we had been posting, we decided to collect data using this survey with the next phase of this project. Institutional Review Board (IRB) approval was obtained for collecting data based on the survey that had been developed using input from the patient community. Participants provided informed consent. Participants were required to be over the age of 18 years old, able to read and write in English, and have a current self-reported diagnosis of ME and/or CFS. Participants completed the questionnaire online using Research Electronic Data Capture (REDCap), a secure online survey tool [18]. Respondents were instructed to save their answers and return to complete the survey at a later time if they were not able to finish the survey in one sitting due to their illness.

2.2. Materials

The first part of the survey assessed demographic characteristics, as well as information about illness/diagnosis status (see Table 1). Following this background assessment, the respondents were asked about the onset of their PEM symptoms (see Table 2), and then asked questions relating to factors that trigger PEM (Table 3). This included examples of triggers beyond physical or cognitive exertion, such as "basic activities of daily living", "positional changes", and "emotional events". The survey also asked specific questions about the relationship between triggers of PEM and other factors, such as participants' individual energy limits or the extent to which they may exert themselves.

Next, the participants were asked to evaluate a list of symptoms that are exacerbated following physical and/or cognitive exertion (Table 4). The symptoms included items which have been assessed through other operationalized measures (e.g., "physical fatigue", "unrefreshing sleep", and "flu-like symptoms"), as well as items suggested by patients (e.g., "physical fatigue while mentally wired", "brain twangs" and "burning sensation all over your skin"). Each item was rated for frequency for the past six months on a 5-point Likert scale: 0 = none of the time, 1 = a little of the time, 2 = about half the time, 3 = most of the time, 4 = all of the time. Symptoms of 2 or higher were considered to be the threshold for PEM, based on past studies [19]. For each symptom, frequency values were multiplied by 25 to convert to 100-point scales, with higher values indicating more frequent symptoms.

Table 5 shows item responses of participant experiences of PEM by asking the question "If you go beyond your energy limits by engaging in pre-illness tolerated exercise or activities of daily living, do you experience any of the following?" Several common phrases used to describe PEM were then listed, including "a severity and duration of symptoms that are out of proportion to the initial trigger" and "global worsening of multi-systemic symptoms (an example of this might be aches all over your body plus cognitive problems plus light and/or sound sensitivity)".

Following the PEM symptom list, the survey included an assessment of duration of PEM and length of recovery time, as well as information about illness course and functioning (Table 6). To better understand the relationship between PEM and exertion, participants were asked if the severity and duration of PEM was out-of-proportion to the type, intensity, frequency, and duration of exertion. Participants were then asked whether they had ever experienced an "adrenaline surge" after going beyond their energy limit, and how long the surge lasts before the onset of PEM. Next, patients were assessed on their illness course and functional status by asking how long ago they began feeling sick with ME or CFS, if the illness has been present for at least 50% of the time, and how they would describe their illness and functioning. Participants were also asked if they are managing their PEM symptoms by pacing or "staying within their energy envelope," one of the few patient recommended treatments for ME and CFS [20].

The survey also requested information about past tests the participant may have completed, such as a cardiopulmonary or tilt table test. Lastly, the survey assessed if the participants felt that this patient-driven survey accurately depicts their PEM experience.

3. Results

The international online convenience sample included 1,534 adults identifying as having ME and/or CFS who completed the questionnaire (347 additional respondents had incomplete surveys and were not included in this analysis). Respondents were from over 35 countries. As indicated in Table 1, 41.1% of participants reported currently living in the United States. The sample consisted of mostly females (84.6%). The majority of participants were white/Caucasian (97.5%), and 2% identified as being of Latino or Hispanic origin. Just over half of the participants were married or living with a partner (56.6%), 39.3% had a standard college degree, and 45.7% were receiving disability payments.

Table 1 indicates that 50.7% of participants had a diagnosis of CFS, 22.0% had a diagnosis of ME, and 27.2% had a diagnosis of both ME and CFS. For our entire sample, 94.4% reported being diagnosed by a medical doctor.

Table 1. Demographic characteristics of patients with myalgic encephalomyelitis (ME) and chronic fatigue syndrome (CFS) (N = 1534).

Age	M (SD)
	51.26 (13.08)
Gender	**% (n)**
Female	84.6 (1,298)
Male	14.9 (229)
Race	**% (n)**
White/Caucasian	97.5 (1,495)
Black/African American	0.3 (4)
American Indian or Alaska Native	0.7 (11)
Asian or Pacific Islander	1.1 (17)
Latino/Hispanic Origin	2.0 (30)
Prefer not to respond	1.4 (22)
Marital Status	**% (n)**
Married or living with partner	56.6 (869)
Never married	23.3 (357)
Divorced	13.9 (213)
Separated	2.6 (40)
Widowed	2.0 (31)
Prefer not to answer	1.2 (19)
Education Level	**% (n)**
Graduate/professional degree	29.1 (446)
Standard college/university degree	39.3 (603)
Partial college	22.1 (339)
High school or General Education Development (GED)	5.9 (91)
Some high school	2.5 (39)
Less than high school	0.8 (12)
Employment Status	**% (n)**
On disability	45.7 (701)
Working full-time	6.8 (104)
Working part-time	13.2 (203)
Homemaker	7.3 (112)
Student	3.3 (50)
Retired	18.1 (278)

Table 1. Cont.

Unemployed	16.0 (245)
Prior to leaving the workforce, did you cut back either in number of hours worked or in responsibilities	57.5 (880)
Diagnosis	**% (n)**
CFS	50.7 (777)
ME	22.0 (338)
Both ME and CFS	27.2 (418)
Who diagnosed you?	**% (n)**
Medical doctor	94.4 (1448)
Was the medical doctor an expert/knowledgeable of ME/CFS?	55.6 (853)
Alternative practitioner	5.5 (85)
Self-diagnosed	7.6 (117)
Current Annual Income (in US dollars)	**% (n)**
Less than $24,999	52.2 (801)
$25,000 to $49,999	14.7 (225)
$50,000 to $99,999	8.3 (128)
$100,000 to $149,999	2.8 (43)
$150,000 to $199,999	0.9 (14)
$200,000 to $249,999	0.2 (3)
$250,000 or more	1.0 (16)
Prefer Not to Respond	18.1 (277)
Annual Income prior to becoming ill (in US dollars)	**% (n)**
Less than $24,999	15.4 (237)
$25,000 to $49,999	25.0 (384)
$50,000 to $99,999	25.4 (390)
$100,000 to $149,999	6.7 (103)
$150,000 to $199,999	1.8 (27)
$200,000 to $249,999	1.2 (18)
$250,000 or more	1.7 (26)
Prefer Not to Respond	19.9 (305)

Note: Percentages may not add up to 100% due to missing data. For employment status, there were also several open response questions asking about what conditions participants received disability for, and for current and past job titles.

Descriptive statistics of PEM onset are reported in Table 2. Over half of participants had experienced onset of symptom exacerbation immediately after exertion (72.3%), while 91.4% had experienced delayed onset after exertion. To determine the length of the delay between exertion and the onset of PEM, participants selected periods for when the onset of PEM might occur when onset is delayed. A delay of between 1–2 days after exertion was experienced by 53.1% of the participants.

Table 2. Onset (N = 1534).

Items	% (n)
Immediate onset of symptom exacerbation	**72.3 (1109)**
All the time	9.9 (152)
Most of the time	21.9 (336)
About half the time	24.1 (369)
A little of the time	15.6 (239)
Delayed onset of symptom exacerbation	**91.4 (1402)**
All the time	21.8 (335)
Most of the time	37.1 (569)
About half the time	23.4 (359)
A little of the time	8.1 (125)
How long after the exertion does your symptom exacerbation occur *	
1 h or less	16.5 (253)
2–6 h	33.1 (508)

Table 2. *Cont.*

Items	% (n)
7–12 h	31.0 (476)
13–24 h	43.2 (662)
1–2 days	53.1 (815)
3–4 days	15.7 (241)
5–6 days	4.5 (69)
More than 1 week	4.2 (65)

Note: * For this item, participants could select more than one answer. There is also an option for participants to describe what activities and which symptoms affect immediate and/or delayed onset.

Table 3 describes PEM triggers, with 78.2% endorsing "basic activities of daily living", 64.5% endorsing "positional changes", and 93.2% endorsing "emotional stress (good or bad)". Additionally, 84.9% said there were some instances in which the specific precipitants could not be identified. The highest endorsed non-exertion triggers reported by participants were as follows: emotional events (88.3%), noise (85.5%), and sensory overload (83.6%).

Table 3. Triggers (*N* = 1534).

Items	% (n)
Basic activities of daily living trigger symptom exacerbation	**78.2 (1199)**
All of the time	20.8 (319)
Most of the time	24.1 (370)
About half the time	17.7 (272)
A little of the time	15.3 (234)
Positional changes lead to symptom exacerbation	**64.5 (990)**
All of the time	14.9 (229)
Most of the time	20.0 (307)
About half the time	15.5 (238)
A little of the time	13.9 (213)
Emotional stress (good or bad) lead to symptom exacerbation	**93.2 (1429)**
All of the time	34.0 (522)
Most of the time	29.2 (448)
About half the time	18.3 (280)
A little of the time	11.5 (177)
Instances in which the specific precipitants cannot be identified	84.9 (1302)
Able to exercise a little as long as you stay within certain limits without symptom exacerbation	37.0 (567)
Takes less exposure than usual to trigger PEM on days you are recovering from symptom exacerbation	94.3 (1447)
Sensitized to particular triggers so they cause an even more abnormal response over time	48.1 (738)
Severity of the PEM reaction proportionate to how far beyond your limits you have gone	80.9 (1241)
Mild overexertion over several days produces an abnormal physical or cognitive response	96.8 (1485)
Multiple occurrences of PEM that cause your overall health status to become worse over weeks/months	84.4 (1295)
Intolerance to stimulation causes worsening in symptoms, but is not prolonged if stimulus is removed	79.5 (1219)
Fighting off an infection (flu, cold, bladder infection) causes a worsening in all/most of your symptoms	82.3 (1262)
Length of time for recovery correlates with the severity of PEM	79.6 (1221)
Do you have other triggers such as	
Emotional events (good or bad)	88.3 (1354)
Noise	85.3 (1308)
Sensory overload	83.6 (1282)
Visual overload	79.7 (1223)
Heat	74.4 (1141)
Light	68.8 (1055)
Cold	66.3 (1017)
Foods	61.0 (935)
Chemicals	58.0 (889)
Watching movement (such as watching a video)	52.5 (806)
Vibration	47.1 (722)
Drugs used for medication	47.4 (727)
Mold	39.4 (605)
Supplements	27.4 (420)

Table 4 reports the proportion of participants who endorsed the worsening of symptoms due to physical or cognitive exertion. The most commonly endorsed symptoms were as follows: reduced stamina and/or functional capacity (99.4%), physical fatigue (98.9%), cognitive exhaustion (97.4%), problems thinking (97.4%), unrefreshing sleep (95.0%), muscle pain (87.9%), insomnia (87.3%), muscle weakness/instability (87.3%), temperature dysregulation (86.9%), and flu-like symptoms (86.6%). The symptoms endorsed by less than half of the sample included the following: loss of appetite (49.0%), migraines (46.2%), cardiac pain and/or arrhythmia (41.2%), brain twangs (29.9%), burning sensation all over your skin (29.7%), paralysis/inability to move (29.4%), pre-menstrual symptoms (21.1%), and decreased heart rate (15.1%).

Table 4. Symptoms made worse due to physical or cognitive exertion (N = 1534).

Items	% (n) "Yes"	% (n) at "2" Threshold	Mean (SD)
1. Reduced stamina and/or functional capacity	99.4 (1525)	98.0 (1504)	90.60 (17.16)
2. Physical fatigue	98.9 (1517)	98.3 (1508)	87.53 (18.26)
3. Cognitive exhaustion	97.4 (1494)	92.0 (1412)	77.64 (24.87)
4. Problems thinking	97.4 (1494)	92.6 (1420)	78.47 (24.87)
5. Unrefreshing sleep	95.0 (1457)	91.1 (1398)	80.57 (27.65)
6. Muscle pain	87.9 (1349)	81.5 (1250)	69.41 (33.95)
7. Insomnia	87.3 (1339)	75.1 (1152)	62.40 (34.30)
8. Muscle weakness/instability	87.3 (1339)	77.2 (1185)	64.03 (33.86)
9. Temperature dysregulation	86.9 (1333)	75.2 (1153)	63.76 (34.75)
10. Flu-like symptoms	86.6 (1329)	74.4 (1142)	59.52 (33.43)
11. Aches all over your body	85.6 (1313)	79.5 (1219)	68.68 (35.58)
12. Physically fatigued while mentally wired	82.1 (1259)	72.8 (1116)	59.00 (35.65)
13. Dizziness	80.7 (1238)	56.0 (859)	46.28 (33.19)
14. Gastro-intestinal problems	78.6 (1206)	59.3 (910)	49.90 (36.02)
15. Headaches	78.0 (1197)	56.5 (866)	46.48 (34.52)
16. Ataxia	77.6 (1191)	57.8 (886)	47.62 (35.18)
17. Increased heart rate/heart palpitations	77.4 (118)	64.9 (996)	52.28 (36.51)
18. Weak or stiff neck	74.6 (1144)	61.0 (936)	51.35 (38.20)
19. Joint pain	73.0 (1120)	59.5 (912)	49.17 (37.86)
20. Problems with speech	72.4 (1110)	50.0 (767)	40.22 (33.14)
21. Sore throats	70.9 (1087)	47.2 (724)	38.92 (33.55)
22. Muscle twitching	68.1 (1045)	40.9 (627)	35.12 (32.38)
23. Night sweats and chills	67.7 (1038)	46.9 (720)	38.48 (34.69)
24. Sore eyes	67.0 (1028)	49.0 (752)	39.91 (35.70)
25. Nerve pain	63.3 (971)	48.8 (748)	40.65 (38.16)
26. Sore lymph nodes	62.9 (965)	44.0 (675)	36.36 (35.28)
27. Nausea	62.2 (954)	38.1 (584)	31.89 (32.13)
28. Tinnitus	60.3 (925)	39.8 (611)	37.42 (38.96)
29. Trouble breathing	57.8 (887)	40.9 (628)	33.97 (35.67)
30. Neurological symptoms	57.0 (875)	42.8 (656)	34.60 (36.14)
31. Excessive sleep	54.4 (835)	44.5 (682)	36.23 (38.58)
32. Loss of appetite	49.0 (752)	30.9 (474)	25.41 (31.62)
33. Migraines	46.2 (708)	24.6 (378)	21.92 (29.27)
34. Cardiac pain and/or arrhythmia	41.2 (632)	24.8 (381)	21.12 (30.30)
35. Brain twangs	29.9 (459)	17.7 (272)	15.00 (26.82)
36. Severe burning sensation all over skin	29.7 (456)	18.3 (280)	15.96 (28.87)
37. Paralysis/inability to move	29.4 (451)	9.4 (144)	11.49 (21.91)
38. Premenstrual symptoms	21.1 (323)	16.4 (251)	13.56 (29.25)
39. Decreased heart rate	15.1 (231)	7.4 (114)	6.88 (19.09)

Note: % endorsed "yes" means they responded yes to experiencing symptom at any level. % endorsed at "2" threshold means that they experience the symptom at least half the time. Means reflect frequency only (0–100 scale).

In order to gauge participant's general experiences of PEM, participants were asked if they experienced any of the common phrases used to describe PEM (listed in Table 5) after exertion. All of the phrases were endorsed by over 90% of the sample.

Table 5. If you go beyond your energy limits by engaging in pre-illness tolerated exercise or activities of daily living, do you experience any of the following? (N = 1534).

Items	% (n)
An onset that is immediate or delayed by hours or days	98.5 (1511)
Post-exertional exhaustion	98.3 (1508)
A loss of functional capacity and/or stamina	98.2 (1506)
Symptom exacerbation	98.1 (1505)
A severity and duration of symptoms that are out of proportion to the initial trigger	97.4 (1494)
An abnormal response to minimal amounts of physical and/or cognitive exertion	97.3 (1492)
Substantial reduction in pre-illness activity level	96.9 (1486)
A prolonged recovery that can last days, weeks, or months	96.2 (1475)
Global worsening of multi-systemic symptoms	94.0 (1442)
Prolonged worsening of symptoms	92.9 (1425)

The findings reported in Table 6 indicate that over half the participants (58.0%) said PEM lasts on average 3–6 days, with 1–2 days (38.9%), 1 week–1 month (46.7%), and 1–6 months (30.3%) also being frequently reported. Additionally, 67.1% of the sample had experienced a "crash" that never resolved. Over half of the sample (57.2%) said they had experienced an adrenaline surge during or after going beyond their energy limits, and the most commonly reported length of time was "a few hours" (35.8%). Further information about the natural history of participants' ME/CFS illness are also provided in Table 6. The majority of subjects have been sick for over 10 years, with 97.1% reporting their illness being present for more than 50% of the time. Additionally, nearly half of participants described the course of their illness as fluctuating, experiencing good periods and bad periods. Lastly, nearly half of participants classified their status as being able to do light house work, but not being able to work part-time.

Table 6 also contains information on how participants were currently managing their PEM symptoms. Only 6% of patients with ME or CFS felt that pacing completely allowed them to avoid PEM, while the majority reported pacing only being effective some of the time and only at a moderate/mild level. Participants also identified the pacing method they used (e.g., 87.1% indicated it was based on their bodies' reactions whereas 10.7% indicated it was with a heart rate monitor, and 17.3% indicated both).

Patients were also asked about tests to assess their cardiovascular health difficulties and orthostatic intolerance, which are common symptoms of ME and CFS and are often made worse after exertion. Almost a quarter (24.5%) indicated they had undergone a cardiopulmonary test and 29.7% indicated they had taken part in a stand lean/tilt table test. Of those patients, 9.3% had normal cardiopulmonary results, whereas 14.9% had abnormal results. Only 4.8% of the sample had completed an exercise test on back-to-back days.

At the end of the questionnaire, participants were asked if they felt this survey accurately captured their experiences of PEM, and 29.8% felt the survey was very accurate, 57.7% reported it was accurate, 10.7% were neutral, 1.2% thought it was not accurate, and 0.1% said it was not at all accurate.

Table 6. Duration of PEM, illness course, and functioning (N = 1534).

Items	% (n)
Length of prolonged, unpredictable recovery period	95.2 (1460)
Within 24 h	14.1 (216)
Between 1 and 2 days	38.9 (596)
Between 3 and 6 days	58.0 (890)
Between 1 week and 1 month	46.7 (717)
Between 1 and 6 months	30.3 (465)
Between 6 months and 1 year	13.6 (209)
Between 1 and 2 years	9.8 (151)
Over 2 years	12.3 (189)
Crash that has never resolved	67.1 (1029)

Table 6. Cont.

Items	% (n)
Severity and duration out-of-proportion to the TYPE of exertion	96.0 (1473)
All of the time	59.0 (905)
Most of the time	26.1 (401)
About half the time	8.7 (133)
A little of the time	2.0 (31)
Severity and duration out-of-proportion to the INTENSITY of exertion	94.8 (1454)
All of the time	59.5 (913)
Most of the time	26.5 (406)
About half the time	6.6 (102)
A little of the time	1.9 (29)
Severity and duration out-of-proportion to the DURATION of exertion	90.4 (1386)
All of the time	56.9 (873)
Most of the time	25.6 (393)
About half the time	5.1 (78)
A little of the time	1.8 (28)
Severity and duration out-of-proportion to the FREQUENCY of exertion	84.9 (1302)
All of the time	51.5 (790)
Most of the time	24.8 (380)
About half the time	5.5 (85)
A little of the time	2.6 (40)
Adrenaline surges during or after going beyond energy limit	57.2 (878)
Length of adrenaline surge before crashing *	
A few minutes	13.0 (200)
A few hours	35.8 (549)
About 24 h	16.5 (253)
Less than a week	6.1 (94)
About 1 week	1.3 (20)
Over 1 week	1.3 (20)
How long ago did your problem with ME/CFS begin?	
6–11 months ago	0.6 (9)
1–2 years ago	2.9 (45)
3–5 years ago	12.1 (186)
6–10 years ago	15.9 (244)
Over 10 years ago	53.7 (823)
Since childhood/adolescence	14.8 (227)
Has your illness been present for more than 50% of the time since you became ill?	97.1 (1489)
How would you describe the course of your illness?	
Constantly getting worse	29.3 (450)
Constantly improving	1.4 (22)
Persisting (no change)	15.4 (237)
Relapsing and remitting	7.4 (113)
Fluctuating	46.2 (708)
Which statement best describes your illness over the last 6 months?	
I can do all work or family responsibilities without any problems with my energy	0.1 (2)
I can work full-time/finish some family responsibilities, but I have no energy left	2.6 (40)
I can work full-time, but I have no energy left for anything else	4.6 (71)
I can only work part-time at work or on some family responsibilities	14.9 (228)
I can do light housework, but I cannot work part-time	43.0 (659)
I can walk around the house, but I cannot do light housework	29.9 (459)

Table 6. *Cont.*

Items	% (n)
I am not able to work or do anything, I am bedridden/completely incapacitated	4.8 (73)
Pacing allows me to completely avoid symptom exacerbation	6.0 (92)
Pacing allows me to avoid symptom exacerbation only to a certain degree	87.7 (1345)
How frequently is pacing effective?	
All the time	2.3 (35)
Most of the time	22.8 (350)
About half the time	34.1 (523)
A little of the time	27.8 (427)
How effective is pacing in reducing the level of severity of symptoms?	
Very effective	7.6 (117)
Moderately effective	37.2 (570)
Mildly effective	34.2 (525)
Barely effective	8.2 (126)
If you are pacing, is it:	
Based on body symptoms and reactions to triggers	87.1 (1336)
With a heart rate monitor	10.7 (164)
Both of the above	17.3 (265)

Note: * For these items, participants could select more than one answer. There is also an option for participants to describe pacing techniques not listed.

4. Discussion

The objective of this study was to use community-based participatory research in an effort to develop a comprehensive way to assess PEM. Based on the comments and items suggested from patients, the following specific aspects of PEM were found to be the most critical domains: the timing of PEM onset, triggers of PEM, symptoms that are exacerbated following exertion or exposure to triggers, phrases used to describe consequences of PEM, duration of PEM, relationship between exertion and length of recovery, and the importance of considering personal characteristics (e.g., how long the patient has had ME/CFS, the course of their illness, their level of functioning, and coping methods used). The patient perspective provided the authors with the critical information to develop this survey of PEM. Of the patients who took part, 87.5% felt that the resulting survey was either very accurate or accurate.

Onset of symptom exacerbation after exertion was found to vary between patients. As shown in Table 2, the majority of patients experienced both immediate and delayed onset of PEM, and the extent of the delay of symptoms varied considerably. In addition to the unpredictability of PEM onset, several factors affect the duration of PEM before recovery, including the type, intensity, frequency, and duration of the exertion (see Table 6). These findings are consistent with patients' reporting of prolonged recovery from PEM symptoms. In one study in which patients and healthy controls participated in a fatiguing exercise test, the patient group's recovery was prolonged [21]. In addition, VanNess et al. [13] found patients with CFS, in comparison to healthy controls, take considerably longer to recover after completing a maximal cardiopulmonary exercise test the next day and a week later. Our findings are also consistent with a study by Chu et al. [11] who found that when comparing PEM symptom onset between those with ME or CFS to healthy controls, 87-95% of controls had recovered within 24 h after completing an exercise test. Among those with ME and CFS, PEM symptoms peaked at 24 to 48 h later, and 45-60% still experienced symptoms up to 5 days later.

Our survey also assessed specific triggers that bring on symptom exacerbation. The effects of physical and cognitive exertion on PEM have been well-established [13,21–23] and these findings are consistent with the current study. For example, only 37% of subjects reported being able to exercise "a little" without PEM-related symptoms, as long as they stay within "certain limits" (see Table 3). Furthermore, basic activities of daily living (e.g., getting dressed, cooking a meal, bathing), positional changes (e.g., going from lying down to standing up), and emotional stress lead to exacerbation in 78.2%, 64.5%, and 93.2% of patients, respectively.

Another issue explored involved whether there are precipitants of PEM beyond physical or cognitive exertion. The highest reported triggers in addition to physical/cognitive exertion were emotional events (88.3%), noise (85.3%), and sensory (83.6%) and visual overload (79.7%). This is consistent with past literature reporting these types of stimuli as exacerbating symptoms [24]. It has also been hypothesized that exposure to mold could trigger illness onset and PEM symptomology [25]. In our sample, 39.4% reported mold triggering their PEM. This is consistent with findings by Brewer, Thrasher, Straus, Madison, and Hooper [26], where 30% of patients with ME and CFS were reported to have multiple mycotoxins present in their bodies.

Partly as a function of this survey and the interactions with the patient community, there have been several additional developments in the assessment of PEM. First, Cotler et al. [27] found that use of the 5 recommended PEM DSQ items was an excellent screen in identifying PEM in patients with ME and CFS. In addition, as a second step in the process of assessing PEM, 5 additional DSQ items (including the assessment of duration of symptoms) were successfully used to differentiate PEM from other chronic illnesses. In addition, the findings from the patient survey reported on in this article were revised in order to construct a briefer, more concise measure of PEM, which was significantly related to physical functioning [28].

There are several limitations to this study. First, we did not obtain confirmation of ME or CFS diagnoses by independent medical personnel. In addition, we do not know what case definitions, if any, were used in their diagnoses. In addition, consistent with other ME and CFS studies, the sample was not demographically diverse. However, having a sample from several geographic regions did increase the generalizability of findings. Another limitation of the study was the length of the questionnaire. Though participants were presented with the option of pausing, it is reasonable that some may have still found it difficult to complete.

The open, participatory nature of this study provided a unique way of both designing the survey and gathering comprehensive information from the ME and CFS community regarding PEM. There are unique benefits that can accrue to the research and patient community by actively collaborating on instrument development as well as other policy issues, such as the selection of a name for the illness as well as the case definition [29]. By collaborating with the ME and CFS community, we have provided a model of community-based participatory research, which has multiple advantages to both the patient and research communities [30]. We close with this quote regarding what needs to occur to further this type of collaborative research in the ME and CFS areas:

"An alternative vision is still possible if those in power are willing to bring all interested parties to the table, including international representatives, historians on the science of illness criteria, and social scientists adept at developing consensus. In a collaborative, open, interactive, and inclusive process, issues may be explored, committees may be charged with making recommendations, and key gatekeepers may work collaboratively and transparently to build a consensus for change. Involve all parties—patients, scientists, clinicians, and government officials—in the decision-making process [31]."

Author Contributions: Investigation, formal analysis, and writing—original draft, C.S.H.; writing—review and editing, S.B. and J.C.; conceptualization, supervision, and writing—review and editing, L.A.J.

Funding: This research received no external funding.

Acknowledgments: The authors thank the ME and CFS patient community for their collaborative efforts.

Conflicts of Interest: The authors declare no conflicts of interest.

References

1. Ramsay, A.M. *Myalgic Encephalomyelitis and Postviral Fatigue States: The Saga of Royal Free Disease*; Gower Medical Publishing for the Myalgic Encephalomyelitis Association: London, UK, 1988.
2. Brurberg, K.G.; Fonhus, M.S.; Larun, L.; Flottorp, S.; Malterud, K. Case definitions for chronic fatigue syndrome/myalgic encephalomyelitis (cfs/me): A systematic review. *BMJ Open* **2014**, *4*. [CrossRef] [PubMed]
3. Fukuda, K.; Straus, S.E.; Hickie, I.; Sharpe, M.C.; Dobbins, J.G.; Komaroff, A. Chronic fatigue syndrome: A comprehensive approach to its definition and study. *Ann. Intern. Med.* **1994**, *121*, 953–959. [CrossRef] [PubMed]
4. Carruthers, B.M.; Jain, A.K.; De Meirleir, K.L.; Peterson, D.L.; Klimas, N.G.; Lerner, A.M.; van de Sande, M.I. Myalgic encephalomyelitis/chronic fatigue syndrome: Clinical working case definition, diagnostic and treatment protocols. *J. Chronic Fatigue Syndr.* **2003**, *11*, 7–115. [CrossRef]
5. Jason, L.A.; Unger, E.R.; Dimitrakoff, J.D.; Fagin, A.P.; Houghton, M.; Cook, D.B.; Snell, C. Minimum data elements for research reports on cfs. *Brain Behav. Immun.* **2012**, *26*, 401–406. [CrossRef] [PubMed]
6. Mateo, L.J.; Chu, L.; Stevens, S.; Stevens, J.; Snell, C.R.; Davenport, T.; VanNess, J.M. Comparing post-exertional symptoms following serial exercise tests. In Proceedings of the 2018 Pacific Undergraduate Research and Creativity Conference (PURCC), Stockton, CA, USA, 28 April 2018.
7. McManimen, S.L.; Sunnquist, M.L.; Jason, L.A. Deconstructing post-exertional malaise: An exploratory factor analysis. *J. Health Psychol.* **2016**, 1–11. [CrossRef] [PubMed]
8. Blomberg, J.; Gottfries, C.G.; Elfaitouri, A.; Rizwan, M.; Rosen, A. Infection elicited autoimmunity and myalgic encephalomyelitis/chronic fatigue syndrome: An explanatory model. *Front. Immunol.* **2018**, *9*, 229. [CrossRef] [PubMed]
9. Racciatti, D.; Vecchiet, J.; Ceccomancini, A.; Ricci, F.; Pizzigallo, E. Chronic fatigue syndrome following a toxic exposure. *Sci. Total Environ.* **2001**, *270*, 27–31. [CrossRef]
10. Stejskal, V. Metals as a common trigger of inflammation resulting in non-specific symptoms: Diagnosis and treatment. *ISR Med. Assoc. J.* **2014**, *16*, 753–758. [PubMed]
11. Chu, L.; Valencia, I.J.; Garvert, D.W.; Montoya, J.G. Deconstructing post-exertional malaise in myalgic encephalomyelitis/chronic fatigue syndrome: A patient centered, cross-sectional survey. *PLoS ONE* **2018**, *13*, e0197811. [CrossRef] [PubMed]
12. Jason, L.A.; Evans, M.; Porter, N.; Brown, M.; Brown, A.; Hunnell, J.; Anderson, V.; Lerch, A.; De Meirleir, K.; Friedberg, F. Development of a revised Canadian myalgic encephalomyelitis chronic fatigue syndrome case definition. *Am. J. Biochem. Biotechnol.* **2010**, *6*, 120–135. [CrossRef]
13. VanNess, J.M.; Stevens, S.R.; Bateman, L.; Stiles, T.L.; Snell, C.R. Postexertional malaise in women with chronic fatigue syndrome. *J. Womens Health* **2010**, *19*, 239–244. [CrossRef] [PubMed]
14. NINDS Common Data Elements (CDE) Group. Post-Exertional Malaise Subgroup Summary. Myalgic Encephalomyelitis/Chronic Fatigue Syndrome. 2018. Available online: https://www.commondataelements.ninds.nih.gov/MECFS.aspx#tab=Data_Standards (accessed on 12 December 2018).
15. Simon, M. Results of the Poll to Inform the NIH/CDC's Definition of PEM in All Their Future ME/CFS Research [msg#1]. Available online: https://www.s4me.info/threads/results-of-the-poll-to-inform-the-nih-cdc%E2%80%99s-definition-of-pem-in-all-their-future-me-cfs-research.2221/ (accessed on 2 February 2018).
16. IOM. Beyond myalgic encephalomyelitis/chronic fatigue syndrome: An iom report on redefining an illness. *JAMA* **2015**, *313*, 1101–1102. [CrossRef] [PubMed]
17. Jason, L.A. Small wins matter in advocacy movements: Giving voice to patients. *Am. J. Community Psychol.* **2012**, *49*, 307–316. [CrossRef] [PubMed]
18. Harris, P.A.; Taylor, R.; Thielke, R.; Payne, J.; Gonzalez, N.; Conde, J.G. Research electronic data capture (REDCap)—A metadata-driven methodology and workflow process for providing translational research informatics support. *J. Biomed. Inform.* **2009**, *42*, 377–381. [CrossRef] [PubMed]
19. Jason, L.A.; Sunnquist, M.; Brown, A.; Evans, M.; Vernon, S.D.; Furst, J.; Simonis, V. Examining case definition criteria for chronic fatigue syndrome and myalgic encephalomyelitis. *Fatigue* **2014**, *2*, 40–56. [CrossRef] [PubMed]

20. Goudsmit, E.M.; Nijs, J.; Jason, L.A.; Wallman, K.E. Pacing as a strategy to improve energy management in myalgic encephalomyelitis/chronic fatigue syndrome: A consensus document. *Disabil. Rehabil.* **2012**, *34*, 1140–1147. [CrossRef] [PubMed]
21. Cook, D.B.; Light, A.R.; Light, K.C.; Broderick, G.; Shields, M.R.; Dougherty, R.J.; Vernon, S.D. Neural consequences of post-exertion malaise in myalgic encephalomyelitis/chronic fatigue syndrome. *Brain Behav. Immun.* **2017**, *62*, 87–99. [CrossRef] [PubMed]
22. Keech, A.; Sandler, C.X.; Vollmer-Conna, U.; Cvejic, E.; Lloyd, A.R.; Barry, B.K. Capturing the post-exertional exacerbation of fatigue following physical and cognitive challenge in patients with chronic fatigue syndrome. *J. Psychosom. Res.* **2015**, *79*, 537–549. [CrossRef] [PubMed]
23. Miller, R.R.; Reid, W.D.; Mattman, A.; Yamabayashi, C.; Steiner, T.; Parker, S.; Patrick, D.M. Submaximal exercise testing with near-infrared spectroscopy in myalgic encephalomyelitis/chronic fatigue syndrome patients compared to healthy controls: A case-control study. *J. Transl. Med.* **2015**, *13*, 159. [CrossRef] [PubMed]
24. Soderlund, A.; Skoge, A.M.; Malterud, K. "I could not lift my arm holding the fork..." Living with chronic fatigue syndrome. *Scand. J. Prim. Health Care* **2000**, *18*, 165–169. [PubMed]
25. Gharibzadeh, S.; Hoseini, S.S. Is there any relation between moldy building exposure and chronic fatigue syndrome? *Med. Hypotheses* **2006**, *66*, 1243–1244. [CrossRef] [PubMed]
26. Brewer, J.H.; Thrasher, J.D.; Straus, D.C.; Madison, R.A.; Hooper, D. Detection of mycotoxins in patients with chronic fatigue syndrome. *Toxins* **2013**, *5*, 605–617. [CrossRef] [PubMed]
27. Cotler, J.; Holtzman, C.S.; Dudun, C.; Jason, L.A. A brief questionnaire to assess post-exertional malaise. *Diagnostics* **2018**, *8*, 66. [CrossRef] [PubMed]
28. Jason, L.A.; Holtzman, C.S.; Sunnquist, M.; Cotler, J. The development of an instrument to assess post-exertional malaise in patients with ME and CFS. *J. Health Psychol.* **2018**. [CrossRef] [PubMed]
29. Jason, L.A.; Richman, J.A.; Friedberg, F.; Wagner, L.; Taylor, R.R.; Jordan, K.M. Politics, science, and the emergence of a new disease: The case of chronic fatigue syndrome. *Am. Psychol.* **1997**, *52*, 973–983. [CrossRef] [PubMed]
30. Jason, L.A. To serve or not to serve: Ethical and policy implications. *Am. J. Community Psychol.* **2017**, *60*, 406–413. [CrossRef] [PubMed]
31. Jason, L.A. IOM's Effort to Dislodge Chronic Fatigue Syndrome. Available online: http://oxford.ly/18LEEiQ (accessed on 4 March 2015).

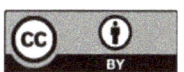

© 2019 by the authors. Licensee MDPI, Basel, Switzerland. This article is an open access article distributed under the terms and conditions of the Creative Commons Attribution (CC BY) license (http://creativecommons.org/licenses/by/4.0/).

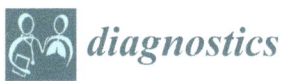

Article

Evidence of Clinical Pathology Abnormalities in People with Myalgic Encephalomyelitis/Chronic Fatigue Syndrome (ME/CFS) from an Analytic Cross-Sectional Study

Luis Nacul [1],*, Barbara de Barros [1], Caroline C. Kingdon [1], Jacqueline M. Cliff [1], Taane G. Clark [1,2], Kathleen Mudie [1], Hazel M. Dockrell [1] and Eliana M. Lacerda [1]

1. Faculty of Infectious and Tropical Diseases, London School of Hygiene & Tropical Medicine, London WC1E 7HT, UK; barbara.de-barros@lshtm.ac.uk (B.d.B.); caroline.kingdon@lshtm.ac.uk (C.C.K.); Jackie.cliff@lshtm.ac.uk (J.M.C.); taane.clark@lshtm.ac.uk (T.G.C.); kathleen.mudie1@lshtm.ac.uk (K.M.); hazel.dockrell@lshtm.ac.uk (H.M.D.); eliana.lacerda@lshtm.ac.uk (E.M.L.)
2. Faculty of Epidemiology and Population Health, London School of Hygiene & Tropical Medicine, London WC1E 7HT, UK
* Correspondence: luis.nacul@lshtm.ac.uk

Received: 27 March 2019; Accepted: 4 April 2019; Published: 10 April 2019

Abstract: Myalgic encephalomyelitis/chronic fatigue syndrome (ME/CFS) is a debilitating disease presenting with extreme fatigue, post-exertional malaise, and other symptoms. In the absence of a diagnostic biomarker, ME/CFS is diagnosed clinically, although laboratory tests are routinely used to exclude alternative diagnoses. In this analytical cross-sectional study, we aimed to explore potential haematological and biochemical markers for ME/CFS, and disease severity. We reviewed laboratory test results from 272 people with ME/CFS and 136 healthy controls participating in the UK ME/CFS Biobank (UKMEB). After corrections for multiple comparisons, most results were within the normal range, but people with severe ME/CFS presented with lower median values ($p < 0.001$) of serum creatine kinase (CK; median = 54 U/L), compared to healthy controls (HCs; median = 101.5 U/L) and non-severe ME/CFS (median = 84 U/L). The differences in CK concentrations persisted after adjusting for sex, age, body mass index, muscle mass, disease duration, and activity levels (odds ratio (OR) for being a severe case = 0.05 (95% confidence interval (CI) = 0.02–0.15) compared to controls, and OR = 0.16 (95% CI = 0.07–0.40), compared to mild cases). This is the first report that serum CK concentrations are markedly reduced in severe ME/CFS, and these results suggest that serum CK merits further investigation as a biomarker for severe ME/CFS.

Keywords: myalgic encephalomyelitis/chronic fatigue syndrome (ME/CFS); energy metabolism; potential biomarkers

1. Introduction

Myalgic encephalomyelitis/chronic fatigue syndrome (ME/CFS) is classified as a neurological disease [1], presenting with long-term fatigue resulting in substantial reductions in occupational, personal, social, and educational activities. Commonly-associated symptoms include impaired memory or concentration, muscle and multi-joint pain, new headaches, unrefreshing sleep, and post-exertional malaise [2,3]. Many patients experience orthostatic intolerance and may complain of dizziness, spatial disorientation, sweating, palpitations, or fainting and generalised weakness [2–4]. Although dysregulation of the nervous, immune and endocrine systems, with impaired cellular energy metabolism and ion transport, has been suggested [2], the pathophysiology of ME/CFS is still not fully understood, and there are no biological markers that are widely used for diagnosis, disease sub-grouping, or prognosis.

ME/CFS is diagnosed using clinical criteria based on detailed clinical history and physical examination; laboratory tests are used to exclude other conditions that can present with fatigue and general ill health [2–5]. A major goal of clinical research in ME/CFS is to improve diagnosis and find clinical and laboratory-based tests that may be used as disease markers. In 2011 we launched the UK ME/CFS Biobank (UKMEB) as a resource to accelerate ME/CFS research [6]. A rigorous assessment, alongside comprehensive clinical phenotyping of UKMEB participants, is essential to ensure that ME/CFS diagnosis is accurate according to recognised clinical criteria. The analysis of these clinical data in relation to molecular markers further supports the better understanding of disease aetiology and pathophysiology. In this study we compared baseline laboratory tests results from UKMEB participants with ME/CFS, including mildly/moderately and severely affected (i.e., house-bound or bed-bound) individuals, and healthy controls, which were collected as part of the routine workup of participants.

2. Materials and Methods

This analytical cross-sectional study was carried out with a sub-cohort of the UKMEB consenting participants. Recruitment—including eligibility criteria, data and sample collection, and handling of biosamples for the UKMEB—are described in detail elsewhere [6]. Adult participants with ME/CFS previously diagnosed by general practitioners and/or ME/CFS specialists and healthy controls were recruited through the UK National Health Service (NHS). Inclusion criteria for participants with ME/CFS included compliance with the Centers for Disease Control and Prevention criteria (CDC, 1994) or Canadian Consensus Criteria [2,3], which was ascertained by the clinical research team. Experienced research nurses assessed all participants, and blood was collected for immediate baseline clinical laboratory tests, as well as for research purposes and long-term storage. Blood collections took place at participating clinics or at the participants' homes (for severely affected cases), and samples were transferred within 6 hours for processing and storage [7]. Data entry, sample transportation, preparation, processing, and storage of the samples followed standard operating procedures (SOPs) [6].

Baseline laboratory tests were used primarily to exclude participants with ME/CFS whose symptoms of chronic fatigue could be explained by other conditions. These tests comprised: full blood count, erythrocyte sedimentation rate (ESR), serum vitamin B12 and folate; biochemical tests including electrolytes, creatinine, urea, serum creatine kinase (CK), liver function tests, C-reactive protein, rheumatoid factor, thyroid function tests; tissue transglutaminase antibodies; and urine analysis for protein, glucose, and blood. CK isoenzymes, mainly produced in skeletal muscle (CK-MM) and heart muscle (CK-MB), and aldolase were analysed in a sub-sample of 50 cases (25 severe and 25 non-severe cases) and 25 controls. According to the proximity of the collection site, blood samples were analysed by the haematology, clinical pathology, and immunology laboratories at the Norfolk and Norwich University Hospital or the Royal Free Hospital in London; standard NHS laboratory protocols were used for all tests [8]. The NHS laboratory staff was blinded to the status of study participants, i.e., if they were cases or controls.

This study included a sample of 272 confirmed ME/CFS cases and 136 healthy controls. ME/CFS cases were further classified as mild/moderate ($n = 216$) or severe ($n = 56$). The definition of severity was made at recruitment based on whether the patient was mainly house-bound or bed-bound (severe) or was ambulatory (mild/moderate cases). We visually inspected the shape of the continuous variables' distributions and, when departure from normality was observed, we used natural log transformation (CK, C-reactive protein (CRP), bilirubin, folate, vitamin B12) or square root transformation (ESR) to produce data that approximated a normal distribution for regression analysis. Figure A1 (Appendix A) shows the CK distribution before and after log transformation, by study group. We used log transformed results to carry out a power calculation of serum CK to detect mean differences of 0.34 (based on a standard deviation (SD) of 0.58 and means of 4.39 and 4.73 for cases and controls, respectively). We established that a sample size of at least 146 cases and 78 controls would be adequate to detect mean differences with a power or 95% and a type I error of 1%. The number of missing values was lower than 5% across all the variables, apart from one blood test (erythrocyte sedimentation rate) whose proportion of missing results was similar among the groups (16.5% to 17.6%); thus, we opted to maintain the variable in the analyses. Univariate analyses were performed using chi-squared tests for comparison of proportions and analysis of variance (ANOVA) for comparison of means of normally distributed continuous variables. For significant departures from normality, Wilcoxon rank sum or Kruskal–Wallis tests [9] were used to compare medians between two or more unmatched study groups respectively.

For putatively interesting results from the univariate analyses (Wilcoxon rank-sum test $p < 0.01$), logistic regression analyses [9] were used, and included the covariates: age-group at the time of recruitment, sex, body mass index (as ascertained during physical examination, in kg/m^2), disease duration (in months, for comparisons between cases only), muscle mass index percentage of total body weight (using a Tanita BC-418 MA body composition analyser), and recent activity levels. Activity levels were estimated from answers to specific questions on the bespoke participant questionnaire: participants were asked to put their perceived activity levels over the 7 days preceding the blood draw into one of five categories, ranging from "not active at all" to "very active". For some analyses, the two categories of activity at the extremes were merged, and the variable used had three resulting categories. The linearity assumption of covariates within the logistic regression models was assessed using generalised additive models (the "mgcv" package in R) [10]. The linearity assumption was satisfied in all models and so activity level was treated as an ordinal categorical variable when adjusting in multivariate analyses. To minimise potential type I errors, due to multiple testing, a Bonferroni-based threshold of $p <0.001$ was conservatively established (i.e., we divided the statistically significant level of 0.05 by the 29 number of individual laboratory tests that were compared, totalling 0.0017). We also used receiver operating characteristic (ROC) curves to assess whether the laboratory test results were able to discriminate people with ME/CFS (PWME) from healthy controls, or people with mild/moderate ME/CFS from those with severe symptoms. This type of analysis produces a curve chart that shows sensitivity vs. specificity, and the resulting area under the curve (AUC) represents how well a laboratory test can distinguish between two groups: diseased versus non-diseased, or having mild/moderate ME/CFS versus severe symptoms [9]. The ROC curves were calculated using the "pROC" package in R. All analyses were performed using Stata® version 15.1 or the R-statistical platform [10].

Ethics approval and consent to participate: Ethical approval was granted by the LSHTM Ethics Committee 16 January 2012 (Ref.6123) and the National Research Ethics Service (NRES) London—Bloomsbury Research Ethics Committee 22 December 2011 (REC ref.11/10/1760, IRAS ID: 77765). All biobank participants provided written consent for questionnaire, clinical measurement, and laboratory test data, and samples to be made available for ethically-approved research, after receiving an extensive information sheet and consent form, which includes an option to withdraw from the study at any time.

Availability of data and material: The datasets used and/or analysed during the current study are available upon request, from the UK ME/CFS Biobank UKMEB Steering Committee, who considers requests from data and/or biosamples, as per UKMEB protocols (https://cureme.lshtm.ac.uk/researchers/protocols-application-documents/).

3. Results

Table 1 shows the distribution of baseline variables by study group. The proportion of women was higher among cases, who were on average less active and had lower body muscle mass. Mild cases had the highest body mass index (BMI) compared to severe cases (lowest) and healthy controls (Table 1).

Table 1. Baseline characteristics of study participants.

Characteristic	Healthy Controls (n = 136) n (%)	Mild/Moderate ME/CFS Cases (n = 216) n (%)	Severe ME/CFS Cases (n = 56) n (%)	P-Value (hc/mm/sa)	P-Value (hc/me)
Female	84 (61.8)	166 (76.9)	43 (76.8)	0.006 [a]	0.001 [a]
Male	52 (38.2)	50 (23.1)	13 (23.2)		
Age (years)				0.900 [a]	0.900 [a]
18–29	23 (16.9)	34 (15.7)	10 (17.8)		
30–39	34 (25)	48 (22.3)	13 (23.2)		
40–49	35 (25.7)	64 (29.6)	12 (21.5)		
50–60	44 (32.4)	70 (32.4)	21 (37.5)		
Level of activity *				<0.0001 [a]	<0.0001 [a]
Very active	33 (25.2)	1 (0.6)	2 (3.5)		
Rather active	59 (45)	25 (12.3)	3 (5.3)		
Neither active nor inactive	22 (16.8)	49 (24.1)	3 (5.3)		
Rather inactive	16 (12.3)	91 (44.8)	15 (26.8)		
Not at all active	1 (0.7)	37 (18.2)	33 (59.1)		
Body mass index (mean) *	25.96	27.17	23.73	0.002 [b]	0.360 [b]
Body muscle (%) *	49.5	46.3	45.7	0.003 [b]	0.001 [b]

[a] χ^2 test; [b] ANOVA; p-values compare healthy controls with mild–moderate cases and with severe cases (penultimate column), and with all myalgic encephalomyelitis (ME) or chronic fatigue syndrome (CFS) cases (last column). * The number of participants with missing data on level of activity was 18 (5 healthy controls, 13 mild/moderate ME/CFS cases); 4 severely-affected ME/CFS cases were missing body mass index (BMI) data; and 5 severely-affected ME/CFS cases were missing data on body muscle. ME/CFS = Myalgic Encephalomyelitis/Chronic Fatigue Syndrome; hc = healthy controls, mm: ME/CFS mild/moderately affected; sa = ME/CFS severely affected; me = ME/CFS cases.

Nineteen biochemical and 10 haematological tests were performed across the participants (Tables 2 and 3). As expected, there were correlations between many of the test results (Spearman's Correlation: median 0.09; range 0.00–0.94), including between: (i) creatinine and urea, and of both with CK (range: 0.35–0.40); (ii) CK and aspartate aminotransferase (AST) (0.40); (iii) albumin and free T4, total protein and globulin (0.35–0.62); (iv) C-Reactive Protein (CRP) and Erythrocyte Sedimentation Rate (ESR) (0.47); (v) monocytes with white blood cells, lymphocytes and neutrophils (0.42–0.91) (Supplementary Figures S1 and S2). In Appendix B (Table A1) we present the reference ranges for the laboratory tests, analysed in this paper. The distributions of the analytes were compared between cases and controls (Table 2), and between severe and non-severe ME/CFS cases (Table 3). ESR, platelets, and CRP were raised in PWME, while CK and urea were reduced (Table 2; Wilcoxon rank sum $p < 0.01$). Compared with mild cases, those with severe disease had raised albumin, free T4 and serum folate, and lower CK, CRP, potassium, creatinine, and bilirubin (Table 3; Wilcoxon rank sum $p < 0.01$).

The reduced CK values were mainly due to low values of CK-MM isoenzyme, for which the mean was 44 U/L (interquartile range (IQR) = 24–86) in severe cases, compared to 73 (IQR = 37–94) in the mild/moderately affected and 90 (IQR = 41–238) in healthy controls ($p = 0.03$). CK-MB and aldolase values were also lowest in severely affected cases (Kruskal–Wallis p-values of 0.27 and 0.09, respectively). The ratio of CK-MB/CK-total was highest in the severe 0.26 (IQR = 0.18–0.39), compared to 0.20 (IQR = 0.10–0.32) in non-severe cases and 0.14 (IQR = 0.09–0.25) in healthy controls ($p = 0.03$), confirming the main contribution of reduced CK-MM values to the low concentration of total CK in cases, and particularly the severely affected (see also Tables 2 and 3). Total CK correlated very strongly with CK-MM ($r = 0.99$) in all study groups, but weaker correlations were found between total (CK) and CK-MB (from $r = 0.22$ in the severely affected, $r = 0.32$ in milder cases, and $r = 0.63$ in controls). This further demonstrates CK-MM as the main driver of reduced total CK concentrations in ME/CFS.

Table 2. Comparison of baseline laboratory haematological and biochemical test results from ME/CFS cases and healthy controls.

Assay	All Cases (n = 272) Median	IQR	Healthy Controls (n = 136) Median	IQR	Wilcoxon p [a]
WBC (10^9/L)	6.1	(5.2,7.3)	5.9	(5.1,6.8)	0.268
Platelets (10^9/L)	**262**	**(226,310)**	**247**	**(206,282)**	**<0.001**
Haemoglobin (g/L)	137	(129,148)	139	(130,149)	0.433
Haematocrit	0.412	(0.391,0.438)	0.418	(0.395,0.446)	0.165
Neutrophils (10^9/L)	3.47	(2.72,4.28)	3.28	(2.56,4.31)	0.374
Lymphocytes (10^9/L)	1.88	(1.61,2.30)	1.815	(1.525,2.140)	0.146
Monocytes (10^9/L)	0.43	(0.34,0.55)	0.43	(0.35,0.55)	0.869
Eosinophils (10^9/L)	0.135	(0.80,0.24)	0.14	(0.09,0.22)	0.701
Basophils (10^9/L)	0.03	(0.02,0.05)	0.03	(0.02,0.04)	0.923
ESR (mm/h)	**7**	**(4,12)**	**5**	**(2,8)**	**<0.001**
Sodium (mmol/L)	140	(139,142)	140	(139,142)	0.336
Potassium (mmol/L)	4.2	(4.0,4.4)	4.2	(4.0,4.4)	0.680
Urea (mmol/L)	**4.3**	**(3.5,5.1)**	**4.8**	**(3.9,5.7)**	**<0.001**
Creatinine (umol/L)	74	(67,85)	77	(66,88)	0.539
Adj. calcium (mmol/L)	2.36	(2.31,2.42)	2.37	(2.32,2.41)	0.900
Inorg. phosphate (mmol/L)	1.03	(0.90,1.16)	1.05	(0.93,1.14)	0.452
Total bilirubin (umol/L)	9	(7,11)	9	(7,13)	0.087
Albumin (g/L)	44	(41,47)	44	(41,47)	0.531
Globulins (g/L)	31	(29,32)	30	(28,32)	0.363
ALP (U/L)	67	(56,80)	63.5	(52,75)	0.055
AST (U/L)	20	(16,23)	20	(18,24)	0.247
Total protein (g/L)	73	(70,76)	72	(68,75)	0.023
CK (U/L)	**80**	**(56,107)**	**101.5**	**(76,152)**	**<0.001**
CK-MM (U/L) *	55	(28,100)	90.0	(41,238)	0.030
CK-MB (U/L) *	17	(14,22)	17	(14,23)	0.780
Aldolase *	3.8	(2.8,4.6)	4.0	(2.8,4.6)	0.620
CRP (mg/L)	2	(1,4)	1	(1,3)	0.007
Free T3 (pmol/L)	4.5	(4.1,4.9)	4.6	(4.2,5.1)	0.238
Free T4 (pmol/L)	14	(13,16)	14	(3,16)	0.242
TSH (mU/L)	1.6	(1.2,2.3)	1.62	(1.15,2.40)	0.637
Serum vitamin B12 (pg/mL)	388	(310,539)	379	(309,462)	0.164
Serum folate (ng/m)	8.6	(5.6,12.6)	9.0	(6.6,12.2)	0.313

[a] Wilcoxon rank sum test; * For CK isoenzymes CK-MM and CK-MB and aldolase, n = 50 cases and 25 controls. WBC = white blood cells; ESR = erythrocyte sedimentation rate; Adj. calcium = adjusted calcium; Inorg. phosphate = inorganic phosphate; ALP = alkaline phosphatase; AST = aspartate aminotransferase; CK = creatine kinase; CK-MM = CK produced in skeletal muscle; CK-MB = CK produced in heart muscle; CRP = C-reactive protein; TSH = thyroid stimulating hormone; IQR = interquartile range. In bold are variables ($p < 0.001$) carried forward for regression analysis.

Table 3. Comparison of baseline laboratory haematological and biochemical test results from severe and mild/moderate ME/CFS cases.

Assay	Severe Cases (n = 56) Median	IQR	Mild Cases (n = 216) Median	IQR	Wilcoxon p [a]
WBC (10^9/L)	5.85	(5.05,7.54)	6.11	(5.2,7.1)	0.744
Platelets (10^9/L)	254.5	(221,305)	266	(229,310)	0.585
Haemoglobin (g/L)	134	(126,144)	137.5	(130,149)	0.038
Haematocrit	0.405	(0.388,0.428)	0.413	(0.391,0.440)	0.156
Neutrophils (10^9/L)	3.44	(2.89,4.20)	3.485	(2.68,4.32)	0.856
Lymphocytes (10^9/L)	1.785	(1.59,2.05)	1.915	(1.62,2.32)	0.061
Monocytes (10^9/L)	0.46	(0.36,0.59)	0.425	(0.34,0.54)	0.078
Eosinophils (10^9/L)	0.165	(0.075,0.265)	0.13	(0.08,0.23)	0.366
Basophils (10^9/L)	0.03	(0.02,0.05)	0.03	(0.02,0.04)	0.697
ESR (mm/h)	5	(2,10)	7	(5,12)	0.057
Sodium (mmol/L)	141	(140,142)	140	(139,141)	0.015
Potassium (mmol/L)	4	(3.8,4.3)	4.2	(4.0,4.4)	**0.003**
Urea (mmol/L)	4.15	(3.4,5.1)	4.3	(3.5,5.2)	0.317
Creatinine (µmol/L)	65	(59,74)	78	(68,86)	**<0.001**
Adj. calcium (mmol/L)	2.35	(2.29,2.41)	2.37	(2.31,2.42)	0.048
Inorg. phosphate (mmol/L)	1.03	(0.93,1.16)	1.03	(0.89,1.16)	0.439
Total bilirubin (µmol/L)	7	(5,9)	9	(7,12)	**<0.001**
Albumin (g/L)	46	(44,49)	43	(40,46)	**<0.001**
Globulins (g/L)	29	(29,29)	31	(29,33)	0.542
ALP (U/L)	64	(54,80)	67	(56,81)	0.388
AST (U/L)	19	(16,22)	20.5	(16.5,24.0)	0.438
Total protein (g/L)	68	(68,68)	73	(70,76)	0.148
CK (U/L)	54	(45,78)	84	(63,113)	**<0.001**
CK-MM (U/L) *	44	(24,86)	73	(37,194)	0.030
CK-MB (U/L) *	16	(13,20)	19	(17,22)	0.080
Aldolase *	3.6	(2.5,4.0)	4.0	(2.8,4.6)	0.040
CRP (mg/L)	1	(1,5)	2	(2,6)	**<0.001**
Free T3 (pmol/L)	4.4	(4.1,4.7)	4.6	(4.2,4.9)	0.073
Free T4 (pmol/L)	16.1	(14.2,18.0)	14.0	(13.0,15.3)	**<0.001**
TSH (mU/L)	1.59	(1.14,2.28)	1.61	(1.16,2.40)	0.795
Serum vitamin B12 (pg/mL)	449	(333,659)	382	(305,532)	0.038
Serum folate (ng/m)	9.8	(8.0,14.7)	7.6	(5.0,12.6)	**0.002**

[a] Wilcoxon rank sum test; * For CK isoenzymes CK-MM and CK-MB and aldolase, 25 cases in each group. WBC = white blood cells; ESR = erythrocyte sedimentation rate; Adj. calcium = adjusted calcium; Inorg. phosphate = inorganic phosphate; ALP = alkaline phosphatase; AST = aspartate aminotransferase; CK = creatine kinase; CK-MM = CK produced in skeletal muscle; CK-MB = CK produced in heart muscle; CRP = C-reactive protein, TSH = thyroid stimulating hormone, IQR = interquartile range. In bold are variables ($p < 0.01$) carried forward for regression analysis.

Table 4 shows results of the multivariate logistic regression, from which (ln) CK levels were shown to be inversely associated with the risk of being a ME/CFS case compared with being a healthy control (odds ratio (OR) 0.36; $p < 0.001$). The same analysis focusing on severe cases (vs. controls) revealed elevated risks associated with lower (ln) bilirubin (OR 0.23; $p < 0.001$) and lower (ln) CK (OR 0.05; $p < 0.001$), as well as with higher albumin (OR 1.20; $p < 0.001$) and T4 (OR 1.42; $p < 0.001$). Similarly, lower levels of creatinine (OR 0.91; $p < 0.001$), (ln) bilirubin (OR 0.15; $p < 0.001$) and (ln) CK (OR 0.16; $p < 0.001$) were associated with increased risk of severe compared to mild ME/CFS. Consistent with the above, increased albumin levels were associated with greater risk of being a severe compared to a mild case (OR 1.25; $p < 0.001$).

Table 4. Laboratory test results in ME/CFS cases and healthy controls (adjusted analysis ***).

	Assay	Odds Ratio	(95% CI)	p-Value
ME/CFS cases vs. healthy controls	Platelets	1.01	(1.00–1.01)	0.007
	Urea	0.78	(0.65–0.94)	0.008
	CK *	0.36	(0.23–0.57)	<0.001
	CRP *	1.37	(0.99–1.90)	0.059
	ERS **	1.33	(1.04–1.71)	0.023
Severe ME/CFS cases vs. healthy controls	Urea	0.71	(0.53–0.96)	0.027
	Creatinine	0.95	(0.91–0.98)	0.001
	Bilirubin *	0.23	(0.10–0.52)	**<0.001**
	Albumin	1.20	(1.08–1.33)	**<0.001**
	CK *	0.05	(0.02–0.15)	**<0.001**
	T4	1.42	(1.21–1.66)	**<0.001**
	Vit. B12 *	4.12	(1.64–10.36)	0.0026
Severe ME/CFS cases vs. mild/moderate ME/CFS cases ****	Potassium	0.38	(0.13–1.13)	0.082
	Creatinine	0.91	(0.87–0.94)	**<0.001**
	Bilirubin *	0.15	(0.06–0.36)	**<0.001**
	Albumin	1.25	(1.13–1.38)	**<0.001**
	CK *	0.16	(0.07–0.40)	**<0.001**
	CRP *	0.56	(0.32–0.97)	0.040
	T4	1.26	(1.09–1.45)	0.0014
	Folate *	1.83	(0.98–3.40)	0.058

* ln transformed; ** Square-root transformed; *** Adjusted for sex, age-group, BMI, and muscle mass, current physical activity level; **** Further adjusted for disease duration; ME/CFS = Myalgic Encephalomyelitis/Chronic Fatigue Syndrome; ESR = erythrocyte sedimentation rate, CK = creatine kinase, CRP = C-reactive protein. Bolded text signifies $p < 0.001$.

Across the analyses, differences in CK were the most consistent; there were marked differences between cases and healthy controls, with severe cases having much lower levels than mild/moderate cases or healthy controls (Figure 1a). By refitting the different outcome models either with urea, creatinine, bilirubin, albumin, T4 and CK, or with CK alone, we could estimate the value of CK as a potential marker for ME/CFS (Figure 1b). The ROC curve analysis for routine serum CK had a limited role in distinguishing ME/CFS cases from healthy controls (AUC = 67%) but had a potential role in distinguishing severely affected participants with ME/CFS from those with mild/moderate ME/CFS (AUC = 75%) and from healthy controls (AUC = 84%) (Figure 1b). A full model adding CK, bilirubin, albumin, T4, creatinine, and CRP, improved predictions, particularly when severe cases were compared to non-severe cases and healthy controls (AUC = 91%; improvement over CK alone $p \ll 0.001$), and a reduced model of CK, bilirubin, albumin and T4 (based on Table 4) had similar performance (AUC = 90%).

We found a cut-off value of 51 U/L for serum CK to have high sensitivity for both ME/CFS groups of severity compared to controls (sensitivity = 96%), and for severe ME/CFS cases compared to mild/moderate cases (sensitivity = 88.7%). However, these have low specificity (<50%).

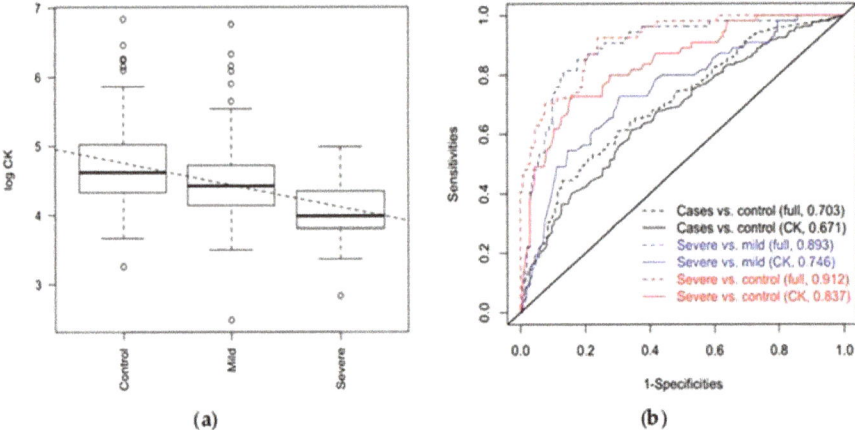

Figure 1. (a) Levels of CK and disease outcome. CK was measured in healthy controls $n = 136$, mild/moderate ME/CFS cases $n = 216$, and severe ME/CFS cases $n = 56$. Intercept 5.07411 (se 0.07907, $p < 0.001$); slope-0.31797 (se 0.04120, $p = 0.001$). (b) ROC curves showing the predictability of a "full" model (including urea, creatinine, bilirubin, albumin, CK, T4; dashed lined) vs CK alone (solid line); areas under the curve (AUC) are presented in the legend. CK = creatine kinase; ME/CFS = Myalgic Encephalomyelitis/Chronic Fatigue Syndrome; ROC = Receiver Operating Curves.

Considering the strong association between activity levels and participant category—either case or control ($p < 0.0001$)—we explored further the association between ln CK values and participant category in three different strata of activity levels, i.e., "not at all active or rather inactive", "neither active nor inactive", and "rather active or very active". The results presented in Table 5, show clear trends towards lower CK values in cases, particularly as those severely-affected are compared with healthy controls. The highest significant levels are seen in those who declared they have been inactive ($p < 0.001$).

Table 5. Median total CK (IQR) according to reported activity levels *.

	Inactive ($n = 190$)	Average ($n = 72$)	Active ($n = 121$)
Healthy controls ($n = 129$)	76(70,157)	98(66,152)	110(84,153)
Mild/moderate ME/CFS cases ($n = 199$)	82(61,110)	92 (68,143)	85(73,108)
Severe ME/CFS cases ($n = 55$)	52(45,77)	46 (44,78)	60(46,91)
p-value **	<0.001	0.200	0.020

* Association between activity levels and case category (chi-squared test) $p < 0.0001$; ** p-value for Kruskal–Wallis statistics comparing CK in healthy controls, mild-moderate, and severe cases within each activity level group.

4. Discussion

Routine laboratory tests are usually reported as normal in PWME, when they are used to exclude other illnesses causing chronic fatigue. Among the routine laboratory tests for ME/CFS is serum CK, with studies typically reporting CK results within normal ranges if, indeed, they are reported [11,12]. We found that PWME had lower CK levels than healthy controls, and that CK was significantly lower in people with severe ME/CFS compared to those who were mild/moderately affected. The associations persisted after adjusting for sex, age-group, BMI, muscle mass, or recent physical activity levels (all of which potentially affect CK concentrations in serum [13,14]), as well as disease duration where appropriate (i.e., when comparing cases of differing severity levels). Creatinine and bilirubin were also found to be significantly lower in severely-affected patients compared to mild/moderate cases, while albumin was higher in severe cases. There was a trend towards higher levels of CRP and ESR in ME/CFS, and particularly in those with mild/moderate disease. CK levels were found to be good predictors of severe ME/CFS cases as compared to those who were less severely-affected or healthy controls; this was enhanced by the inclusion of other laboratory tests results in the model.

4.1. The Physiological and Clinical Importance of CK

CK is a key enzyme involved in energy production and homeostasis processes, particularly in tissues with highly dynamic and fluctuating energy demands which must be quickly satisfied, such as the brain, skeletal muscle, and heart [15]. It is also present in many other cells, such as immune and epithelial cells, where it also plays a crucial role in energy production [16,17].

Cellular energy is mainly generated from the breakdown of the high-energy molecule, adenosine triphosphate (ATP). Although the complex mechanisms of cellular energy balance are not fully understood, there is evidence that muscle cells depend on several processes to increase energy availability and to avoid complete energy depletion by drawing on stores of ATP. CK plays a crucial role in these processes: firstly, by establishing an efficient cytosolic storage of high-energy phosphates for rapid ATP replenishment [13], it catalyses the relocation of γ-phosphate from ATP to creatine to generate phosphocreatine and adenosine diphosphate (ADP), in a reversible process [18]; and secondly, it is involved in the transfer of high-energy phosphate from the mitochondria to the muscle cell cytoplasm, where it is used during muscle contraction [19]. Thus, measures of CK in serum may indicate the availability of cellular energy [13].

CK serum concentrations are widely used to diagnose and monitor a range of muscle diseases when high levels are clinically relevant. CK levels are known to increase with muscle injury and inflammation [13], and may also be high in hypothyroid myopathy and secondary to treatment with statins [14]; increased levels of serum CK can be seen in trained athletes and in individuals after extreme exercise [20]. There are three types of CK, called isoenzymes: CK-MM (found in muscle and raised in many muscle diseases), CK-MB (present in heart muscle in particular), and CK-BB (found mostly in the brain but usually undetectable in peripheral blood) [13]. CK-MB used to be widely used in the diagnosis of ischaemic heart disease, though it has now been superseded by other disease markers [21].

Low serum CK concentrations have been reported less frequently, but they may be of clinical significance in some rheumatological [22,23] and connective tissue diseases [24]. The causes and significance of these findings are unclear, but it has been suggested that serum CK may be inversely related to inflammatory processes [24,25], and low CK levels have been associated with muscle weakness, independently of muscle atrophy [23]. A study on patients with severe renal failure reported a significant association between lower serum CK and an increased risk of death, and suggested that their serological findings might be explained by the patients' wasted muscle mass and poor nutritional status [26], but there was no subsequent suggestion of using serum CK for diagnosis or management of these conditions. In studies on Huntington's disease, a severe degenerative neurological disease [27], it has been suggested that reduced brain energy may result from the reduced activity of the CK system, and that loss of CK-BB may be an important unrecognized biomarker of this disease.

The low concentrationsof serum CK found in people with ME/CFS suggests an abnormality in energy metabolism, which have been reported by distinct authors (e.g., references [28–32]) and could explain the intolerance to exertion commonly reported by patients, and consequent reduction in activity levels [2]. An alternative or additional explanation is that the lower serum CK resulted, at least partially, from physical inactivity. Nevertheless, the persistent significant association between lower serum CK and disease severity in the multivariate model that controls for activity suggests that these results cannot be fully explained by reduced physical activity, but that there are other factors involved. To explore further a potential confounding role of activity levels, we compared median serum values of CK in different strata of activity category. The values were reduced in severely affected cases in all strata Nevertheless, the potential for residual confounding is still present, and differential misclassification on activity levels, with over-estimation of activity in severe ME/CFS cases, remains a possible (and at least partial) explanation, for the difference in the levels of CK observed. However, with the increasing number of reports on energy metabolism abnormalities in people with ME/CFS, further exploration of this association is warranted.

In addition to intolerance to physical exercise, patients with ME/CFS usually also report mental fatigue and "brain fog", as well as subjective muscle weakness [2,4,33]. Considering the importance of CK in both muscle and brain metabolism, the low concentrations of this enzyme could, at least partially, explain those symptoms.

Some researchers have previously reported intriguing findings on serum CK in PWME. For example, two studies with 30 and 33 individuals, compared the CK serum concentration of ME/CFS patients (diagnosed by the CDC-1994 criteria [3]) with those of healthy controls before and after exercise, in order to evaluate physical capacity [34,35]. The mean CK in PWME was lower, though not significantly, than in controls, and did not increase with exertion in those with ME/CFS (as seen in healthy individuals). The results suggests that lack of acute physical effort was not the main factor determining CK levels in PWME [34,35]. Another study on PWME found higher serum CK in participants with enterovirus-specific RNA detected in muscle by biopsy, than in those with no evidence of enteroviral infections. That study suggested that a sub-group of PWME might have muscle damage secondary to enterovirus infection, but unfortunately, the authors did not specify the concentrations of CK in the group of patients with lower values [36].

Other studies have considered possible mitochondrial function impairment in ME/CFS, which reinforces the plausibility of metabolic dysfunction in the energy system (e.g., references [28–30]) as our findings indicate.

4.2. Other Study Findings

Creatinine levels were found to be significantly lower in severe ME/CFS. Creatine phosphate (CP) is converted to creatinine in muscle and creatinine is excreted in urine [13], so low CP resulting from poor conversion of creatine to CP by CK could explain the low levels of creatinine found in severe ME/CFS. Low urine concentration of creatinine have also been reported [37].

We also found that urea was reduced and platelets, CRP and ESR increased in PWME, although this was not significant in the multivariate analysis. An inverse relationship between platelets and CK was found in one study on rheumatoid arthritis, together with increases in inflammatory clinical markers such as ESR and CRP [25]. Platelets also tend to increase in inflammatory processes [38]. Nevertheless, the pattern of inflammatory markers in our study leads us to speculate that some degree of inflammation may be related to symptoms in people with mild/moderate ME/CFS. For people with severe disease, it seems that the inflammatory response may have been inhibited, either due to a lack of a persistent stimuli or to impairment of some aspects of the inflammatory response, which may indicate chronic disease with established complications. However, it is important to note that changes in inflammatory markers were relatively modest, and any further assumptions would need to be appropriately tested and confirmed in a further set of samples. We found lower levels of urea in mild/moderate cases, but not in those who were severely-affected. This could relate to creatinine levels, which were also lower in ME/CFS compared to controls; however, for creatinine, the lowest values were present in the most severely-affected. Abnormalities in the urea cycle have been reported in ME/CFS (e.g., [39,40])

Other findings including raised albumin and T4 are more difficult to explain. Raised albumin suggests malnutrition is not a main factor in ME/CFS in this study. The mildly raised T4 could suggest minor changes related to thyroid hormone metabolism, such as in its peripheral conversion, as previously suggested [41]. However, this hypothesis was not corroborated by other findings, which showed similar T3 and TSH levels between the groups, neither do our findings are typical of euthyroid sick syndrome. A higher prevalence of Gilbert's syndrome in ME/CFS has been proposed in the past [42], but this was not found in this study, which showed similar bilirubin levels in cases and controls, with reduced bilirubin levels in people with severe ME/CFS compared to non-severe cases.

Further investigations with a larger sample size and more detailed explorations of metabolic pathways will be needed to confirm whether low CK activity is a primary or secondary event in ME/CFS or, indeed, whether it reflects some other metabolic dysfunction. This could benefit from the use of "diseased" controls groups, such as selected orthopaedic patients with prolonged immobility. Meanwhile, we suggest that CK could be used as a potential marker of severe ME/CFS. It is important to consider the clinical history and physical examination findings, as well as measures of activity (e.g., outputs from accelerometers) at the time of the blood draws for serum CK. Moreover, a "high-normal" result in people who are often sedentary or bedbound, particularly those with severe ME/CFS, should be interpreted with caution, as it could indicate the presence of muscle injury.

4.3. Study Strengths and Limitations

The study investigated a group of people with well-characterised ME/CFS using robust standards of data and sample collection as described in the UK ME/CFS Biobank protocol [6]. In terms of ME/CFS research, this was a large sample: 272 PWME were tested, including 56 who were severely-affected. However, the assessment of activity level was by self-report [6]. If this resulted in overestimation of activity levels in some groups, then differential misclassification may have resulted e.g., if the less active and the severely-affected ME/CFS cases may have overestimated their activity levels [43].

The inclusion of severely-affected ME/CFS participants, typically absent from most previous studies, may have been key to demonstrating abnormalities not previously reported. The results presented here come from routine laboratory tests in PWME and healthy controls. The purpose of the blood tests was primarily to exclude other diseases which could present with similar symptoms; the examination of muscle-related biochemical abnormalities was not in response to a specific hypothesis but was noted when all results were examined to test null hypotheses of no group differences between study groups in laboratory test findings. This means that we were not able to examine abnormalities in muscle/energy metabolism in more detail. However, our ability to investigate our findings further, e.g., through enhanced metabolomic studies and by accessing additional biobanked samples from the cohort, including at different time-points, will be instrumental in further understanding the changes reported here.

5. Conclusions

This is the first study to find significant lower concentrations of CK in PWME. Some indications of low CK values seem to have been overlooked previously when the trend towards lower values was discarded as not significant and was not investigated further. A single measurement of serum CK may not have enough sensitivity and specificity to be used as a biomarker for ME/CFS diagnosis, but, used alongside other clinical and laboratory markers, routine CK blood tests could not only help to diagnose ME/CFS accurately, but also to sub-group cases according to disease severity. It could potentially also be used as a prognostic marker, and as an outcome measurement for observational studies and clinical trials, as well as in clinical practice, pending further longitudinal studies examining the correlation of clinical and laboratory-based phenotypes over time. Whether people with severe ME/CFS featuring low CK constitute a unique sub-group of patients with distinct patterns of biochemical/pathophysiological abnormalities and symptoms, or whether they represent a different phase or an extreme spectrum of the disease, still needs to be clarified.

Our findings give significant support to the growing body of evidence on metabolic abnormalities in ME/CFS, and we suggest further adequately-powered studies that include a fuller investigation of specific metabolic pathways to elucidate whether CK is a primary or secondary abnormality in all or in a sub-group of ME/CFS cases. Such studies should also help to elucidate the causes of such abnormalities. Correlating serum CK concentrations with objectively measured activity levels and other energy metabolism parameters could lead to a better understanding of the pathophysiological abnormalities involved in muscle use and recovery, and their relationship to symptoms such as post-exertional malaise and fatigue.

Supplementary Materials: The following are available online at http://www.mdpi.com/2075-4418/9/2/41/s1. Figure S1: (Absolute) Spearman's correlations between laboratory tests across all samples; Figure S2: Laboratory tests across all samples.

Author Contributions: L.N. conceptualised the study, carried out the analysis, and drafted the manuscript. B.d.B. was involved in the literature review, analysis, and manuscript drafting. E.M.L. and T.G.C. were involved in the analysis, and with all other co-authors (L.N., B.d.B., C.C.K., J.M.C., H.M.D., K.M.) critically revised the manuscript and approved the final version to be published.

Funding: All authors are funded by the National Institutes of Health (NIH/NIAID, Grant R01AI103629). E.M.L., C.C.K. and L.N. are also funded by the ME Association (Grant PF8947_ME Association). T.G.C. is also funded by the Medical Research Council UK (Grants MR/K000551/1, MR/M01360X/1, MR/N010469/1, and MC_PC_15103). The content is solely the responsibility of the authors and does not necessarily represent the official views of the National Institutes of Health.

Acknowledgments: We wish to thank the participants in the UK ME/CFS Biobank and this study, and all those who contributed to the selection, recruitment and assessment of participants. We thank C. Armstrong for reviewing a paper draft.

Conflicts of Interest: The authors declare no conflict of interest.

Abbreviations

ACTN2	actinin alpha 2
ADP	adenosine diphosphate
ALP	alkaline phosphatase
ATP	adenosine triphosphate
AUC	Area Under the Curve
BMI	body mass index
CDK8	cyclin-dependent kinase 8
CI	Confidence Interval
CK	creatine kinase
CK-MM	skeletal muscle expressed-CK
CK-MB	and muscle/brain expressed-CK
CP	creatinine phosphate
CRP	C-reactive protein
ESR	erythrocyte sedimentation rate
HC	healthy controls
ME/CFS	Myalgic Encephalomyelitis/Chronic Fatigue Syndrome
NHS	National Health Service (UK)
OR	odds ratio
PWME	people with ME/CFS
RNA	ribonucleic acid
ROC curve	receiver operating characteristic curve
UKMEB	UK ME/CFS Biobank
WBC	white blood cells

Appendix A

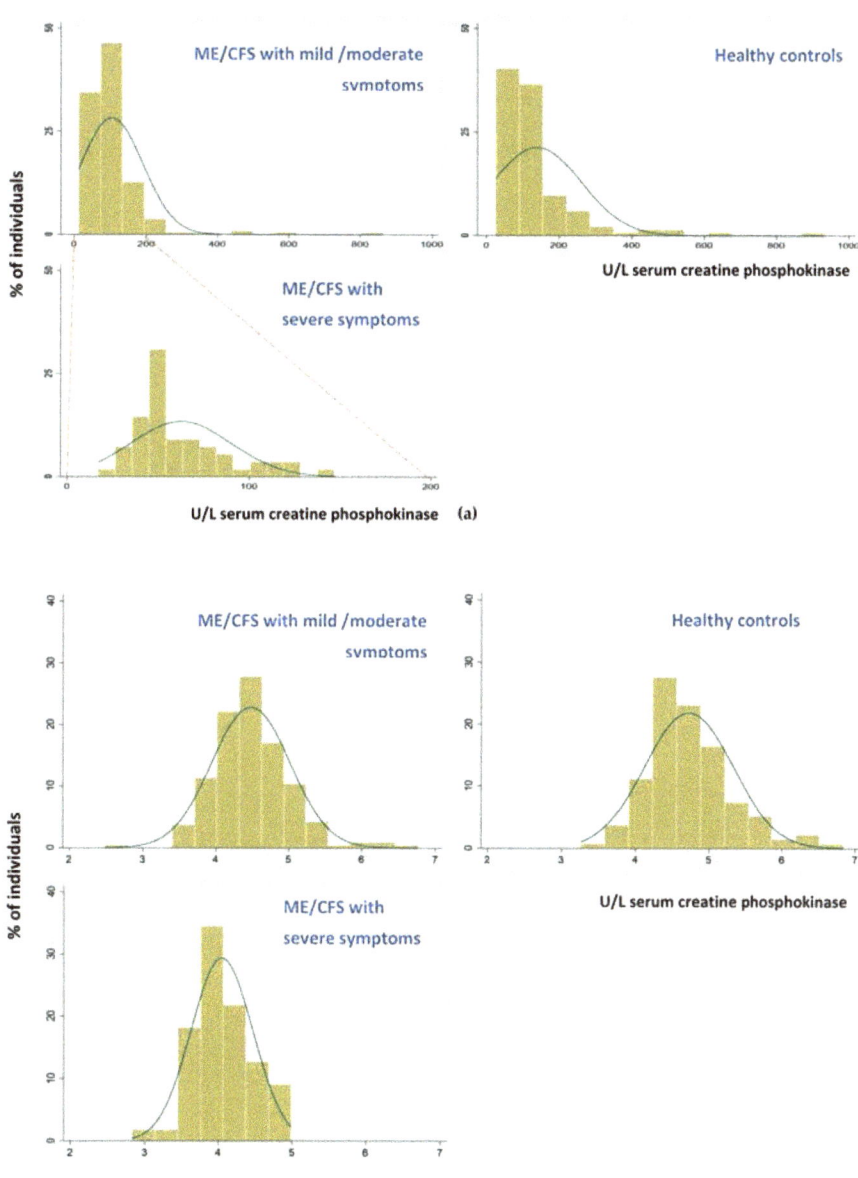

Figure A1. Histograms of serum creatine phosphokinase (CK) results from the UK ME/CFS Biobank participants, by category of recruitment. (**a**) Distribution of CK results (U/L); (**b**) Distribution of transformed lnCK.

Appendix B

Table A1. Blood tests reference ranges used by NHS laboratories.

Blood Tests	Normal Ranges [1]
White blood count (WBC)	$(3.5–11.0) \times 10^9$/L
Platelets (PLT)	$(140–400) \times 10^9$/L
Haemoglobin	110–150 g/L
Haematocrit	0.34–0.50 L/L
Neutrophils	$(1.7–7.5) \times 10^9$/L
Lymphocytes	$(1.0–4.0) \times 10^9$/L
Monocytes	$(0.2–1.5) \times 10^9$/L
Eosinophils	$(0.0–0.5) \times 10^9$/L
Basophils	$(0.0–0.1) \times 10^9$/L
Erythrocyte Sedimentation Rate (ESR)	0–20 mm/h
Sodium	135–145 mmol/L
Potassium	3.5–5.1 mmol/L
Urea	2.1–7.1 mmol/L
Creatinine	49–92 µmol/L
Adjusted calcium	2.20–2.60 mmol/L
Inorganic phosphate	0.80–1.45 mmol/L
Total bilirubin	<21 µmol/L
Albumin	35–50 g/L
Globulins	21–35 g/L
Alkaline Phosphatase (ALP)	<129 U/L
Aspartate aminotransferase (AST)	<31 U/L
Total protein	63–82 g/L
Creatine phosphokinase (CK)	<320 U/L
C Reactive protein (CRP)	0–5 mg/L
Free T3	3.8–6.0
Free T4	12.0–22.0 pmol/L
Thyroid stimulant hormone (TSH)	0.30–4.20 mU/L
Serum vitamin B12	160–925 ng/L
Serum folate	>2.9 µg/L
Aldolase	1–7.5 U/L

[1] Normal reference ranges applied by the specific NHS laboratories, from the NHS collaboration hospitals, i.e., Royal Free Hospital and Norfolk and Norwich University Hospital in the UK.

References

1. WHO. *ICD-10: International Classification of Statistical Classification of Diseases and Related Health Problems*; World Health Organization: Geneva, Switzerland, 2001.
2. Carruthers, B.M.; Jain, A.K.; De Meirleir, K.L.; Peterson, D.; Klimas, N.G.; Lerner, A.M.; Bested, A.C.; Flor-Henry, P.; Joshi, P.; Powles, A.C.P.; et al. Myalgic Encephalomyelitis/Chronic Fatigue Syndrome: Clinical Working Case Definition, Diagnostic and Treatment Protocols. *J. Chronic Fatigue Syndr.* **2003**, *11*, 7–36. [CrossRef]
3. Fukuda, K.; Straus, S.E.; Hickie, I.; Sharpe, M.C.; Dobbins, J.G.; Komaroff, A. The chronic fatigue syndrome: A comprehensive approach to its definition and study. International Chronic Fatigue Syndrome Study Group. *Ann. Intern. Med.* **1994**, *121*, 953–959. [CrossRef] [PubMed]
4. Institute of Medicine (IOM). *Beyond Myalgic Encephalomyelitis/Chronic Fatigue Syndrome: Redefining an Illness*; The National Academies Press: Washington, DC, USA, 2015.
5. Carruthers, B.M.; van de Sande, M.I.; De Meirleir, K.L.; Klimas, N.G.; Broderick, G.; Mitchell, T.; Staines, D.; Powles, A.C.; Speight, N.; Vallings, R.; et al. Myalgic encephalomyelitis: International Consensus Criteria. *J. Intern. Med.* **2011**, *270*, 327–338. [CrossRef] [PubMed]

6. Lacerda, E.M.; Bowman, E.W.; Cliff, J.M.; Kingdon, C.C.; King, E.C.; Lee, J.-S.S.; Clark, T.G.; Dockrell, H.M.; Riley, E.M.; Curran, H.; et al. The UK ME/CFS Biobank for biomedical research on Myalgic Encephalomyelitis/Chronic Fatigue Syndrome (ME/CFS) and Multiple Sclerosis. *Open J. Bioresour.* **2017**, *4*, 4. [CrossRef] [PubMed]
7. University College London. Human Tissue—UCL and associated NHS Trust HTA-licensed Biobanks. 2018. Available online: https://www.ucl.ac.uk/human-tissue/hta-biobanks/UCL-HTA-licensed-Biobanks (accessed on 14 March 2019).
8. NHS Digital. NHS National Laboratory Medicine Catalogue. 2018. Available online: https://isd.digital.nhs.uk/trud3/user/guest/group/0/pack/25/subpack/77/releases (accessed on 26 March 2019).
9. Kirkwood, B.R.; Sterne, J.A.C. *Essential Medical Statistics*, 2nd ed.; Blackwell: Oxford, UK, 2003.
10. R Development Core Team. *R: A Language and Environment for Statistical Computing*; R Foundation for Statistical Computing: Vienna, Austria, 2010; Available online: https://www.r-project.org/ (accessed on 26 March 2019).
11. Bates, D.W.; Buchwald, D.; Lee, J.; Kith, P.; Doolittle, T.; Rutherford, C.; Churchill, W.H.; Schur, P.H.; Wener, M.; Wybenga, D.; et al. Clinical Laboratory Test Findings in Patients With Chronic Fatigue Syndrome. *Arch. Intern. Med.* **1995**, *155*, 97–103.
12. Swanink, C.; Vercoulen, J.H.M.M.; Bleijenberg, G.; Fennis, J.F.M.; Galama, J.M.D.; van der Meer, J.W.M. Chronic fatigue syndrome: A clinical and laboratory study with a well matched control group. *J. Intern. Med.* **1995**, *237*, 499–506. [CrossRef]
13. Baird, M.F.; Graham, S.M.; Baker, J.S.; Bickerstaff, G.F. Creatine-kinase- and exercise-related muscle damage implications for muscle performance and recovery. *J. Nutr. Metab.* **2012**, *2012*, 960363. [CrossRef]
14. Brewster, L.M.; Mairuhu, G.; Sturk, A.; van Montfrans, G.A. Distribution of creatine kinase in the general population: Implications for statin therapy. *Am. Hear. J.* **2007**, *154*, 655–661. [CrossRef]
15. Wallimann, T.; Wyss, M.; Brdiczka, D.; Nicolay, K.; Eppenberger, H.M. Intracellular compartmentation, structure and function of creatine kinase isoenzymes in tissues with high and fluctuating energy demands: The "phosphocreatine circuit" for cellular energy homeostasis. *Biochem. J.* **1992**, *281 Pt 1*, 21–40. [CrossRef]
16. Kitzenberg, D.; Colgan, S.P.; Glover, L.E. Creatine kinase in ischemic and inflammatory disorders. *Clin. Transl. Med.* **2016**, *5*, 31. [CrossRef]
17. Wallimann, T.; Hemmer, W. Creatine kinase in non-muscle tissues and cells. *Mol. Cell Biochem.* **1994**, *133–134*, 193–220. [CrossRef]
18. Baker, J.S.; McCormick, M.C.; Roberg, R.A. Interaction among Skeletal Muscle Metabolic Energy Systems during Intense Exercise. *J Nutr Metab.* **2010**, *2010*, 905612. [CrossRef]
19. Bessman, S.P.; Carpenter, C.L. THE CREATINE-CREATINE PHOSPHATE ENERGY SHUTTLE. 1985. Available online: www.annualreviews.org (accessed on 26 March 2019).
20. Young, A. Plasma creatine kinase after the marathon-a diagnostic dilemma. *Brit. J. Sports Med.* **1984**, *18*, 269–272. [CrossRef]
21. Antman, E.; Bassand, J.-P.; Klein, W.; Ohman, M.; Lopez Sendon, J.L.; Rydén, L.; Simoons, M.; Tendera, M. Myocardial infarction redefined—A consensus document of The Joint European Society of Cardiology/American College of Cardiology committee for the redefinition of myocardial infarction: The Joint European Society of Cardiology/American College of Cardiology Committee. *J. Am. Coll. Cardiol.* **2000**, *36*, 959–969.
22. Lee, Y.H.; Choi, S.J.; Ji, J.D.; Song, G.G. Serum creatine kinase in patients with rheumatic diseases. *Clin. Rheumatol.* **2000**, *19*, 296–300. [CrossRef]
23. Stucki, G.; Brühlmann, P.; Stoll, T.; Stucki, S.; Willer, B.; Michel, B.A. Low serum creatine kinase activity is associated with muscle weakness in patients with rheumatoid arthritis. *J. Rheumatol.* **1996**, *23*, 603–608.
24. Wei, N.; Pavlidis, N.; Tsokos, G.; Elin, R.J.; Plotz, P.H. Clinical Significance of Low Creatine Phosphokinase Values in Patients With Connective Tissue Diseases. *J. Am. Med. Assoc.* **1981**, *246*, 1921. [CrossRef]
25. Sanmartí, R.; Collado, A.; Gratacós, J.; Bedini, J.L.; Pañella, D.; Filella, X.; Llena, J.; Muñoz-Gomez, J. Reduced activity of serum creatine kinase in rheumatoid arthritis: A phenomenon linked to the inflammatory response. *Br. J. Rheumatol.* **1994**, *33*, 231–234. [CrossRef] [PubMed]
26. Flahault, A.; Metzger, M.; Chasse, J.F.; Haymann, J.P.; Boffa, J.J.; Flamant, M.; Vrtovsnik, F.; Houillier, P.; Stengel, B.; Thervet, E.; et al. Low Serum Creatine Kinase Level Predicts Mortality in Patients with a Chronic Kidney Disease. *PLoS ONE* **2016**, *11*, e0156433. [CrossRef] [PubMed]

27. Kim, J.; Amante, D.J.; Moody, J.P.; Edgerly, C.K.; Bordiuk, O.L.; Smith, K.; Matson, S.A.; Matson, W.R.; Scherzer, C.R.; Rosas, H.D.; et al. Reduced creatine kinase as a central and peripheral biomarker in Huntington's disease. *Biochim. Biophys. Acta.* **2010**, *1802*, 673–681. [CrossRef] [PubMed]
28. Vernon, S.D.; Whistler, T.; Cameron, B.; Hickie, I.B.; Reeves, W.C.; Lloyd, A. Preliminary evidence of mitochondrial dysfunction associated with post-infective fatigue after acute infection with Epstein Barr virus. *BMC Infect. Dis.* **2006**, *6*, 15. [CrossRef]
29. Schoeman, E.M.; Van Der Westhuizen, F.H.; Erasmus, E.; van Dyk, E.; Knowles, C.V.; Al-Ali, S.; Ng, W.F.; Taylor, R.W.; Newton, J.L.; Elson, J.L. Clinically proven mtDNA mutations are not common in those with chronic fatigue syndrome. *BMC Med. Genet.* **2017**, *18*, 29. [CrossRef]
30. Tomas, C.; Brown, A.; Strassheim, V.; Elson, J.; Newton, J.; Manning, P. Cellular bioenergetics is impaired in patients with chronic fatigue syndrome. *PLoS ONE* **2017**, *12*, e0186802. [CrossRef]
31. Armstrong, C.W.; McGregor, N.R.; Lewis, D.P.; Butt, H.L.; Gooley, P.R. Metabolic profiling reveals anomalous energy metabolism and oxidative stress pathways in chronic fatigue syndrome patients. *Metabolomics* **2015**, *11*, 1626–1639. [CrossRef]
32. Germain, A.; Ruppert, D.; Levine, S.M.; Hanson, M.R. Metabolic profiling of a myalgic encephalomyelitis/chronic fatigue syndrome discovery cohort reveals disturbances in fatty acid and lipid metabolism. *Mol. Biosyst.* **2017**, *12*, 371–379. [CrossRef]
33. Gandevia, S. Spinal and Supraspinal Factors in Human Muscle Fatigue. *Physiol. Rev.* **2001**, *81*, 1725–1789. [CrossRef]
34. Riley, M.S.; O'Brien, C.J.; McCluskey, D.R.; Bell, N.P.; Nicholls, D.P. Aerobic work capacity in patients with chronic fatigue syndrome. *BMJ* **1990**, *301*, 953–956. [CrossRef]
35. Vermeulen, R.C.W.; Kurk, R.M.; Visser, F.C.; Sluiter, W.; Scholte, H.R. Patients with chronic fatigue syndrome performed worse than controls in a controlled repeated exercise study despite a normal oxidative phosphorylation capacity. *J. Transl. Med.* **2010**, *8*, 93. [CrossRef]
36. Archard, C.; Bowles, N.; Behan, P.; Bell, E.; Doyle, D. Postviral fatigue syndrome: persistence of enterovirus RNA in muscle and elevated creatine kinase. *J. Royal Soc. Med.* **1988**, *81*, 326–329. [CrossRef]
37. Lidbury, B.A.; Kita, B.; Lewis, D.P.; Hayward, S.; Ludlow, H.; Hedger, M.P.; de Kretser, D.M. Activin B is a novel biomarker for chronic fatigue syndrome/myalgic encephalomyelitis (CFS/ME) diagnosis: A cross sectional study. *J. Transl. Med.* **2017**, *15*, 1–10. [CrossRef]
38. Shattil, S.J.; Newman, P.J. Integrins: Dynamic scaffolds for adhesion and signaling in platelets. *Blood* **2004**, *104*, 1606–1615. [CrossRef]
39. Yamano, E.; Sugimoto, M.; Hirayama, A.; Kume, S.; Yamato, M.; Jin, G.; Tajima, S.; Goda, N.; Iwai, K.; Fukuda, S. Index markers of chronic fatigue syndrome with dysfunction of TCA and urea cycles. *Sci. Rep.* **2016**, *6*, 34990. [CrossRef]
40. Armstrong, C.W.; McGregor, N.R.; Butt, H.L.; Gooley, P.R. Metabolism in chronic fatigue syndrome. *Adv. Clin. Chem.* **2014**, *66*, 121–172.
41. Ruiz-Núñez, B.; Tarasse, R.; Vogelaar, E.F.; Dijck-Brouwer, D.A.J.; Muskiet, F.A.J. Higher prevalence of "low T3 syndrome" in patients with chronic fatigue syndrome: A case-control study. *Front. Endocrinol.* **2018**, *9*, 1–13. [CrossRef]
42. Cleary, K.J.; White, P.D. Gilbert's and chronic fatigue syndromes in men. *Lancet* **1993**, *341*, 842. [CrossRef]
43. Ronda, G.; van Assema, P.; Brug, J. Stages of change, psychological factors and awareness of physical activity levels in the Netherlands. *Health Promot. Int.* **2001**, *16*, 305–314. [CrossRef]

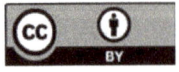

© 2019 by the authors. Licensee MDPI, Basel, Switzerland. This article is an open access article distributed under the terms and conditions of the Creative Commons Attribution (CC BY) license (http://creativecommons.org/licenses/by/4.0/).

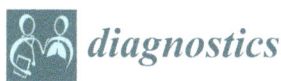

Article

Rethinking ME/CFS Diagnostic Reference Intervals via Machine Learning, and the Utility of Activin B for Defining Symptom Severity

Brett A. Lidbury [1,*], Badia Kita [2], Alice M. Richardson [1], Donald P. Lewis [3], Edwina Privitera [3], Susan Hayward [4], David de Kretser [2,5] and Mark Hedger [4]

1. National Centre for Epidemiology and Population Health, RSPH, College of Health and Medicine, The Australian National University, Canberra, ACT 2601, Australia
2. Paranta Biosciences Limited, Suite 549, 1 Queens Rd, Melbourne, VIC 3004, Australia
3. CFS Discovery, Donvale Specialist Medical Centre, Donvale, VIC 3111, Australia
4. Centre for Reproductive Health, Hudson Institute of Medical Research, Clayton, VIC 3168, Australia
5. Department of Anatomy and Developmental Biology, School of Biomedical Sciences, Monash University, Clayton, VIC 3800, Australia
* Correspondence: brett.lidbury@anu.edu.au

Received: 28 May 2019; Accepted: 15 July 2019; Published: 19 July 2019

Abstract: Biomarker discovery applied to myalgic encephalomyelitis/chronic fatigue syndrome (ME/CFS), a disabling disease of inconclusive aetiology, has identified several cytokines to potentially fulfil a role as a quantitative blood/serum marker for laboratory diagnosis, with activin B a recent addition. We explored further the potential of serum activin B as a ME/CFS biomarker, alone and in combination with a range of routine test results obtained from pathology laboratories. Previous pilot study results showed that activin B was significantly elevated for the ME/CFS participants compared to healthy (control) participants. All the participants were recruited via CFS Discovery and assessed via the Canadian/International Consensus Criteria. A significant difference for serum activin B was also detected for ME/CFS and control cohorts recruited for this study, but median levels were significantly lower for the ME/CFS cohort. Random Forest (RF) modelling identified five routine pathology blood test markers that collectively predicted ME/CFS at ≥62% when compared via weighted standing time (WST) severity classes. A closer analysis revealed that the inclusion of activin B to the panel of pathology markers improved the prediction of mild to moderate ME/CFS cases. Applying correct WST class prediction from RFA modelling, new reference intervals were calculated for activin B and associated pathology markers, where 24-h urinary creatinine clearance, serum urea and serum activin B showed the best potential as diagnostic markers. While the serum activin B results remained statistically significant for the new participant cohorts, activin B was found to also have utility in enhancing the prediction of symptom severity, as represented by WST class.

Keywords: myalgic encephalomyelitis; chronic fatigue syndrome; activin; pathology; biomarker; cytokine; machine learning; reference intervals

1. Introduction

The quest for a quantitative diagnostic and a specific marker for ME/CFS has yet to identify a reliable candidate, whether through routine pathology markers, or research efforts in immunology, microbiology, neuroscience and elsewhere. A number of cytokines, for example transforming growth factor-beta (TGF-β) and interleukin-10 (IL-10), have shown previous promise, but have not ultimately delivered a validated diagnostic test [1–7]. To the list of potential serum markers, we have recently added activin B, which was detected in a pilot research study involving volunteers recruited via CFS Discovery (Donvale Victoria) [8].

Activin B, along with activin A, is a member of the activin family of proteins, which belong to the TGF-β superfamily of growth and differentiation factors. Follistatin is a high-affinity binding protein for both activins, with diverse roles in physiology that include reproduction, haematopoiesis, immune cell development, as well as inflammation and immunity. The biology of activin A, at the time of writing, is better understood than that of activin B, although there is evidence of differences in relation to hepcidin regulation, associated receptor binding and SMAD signalling [9–11].

Following the activin findings from preliminary studies [8], this investigation aimed to validate these previous observations on a separate and larger population recruited by the same ME/CFS clinic in Melbourne. As well as the activin focus, other aims included applying the results from pathology and clinical testing, with and without activin B, to the pattern recognition algorithm random forest (RF), to identify wider marker patterns that separate ME/CFS cases from healthy controls. In addition to the development of activin B as a serum biomarker, a longer-term aim is to develop simpler diagnostic tools from routine data to assist health professionals diagnose ME/CFS.

The report herein examines the diagnostic potential of serum activin B, both individually and in combination with other blood, serum and urine markers considered for the assessment of research participants. The investigation directly compared the ME/CFS cases to healthy controls, but also examined the application of the weighted standing time (WST), as a measure of symptom severity, to stratify the ME/CFS cohort into mild to severe classes prior to analysis.

2. Materials and Methods

2.1. Participant Recruitment and Ethics Approval

The recruitment of research participants and associated procedures were described previously [8]. All the participants were recruited via CFS Discovery (Donvale, VIC, 3111), either via direct invitation to existing patients, or responses to advertising locally, and via social networking sites. Only participants with a previous ME/CFS diagnosis were recruited.

Human Ethics approval was granted by the ANU Human Research Ethics Committee (Approval No. 2015/193, approval date 29 June 2015), with approved consent forms and participant information provided to each potential participant. Inclusion in the study was allowed after signed consent was received by the researchers. Specific participant identifiers were not supplied to the researchers, and only known to the clinicians and clinic staff. Each research participant was given an identification code by the clinic, with age (at time of the appointment) and sex also provided. Eighty-five (85) participants were initially recruited for the ME/CFS cohort, with five eventually excluded due to comorbidities and/or difficulties attending the required appointments. Seventeen (17) healthy control (HC) participants were recruited too and underwent the same assessment as the ME/CFS cohort, giving a total study cohort size of 97 participants.

2.2. ME/CFS Assessment, Sample Collection and Tests

Each participant was examined by the CFS Discovery clinicians using the International Consensus Criteria to guide ME/CFS diagnosis [12] (NB: the earlier pilot study used the Canadian Criteria, which was replaced by the International Criteria in 2011–12). To be included in the ME/CFS participant cohort, the International Consensus Criteria must have been satisfied.

All participants performed a test for orthostatic intolerance (standing test—see section on weighted standing time for details) that included the collection of autonomic data during repose and the standing task [13]. After the standing test, non-fasting venous blood samples were collected for routine pathology testing, in addition to a parathyroid hormone (PTH), thyroid function testing (TFT), vitamin D and serum activin B [8]. For participants who were able, 24-h urine samples were collected and the volume, sodium (Na^+), potassium (K^+) and creatinine 24-h excretion rates were calculated.

Qualitative symptom inventories and questionnaires were also conducted for each participant, including the Epworth Sleep Scale [14] and the DASS-42 [15,16].

For the range of tests conducted, please refer to previous publications describing the CFS Discovery pilot studies [8,13].

2.3. Data Cleaning, Organisation and Structure

Data were collected for each participant as standard practice for the CFS Discovery staff and stored electronically in the secure clinic database. Each participant/patient file contained all the questionnaire and survey data, the printed pathology results (Australian Clinical Laboratories, South Australia), the standing test (orthostatic intolerance) data, including blood pressure (BP), heart rate (HR) and associated autonomic measurements and calculations, the standing time and standing difficulty, as well as clinical notes recording patient details (age, sex, weight, height).

An identification code was assigned to each research participant by CFS Discovery staff, after which data were matched and added to a spreadsheet for researcher interrogation. Heart rate (HR) data collected during the standing test was assessed for evidence of POTS (postural orthostatic tachycardia syndrome), with a HR increase of ≥30 beats per minute (bpm) upon standing from a lying position accepted as positive for co-morbid POTS [13,17]. The final data collection included the standing time and difficulty scores, WST calculations, POTS (yes or no), blood, serum and urine pathology results, serum activin B, DASS and Epworth Sleep scale results, along with notes on other conditions or comorbidities.

After the clinic appointment, the participants were asked to collect a 24-h urine sample within a week of the clinic visit. A minority of participants did not collect this sample, resulting in a number of missing values for urinary Na^+, K^+, creatinine and their 24-h excretion rates. With small to medium samples sizes, the median for each WST class was calculated and used to fill the missing values for each specific class.

2.4. Orthostatic Intolerance (OI) Assessment

Standing difficulty is a subjective ordinal scale developed by CFS Discovery clinicians, which with standing time (maximum of 20 min, recorded at two-minute intervals with autonomic measurements, as well as at repose before and after standing) is used to calculate the weighted standing time (WST). The standing difficulty scale ranges from 0 (no difficulty standing during 20 min upright) to 10 (extreme difficulty to maintain an upright stance). If the participant was not able to stand for at least 10 min, they were given a standing difficult score of 14. The participants who could maintain an upright stance for longer than 10 min, but not stand for the entire 20 min, were scored at 12 for standing difficulty. The standing difficulty scale has not been validated on other patient/participant populations.

2.5. Weighted Standing Time (WST)

The standing test procedure to assess orthostatic intolerance and detect POTS has been published previously [13], with a British study finding similar rates of POTS in a cohort from northern England [17]. Furthermore, the WST and its capacity to stratify ME/CFS severity, along with identify useful patterns in diagnostic markers, was recently published [18].

In brief, the WST takes the standing time (0–20 min, recorded at 2-min intervals) and weights this time with the subjective standing difficulty score, as described by the following equation:

$$\text{Weighted standing time (WST)} = \text{Time standing (mins)} \times (1 - (\text{Difficulty}/14)) \quad (1)$$

The WST, therefore, provides a proxy for ME/CFS severity and a response variable with which to investigate the significance of the predictor (independent) variables and their interactions. The results presented herein were generated from the analyses of WST severity classes, as summarised in Table 1. With the majority of the study participants able to stand for the entire 20 min of the orthostatic intolerance (OI) test, standing time alone was not an effective response variable.

Table 1. Definitions of ME/CFS symptom severity classes by Weighted Standing Time (WST), with reference to standing time and difficulty. (**a**) Four categories featuring a healthy control category, and a severity scale from mild to severe symptoms. (**b**) Three severity classes where the healthy control cohort (0) was combined with the mild category (1) from Table (**a**) to increase sample size for random forest algorithm interrogation (WST). All ME/CFS cases fulfilled the ICC diagnostic criteria.

(a)			
Category	n	WST	Definition of ME/CFS Symptom Severity Class (Post ICC)
0	17	14.29–18.57	Healthy—No disease; All stood 20 min at Difficulty 1–4
1	19	15.71–18.57	Mild severity; All stood 20 min at Difficulty 1–3
2	38	6.43–14.29	Moderate Severity; All stood 20 min at Difficulty 4–10
3	23	0.0–2.57	Severe; All <20 min standing + Difficulty 12 or 14
(b)			
Category	n	WST	Definition of ME/CFS Symptom Severity Class (Post ICC)
0 *	36	14.29–18.57	Healthy + Mild symptoms; All stood 20 min at Difficulty 1–4
1	38	6.43–14.29	Moderate Severity; All stood 20 min at Difficulty 4–10
2	23	0.0–2.57	Severe; All <20 min standing + Difficulty 12 or 14

ICC—International Consensus Criteria (Diagnostic criteria for ME/CFS [12]). Standing time scale—0 to 20 min, with measurements at every two minutes; Standing difficulty scale—0 represents no difficulty, 14 represents extreme difficulty resulting in the inability to stand upright for a minimum of 10 min. * (0 + 1 from Table 1a).

2.6. Statistics and Machine Learning

2.6.1. Statistical Analyses

All descriptive statistics, test (inferential) statistics and regression/correlation analyses were performed using SPSS (Version 22—IBM SPSS software, Chicago, IL, USA).

Prior to conducting the appropriate statistical analyses, all raw data collected for investigation were subject to a one-sample Kolmogorov–Smirnov (K-S) test to assess whether they fulfilled a normal distribution, with K-S results of $p \leq 0.05$ indicating that the specific marker distribution was significantly different from a normal curve. Based on the K-S results (Table 2), statistical significance between two groups was estimated by a Mann–Whitney U test, and three or more groups by Kruskal–Wallis non-parametric tests. Jonckheere–Terpstra non-parametric tests were also applied where the groups were clearly ordinal. Descriptive results were presented as the median and 25th–75th interquartile range (IQR).

Significance was set at $p < 0.05$ for the two group comparisons using the Mann–Whitney U test, and also for comparisons across more than two classes in the Kruskal–Wallis (KW) test.

2.6.2. Machine Learning

R statistical programming version 3.5.1 was used to run the recursive partitioning algorithms random forest (R library randomForest) and decision trees (R library rpart) [19,20]. Algorithm tuning was performed via the R caret package [21].

Table 2. Comparison of ME/CFS and healthy control participants via a range of pathology markers, questionnaire results, and serum Activin B. Results summarised as medians and 25th–75th IQR for a ME/CFS cohort diagnosed by the International Clinical Criteria, and a control cohort of healthy participants.

Blood/Serum/Urine Marker	Median (25–75%) ME/CFS (n)	Median (25–75%) Healthy Control (n)	p-Value *	K-S (p-Value) **
MCH (pg)	30.80 (79) (29.40–31.50)	30.35 (17) (29.55–31.40)	0.44	0.025
Lymphocytes ($\times 10^9$/L)	2.00 (80) (1.50–2.30)	2.30 (17) (1.90–2.60)	0.08	0.009
Neutrophils ($\times 10^9$/L)	3.70 (80) (2.80–4.78)	4.30 (17) (3.35–5.35)	0.16	0.076
Platelets ($\times 10^9$/L)	260.5 (80) (232.0–303.8)	264.0 (17) (234.5–297.0)	0.76	0.200
Serum Sodium (mmol/L)	141 (79) (140–142)	141 (17) (139.5–142)	0.15	<0.001
Serum Bicarbonate (mmol/L)	29 (79) (27–32)	29 (17) (28–30.5)	0.32	0.016
Serum Urea (mmol/L)	4.9 (79) (3.9–5.7)	5.5 (17) (4.8–7.9)	0.04	0.002
Serum Creatinine (μmol/L)	74.0 (79) (66.0–82.0)	76.0 (17) (67.5–82.5)	0.67	0.001
ALP (U/L)	67.5 (80) (56.0–80.5)	65.0 (17) (52.0–77.5)	0.49	0.200
PTH (pmol/L)	5.45 (80) (3.33–6.78)	7.70 (15) (5.20–8.80)	0.03	0.001
Urinary Creatinine Excretion Rate (mmol/24 h)	9.9 (68) (8.1–11.7)	13.1 (13) (10.8–17.2)	0.004	0.020
Activin B (pg/mL)	85.95 (80) (70.48–125.76)	114.19 (17) (92.21–162.24)	0.013	<0.001
Survey Results	**ME/CFS (n)**	**Healthy Control (n)**	**p-Value ***	**K-S (p-Value) ***
DASS (Total) ^	28.0 (54) (14.8–47.0)	8.0 (17) (4.0–11.5)	<0.001	0.001
Epworth Sleep Scale	5.5 (54) (3.0–9.3)	4.00 (17) (3.0–6.5)	0.09	<0.001
Age (Years)	48.0 (80) (39.3–56.0)	41.0 (17) (29.0–51.0)	0.02	0.200

* Median and 25–75% IQR (Inter-Quartile Range) - Mann–Whitney U test - Significance at $p < 0.05$.
** Kolmogorov–Smirnoff test (one sample) for Normal data distribution. ^ DASS-42 (Depression, Anxiety, Stress total score).

Random forest analysis (RFA) was performed using the WST classes summarised in Table 1b. Due to class imbalance and the relatively small overall sample size, the healthy controls were combined with mild ME/CFS cases (Table 1a) to create an adjusted WST class 0, and therefore provide a larger class sample size for subsequent RFA. Running the original WST classes (Table 1a) as the response of interest resulted in very poor class prediction, and as such, an ineffective model, in spite of attempts to compensate with class balancing R script. Future studies will benefit from larger sample sizes, particularly for healthy control cases.

All the RFA results presented herein used the three-class (WST) model to detect predictors of absent or mild ME/CFS symptoms (0), compared to moderate (1) or severe (2) symptoms (Table 1b).

Severe cases were characterised by their inability to remain upright for the full twenty minutes of the standing test for orthostatic intolerance. Missing values in the raw data were filled by the median for each WST category, prior to RFA. Missing data was most pronounced for the 24-h urine markers, with 15–20% missingness found due to test non-compliance after the CFS Discovery initial appointment. The total case numbers for the ME/CFS and healthy cohorts are summarised in Table 2. Individual missing values were also found for serum urea and electrolytes, and MCH.

Via algorithm tuning (caret), all RFA had the following features:

mtry = 4 (4 predictor variables tried for splitting at each node); *ntree* = 5000 (5000 decision trees grown to determine predictor variable rankings). With the following features included—*replace* = *TRUE* (cases are replaced during algorithm bootstrapping), and *importance* = *TRUE* (as well as Gini Index ranking, scores based on permutation ranking).

As well as the primary RFA to detect and rank predictors of ME/CFS severity via WST, bagging and boosting ensembles for a variety of algorithms were tested in parallel using R statistical programming via the caret and caretEnsemble packages [21,22]. Bagging and boosting are resampling methods used by the algorithm of interest to increase prediction accuracy through reducing variation, or correcting errors during the analysis. The analyses presented allowed for the comparison of machine learning methods, and therefore the assessment of the best analytical strategy for the dataset of interest.

A number of machine learning options are available for the training and testing of data to reveal outcome predictors. To examine the best machine learning option, ensemble analyses that compared random forest analyses (RFA) to support vector machines (SVM), gradient boosting and decision trees, were conducted with the aims of assessing the comparative predictive accuracy of various machine learning techniques. The relationships between the various machine learning algorithm ensembles, presented as accuracy measures and kappa statistics, are summarised in Figure 1.

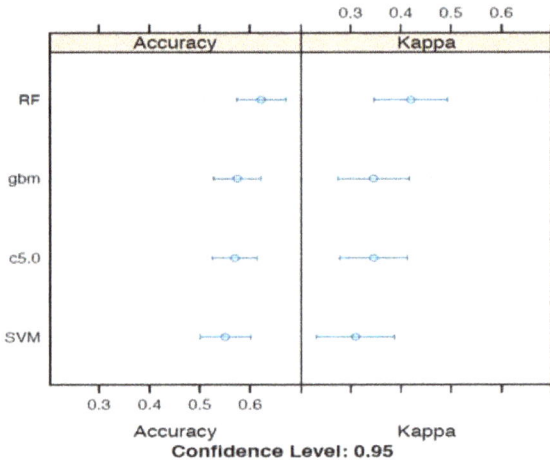

Figure 1. A variety of machine learning ensembles compared to assess performance for ME/CFS WST (0, 1, 2) class prediction, as measured by percentage accuracy and the Kappa statistic. Boosting strategies applied to enhance machine learning performance for ensemble random forest (RF), gradient boosting (gbm), c5.0 tree construction and support vector machines (SVM).

For the WST analyses, RFA produced the best accuracy and kappa results, suggesting this as the most suitable ML method to apply. For a comparatively small data set (for this study, 97 in total), RFA provides a method whereby hundreds to thousands of trees can be propagated as one analysis, and therefore introduce extra robustness into the analysis, which likely explains the superior performance for this data set. Nevertheless, the limitations of the total sample size did reflect in the large differences in accuracy and kappa statistic results. Receiver operating curves (ROC) and associated results were calculated by RFA modelling of MCH, ALP, serum urea, blood lymphocytes, 24-h urinary creatinine and activin B.

Random Forest Analyses (RFA) were subsequently applied to binary outcomes representing the direct comparison of ME/CFS to HCs, as well as the stratification of ME/CFS severity by WST (Table 1). Early investigations did not produce a model because of class imbalance between ME/CFS and HC categories, in spite of introducing class balancing script into the R code for RFA. Combining Healthy Controls with mild ME/CFS cases (Table 1b) solved this problem, allowing the building of

RFA predictive models of disease categories. All the results presented hereafter are on the adjusted WST classes, as summarised in Table 1b.

To calculate the marker thresholds (e.g., ALP > or < 60 U/L), the recursive partitioning algorithm, decision trees, was used on the same dataset classified by WST, with trees developed also for the direct comparison ME/CFS to healthy controls, and the full WST classification from class 0–3 (Table 1a). For all the trees, the minimum split was 20 and the complexity parameter (cp) ranged from 0.01 to 0.085. The direct comparison of ME/CFS cases to healthy controls required a cp of 0.14. Due to the small to moderate starting sample sizes for each WST class, and that the final decision thresholds involved the loss of cases, results must be ascertained with caution, as the final decisions were often drawn from fewer than 10 cases.

2.7. Receiver Operating Characteristics

With the recognition of a predictor variable pattern by RFA, associated with the WST class, the diagnostic potential of the multi-marker profile to accurately separate ME/CFS severity was examined by receiver operating characteristic (ROC) curves, supported by an area under curve (AUC) calculation. A ROC curve plots assay sensitivity (rate of true positives) against the false positive rate (100—Specificity), with AUC estimating the accuracy of separating the two classes. As this suggests, only two WST classes were compared at one time, namely classes 0 versus 1, 0 versus 2, and class 1 versus class 2.

ROC plots were generated and AUC was calculated by the R statistical programming package ROCR [23].

Examples of R code and primary results generated by machine learning and ROC are available in the Supplementary Materials.

2.8. Activin B Assay

The development and optimisation of the activin B assay in human populations have been published previously [24,25]. However, for this study, the established assay for activin B was modified after it was discovered that non-specific interference was impacting the capacity of the assay to accurately measure lower activin B concentrations in human serum. The assay, which was used to measure serum activin B concentrations in the previous pilot study [8,18], was modified by the addition of activin-free gelding serum, as a carrier to remove the interference and enhance the accuracy of activin B detection.

3. Results

3.1. Direct Comparison of ME/CFS and Healthy Cohorts

The direct comparison of a range of pathology (blood, urine, serum) markers, questionnaire results and activin B are summarised in Table 2. The subset of pathology markers included were informed by exploratory data interrogation by machine learning (Figures 1 and 2), with additional serum electrolytes, platelets, neutrophils and parathormone (parathyroid hormone—PTH) also included because of clinical interest in the potential importance of these markers, as well as for the association with renal function suggested by other results. Red cell indices and TFTs showed no anaemia or thyroid deficiency associated with chronic fatigue symptoms, and in general all individual pathology results from ME/CFS and HC were within the laboratory reference interval, with exceptions outside of the reference interval excluded from the analyses if clinically indicated as a diagnostic confounder.

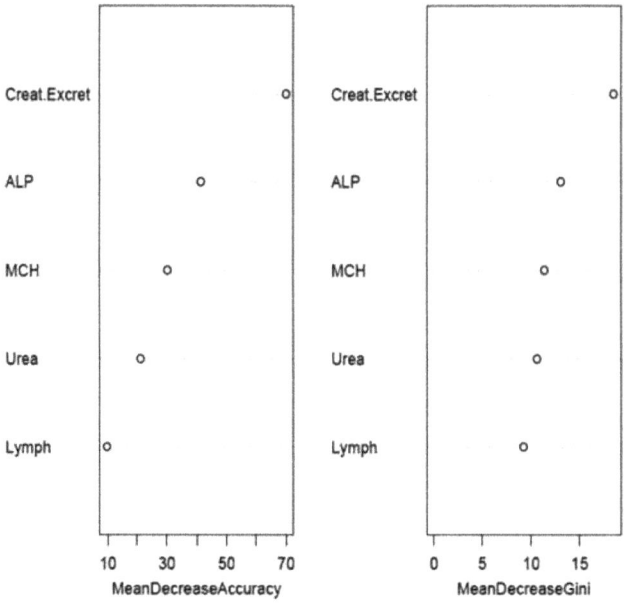
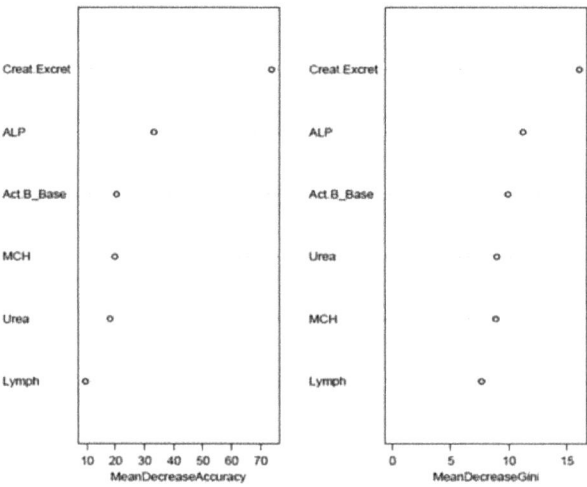

Figure 2. Random Forest plots of (**a**) a model using basic blood and urine test pathology markers to predict Weighted Standing Time (WST) classes (0, 1, 2) of ME/CFS, (**b**) the same model with Activin B results added. The left column represents the RFA Importance measure, and the right column the ranking of predictors by Gini Index. Refer to Table 1b for WST Class definitions. OOB—Out of Bag (Error Rate). Creat.Excret (24-h urinary creatinine excretion rate); ALP (serum alkaline phosphatase); Act.B_Base (first appointment, serum activin B assay); MCH (mean corpuscular haemoglobin); Urea (serum urea); Lymph (blood lymphocyte count).

As summarised in Table 2, the results of Kolmogorov–Smirnov (K-S) testing showed that platelets, ALP, neutrophils and age were assessed as being normally distributed, with the majority of markers at $p \leq 0.025$, which therefore did not follow a normal distribution. For this reason, non-parametric statistics were used for all markers and survey results to determine whether statistical significance was achieved for comparisons between ME/CFS classes. The small loss of power due to nonparametric testing was regarded as clinically unimportant.

Statistically significant differences in median pathology results from the comparison of ME/CFS to HC cases were observed for serum urea, parathyroid hormone (PTH) and 24-h urinary creatinine excretion rate, with each of these significantly decreased for ME/CFS ($p \leq 0.05$). The median age was significantly higher for the ME/CFS group, with the median total DASS score significantly elevated (separate depression and anxiety scores were significantly increased for the ME/CFS group, but not the stress score). Although sleep problems are often reported during ME/CFS assessment, the Epworth Sleep score did not differ significantly between the groups.

Activin B

An objective of this study was to validate a previous (pilot) study result, which found that activin B is a serum biomarker that significantly ($p < 0.05$) separates ME/CFS patients from healthy controls (HC). On direct comparison of the medians (Table 2), activin B was significantly lower ($p = 0.013$) for the ME/CFS cohort compared to results from the HC participant cohort. This is an inversion of the previous results, which found that activin B was significantly elevated in ME/CFS participants [8]. As described in the Materials and Methods, the activin B assay had been re-optimised prior to these analyses.

3.2. Analyses of Markers Stratified by Weighted Standing Time (WST)

3.2.1. Four Severity Categories

Marker variation and survey results were investigated after the ME/CFS cohort was stratified by WST for symptom severity (classes 1–3) and compared to healthy controls (class 0) (Table 3). Median (25th–75th IQR—interquartile range) results were presented and statistical significance assessed by Kruskal–Wallis tests.

Serum urea, ALP and 24-h urinary creatinine excretion rate were statistically significant at $p < 0.05$. The difference between WST classes for DASS (Total) also achieved statistical significance, with increases in total DASS scores obvious for of the WST ME/CFS classes (1–3), when compared to HC (class 0).

Significance at $p < 0.05$ was not observed for activin B when comparing healthy controls (class 0) to the WST stratified ME/CFS cohort (classes 1–3) (Table 3). As seen in Table 3, apart from WST class 2 (moderate severity), the 25–75 IQR were large, suggesting high variations in the activin B results. When the healthy controls (WST 0) were compared directly to WST 2 by the Mann–Whitney U test, a significant result at $p = 0.005$ was found, whereas the comparison of WST 0 to WST 1 and 3 was not significantly different ($p > 0.05$). Based on this observation, activin B is most useful for separating healthy individuals from patients experiencing moderate ME/CFS symptoms, as defined by WST.

Table 3. Comparison of pathology markers, questionnaire results and serum Activin B for ME/CFS sub-cohorts stratified by the Weighted Standing Time (WST) symptom severity scale, compared with a control cohort of healthy participants. Results summarised as medians and 25th–75th IQR.

Blood/Serum/Urine Marker	Weighted Standing Time Median (25th–75th)				p-Value *
	WST 0 (n)	WST 1 (n)	WST 2 (n)	WST 3 (n)	
MCH (pg)	30.8 (17) (29.4–31.5)	30.6 (19) (30.0–31.2)	30.3 (38) (28.7–31.0)	30.9 (23) (30.2–31.6)	0.08
Lymphocytes (×10⁹/L)	2.3 (17) (1.9–2.6)	1.8 (19) (1.5–2.8)	2.0 (38) (1.5–2.3)	2.1 (23) (1.8–2.5)	0.10
Neutrophils (×10⁹/L)	4.3 (17) (3.4–5.4)	3.6 (19) (2.6–4.8)	4.1 (38) (2.9–4.9)	3.5 (23) (2.5–4.5)	0.24
Platelets (×10⁹/L)	264 (17) (235–297)	244 (19) (203–308)	258 (38) (227–307)	273 (23) (251–300)	0.50
Serum Sodium (mmol/L)	141 (17) (139.5–142)	140.8 (18) (141.5–142)	141 (38) (141–142)	140 (23) (141–142)	0.08
Serum Bicarbonate (mmol/L)	29 (17) (28–30.5)	30 (18) (27–32.3)	29 (38) (28–31.5)	29 (23) (27–30)	0.46
Serum Urea (mmol/L)	5.5 (17) (4.75–7.9)	5.1 (18) (3.8–5.6)	5.4 (38) (4.0–6.1)	4.5 (23) (4.0–5.1)	0.04
Serum Creatinine (μmol/L)	76 (17) (67.5–82.5)	73.5 (18) (68–93)	76 (38) (66.5–85.5)	71 (23) (65–77)	0.26
ALP (U/L)	65 (17) (52–77.5)	64 (19) (53–78)	72 (38) (62–84.5)	60 (23) (45–74)	0.035
PTH (pmol/L)	7.7 (15) (5.2–8.8)	5.7 (19) (3.7–6.8)	5.6 (38) (3.7–7.5)	5.2 (23) (2.9–6.5)	0.12
Urinary Creatinine Excretion Rate (mmol/24 h)	13.1 (13) (10.8–17.2)	10 (16) (7.8–14.4)	9.4 (37) (7.7–12.2)	10.2 (21) (9.2–10.9)	0.035
Activin B (pg/mL)	114.19 (17) (92.21–162.24)	89.48 (19) (59.97–147.17)	79.97 (38) (71.00–106.97)	89.74 (23) (70.48–133.19)	0.07
Survey Results	WST 0 (n)	WST 1 (n)	WST 2 (n)	WST 3 (n)	p-Value *
DASS (Total) ^	8 (17) (4–11.5)	25 (16) (10.3–36.3)	28 (26) (15.3–47.3)	28 (12) (16.3–54.5)	<0.001
Epworth Sleep Scale	4 (17) (3–6.5)	4 (16) (1.5–5.8)	7 (26) (3–12)	6.5 (12) (3.3–10.8)	0.04
Age (Years)	41 (17) (29–51)	45 (19) (39–50)	55 (38) (43–61.5)	42 (23) (36–53)	0.01

Weighted Standing Time (symptom severity scale during standing test)—WST 0 (Healthy Controls); WST 1 (ME/CFS - Mild); WST 2 (ME/CFS - Moderate); WST 3 (ME/CFS - Severe)—See Table 1a. IQR (Inter-Quartile Range). * p-value set at $p < 0.05$ (Bonferroni correction not required for Kruskal–Wallis tests). ^ DASS-42 (Depression, Anxiety, Stress total score).

3.2.2. Three Severity Categories

WST classes 0 and 1 were combined to increase sample size for subsequent machine learning (ML), resulting in adjusted WST classes representing categories defining absent or mild symptoms (0), moderate (1) or severe ME/CFS symptoms (2), as reflected by orthostatic intolerance. This adjusted WST classification (Table 1b) was used for all the following RFA and ROC investigations.

Age, Epworth Sleep Scale and total DASS score showed significant variations between WST classes (Table 4—Kruskal–Wallis test). Age was significantly higher for the ME/CFS cohort compared to healthy controls (Table 2). Comparison across WST classes indicated that the participants with moderate symptom severity were responsible for this age difference, which will require further investigation. Of the serum/blood markers, only MCH and ALP were significantly different, with ALP WST class 1 of a higher median compared to WST 0 and 3. Age can impact serum ALP levels; therefore, caution must be exercised when interpreting this result.

Table 4. Comparison of pathology markers, questionnaire results and serum Activin B for ME/CFS sub-cohorts stratified by the Weighted Standing Time (WST) symptom severity scale, including a control cohort of healthy participants. WST 0 and 1 (Table 2) data were pooled prior to analysis. Results summarised as medians and 25th–75th IQR.

Blood/Serum/Urine Marker	Weighted Standing Time Median [25th–75th]			p-Value *
	WST 0 (n)	WST 1 (n)	WST 2 (n)	
MCH (pg)	30.8 (36) (29.9–31.4)	30.2 (38) (28.8–30.9)	30.9 (23) (30.2–31.6)	0.03
Lymphocytes (×10^9/L)	2.0 (36) (1.6–2.6)	1.95 (38) (1.5–2.2)	2.1 (23) (1.8–2.5)	0.15
Neutrophils (×10^9/L)	3.9 (36) (2.8–5.2)	4.1 (38) (2.9–4.9)	3.5 (23) (2.5–4.5)	0.34
Platelets (×10^9/L)	254.5 (36) (214.3–305.0)	256.5 (38) (219.5–305.8)	273.0 (23) (251.0–300.0)	0.45
Serum Sodium (mmol/L)	141 (35) (140–142)	141.5 (38) (141–142)	141 (23) (140–142)	0.07
Serum Bicarbonate (mmol/L)	29 (35) (28–31)	29.5 (38) (28–31.3)	29 (23) (27–30)	0.52
Serum Urea (mmol/L)	5.1 (35) (4.6–6.4)	5.4 (38) (3.9–6.1)	4.5 (23) (4.0–5.1)	0.08
Serum Creatinine (μmol/L)	74 (35) (69–84)	76 (38) (66.8–84.8)	71 (23) (65–77)	0.13
ALP (U/L)	64 (36) (53.3–77.5)	72.5 (38) (62–85.3)	60 (23) (45–74)	0.014
PTH (pmol/L)	5.9 (34) (4.7–8.4)	5.6 (38) (3.7–8.4)	5.2 (23) (2.9–6.5)	0.19
Urinary Creatinine Excretion Rate (mmol/24 h)	12.7 (29) (8.3–15.3)	9.4 (31) (7.7–12)	10.2 (21) (9.2–10.9)	0.13
Activin B (pg/mL)	103.36 (36) (78.57–148.78)	80.73 (38) (71.27–107.81)	89.74 (23) (70.48–133.19)	0.15
Survey Results	WST 0 (n)	WST 1 (n)	WST 2 (n)	p-Value *
DASS (Total) ^	11 (33) (6.5–29.5)	28 (26) (15.3–47.3)	28 (12) (16.3–54.5)	0.004
Epworth Sleep Scale	4 (33) (3–6)	7 (26) (3–12)	6.5 (12) (3.3–10.8)	0.015
Age (Years)	43 (36) (36.3–50)	54.5 (38) (43–61.3)	42.00 (23) (36–53)	0.007

Weighted Standing Time (symptom severity scale during standing test)—WST 0 (Healthy Controls + mild symptoms - WST 1, Table 3); WST 1 (ME/CFS - Moderate); WST 2 (ME/CFS - Severe)—See Table 1b. IQR (Inter-Quartile Range). * p-value set at $p < 0.05$ (Bonferroni correction not required for Kruskal–Wallis tests). ^ DASS-42 (Depression, Anxiety, Stress total score).

A significant difference between WST classes was not observed for activin B. The combination of healthy controls with mild cases increased the WST 0 median, and therefore statistically significant separation from WST classes 1 and 2 was not achieved.

3.3. Exploratory Machine Learning Analyses of ME/CFS and Healthy Control Data

As assessed by algorithm ensembles that calculated percentage accuracy and the kappa statistic (Figure 1), Random Forest Analysis (RFA) was chosen as the machine learning method to conduct deeper analyses of the ME/CFS results. Two sampling methods were tested for each ensemble, namely (a) boosting and (b) bagging. In general, similar accuracy and kappa results were found for both sampling strategies (bagging results not shown).

Figure 2 presents the results of two RFA, one with five routine pathology markers, and the other with activin B included in the same pathology model. The pathology markers represent the most effective constellation of blood or urine test results that most successfully predicted WST categories 0, 1 and 2, with an overall predictive accuracy of 62–65%. The addition of extra pathology variables either did not improve the accuracy of the model or reduced overall WST class predictive accuracy.

The addition of Activin B to the model did not change the overall accuracy of the RFA model, but did slightly improve the prediction accuracy for WST class 2 (severe), at the expense of a poorer WST class 0 prediction (Figure 2b). Activin B ranked as the third most important predictor of ME/CFS-WST categories, behind 24-h urinary creatinine excretion rate and ALP, both on the importance ranking and mean decrease Gini index (Figure 2).

RFA emphasised 24-h urinary creatinine clearance as a key predictor of WST classes, with ALP ranking as the second most important predictor from among the pathology markers. The subsequent analysis of the same data by a tuned ($cp = 0.01$, $minsplit = 20$) single decision tree confirmed the leading role of urinary creatinine as a ME/CFS predictor (decision tree code and results are available in the Supplementary Materials).

3.4. Receiver Operating Characteristic (ROC) Analyses and Discrimination of WST Categories by Activin B and Pathology Markers Post Random Forest

To assess the predictive value of the RFA models applying activin B, mean corpuscular haemoglobin (MCH), serum urea, lymphocytes, alkaline phosphatase (ALP) and urinary creatinine excretion rate to the prediction of ME/CFS, ROC curves were plotted and the area under curve (AUC) was calculated.

ROC curves and AUC calculations were examined as pairwise comparisons between WST classes (0-1, 0-2, 1-2). RFA and ROC were not reliable for the direct comparison of ME/CFS to healthy controls, due to data imbalance issues described elsewhere.

Figure 3 presents the RFA and ROC results for the comparison of WST classes 0 and 1 (Table 1b). Figure 3a shows the Gini Index and Importance (Mean Decrease Accuracy) weighting of predictor variables to discriminate between WST classes 0 and 1 (mild symptoms and healthy cases combined versus moderate ME/CFS symptoms). The rate of urinary creatinine excretion was the top-ranked predictor, followed by serum activin B. For the total constellation of markers, the 0 versus 1 AUC was calculated at 0.755, with the ROC curve showing a clear separation from 0.50 (Figure 3b).

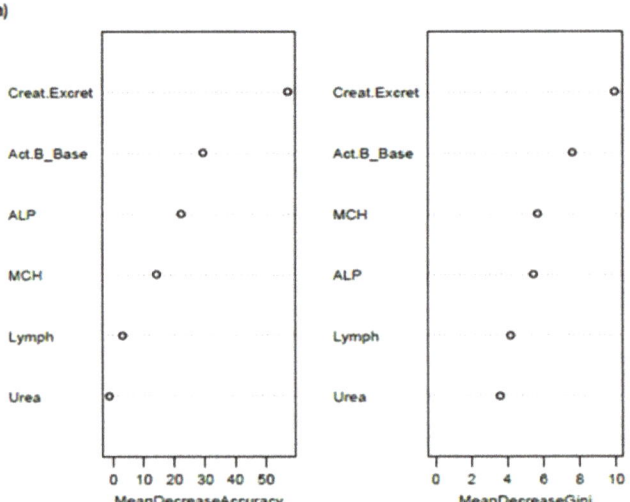

Figure 3. *Cont.*

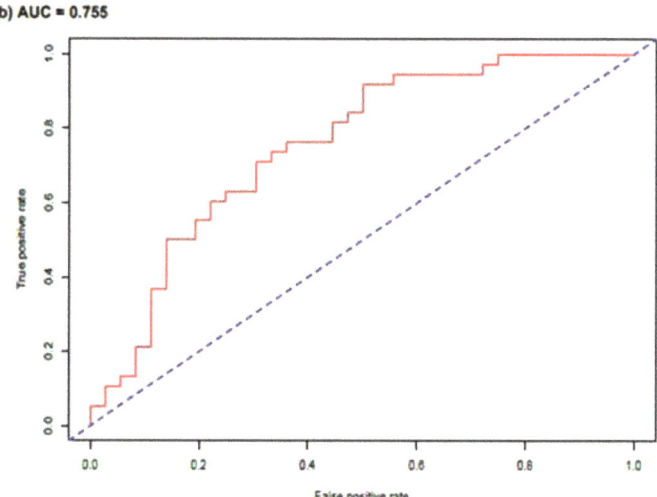

Figure 3. (**a**) Random Forest Analysis (RFA) and (**b**) Receiver Operating Characteristic (ROC) investigations on the prediction of Weighted Standing Time (WST) classes 0 versus 1, and the relative importance of activin B and pathology markers in separating the two WST classes of ME/CFS severity. AUC—area under curve (accuracy calculation from true and false positive rates).

For the ROC-AUC analysis of class 0 versus class 2 (mild ME/CFS symptoms and healthy controls versus severe ME/CFS), urinary creatinine excretion rate was again the top-ranked predictor, with the impact of activin B reduced as determined by Gini Index and Importance scale, and serum urea and ALP elevated in predictive importance (AUC = 0.795). For classes 1 versus class 2, representing moderate versus severe ME/CFS symptoms, ALP, MCH, lymphocytes and serum urea ranked higher on both the Gini Index and Importance scale than urinary creatinine excretion and activin B, inverting the ranking observed for comparisons against class 0 (AUC = 0.704) (Results not shown).

3.5. Correct Prediction of ME/CFS Cases by RFA

As well as ranking predictors, the RF algorithm allowed the prediction of case category (WST class) based on the variables entered into the model. To understand the power of correctly predicted cases as a data modelling method to refine decisions on the diagnostic acuity of marker patterns, ROC was repeated for WST classes 0 versus 1, with only correctly RFA predicted 0 or 1 cases included (Figure 4). The importance ranking of predictors (Figure 4a) resembled that found for the all data general model (Figure 3), with urinary creatinine excretion rate, activin B and ALP the top three predictors of WST classes 0 or 1. The ROC curve showed an excellent separation from the 0.50 threshold, with an AUC of 0.963, which was clearly superior to AUC 0.755 found for the general model of the same WST classes that included all cases, regardless of correct prediction (Figure 3).

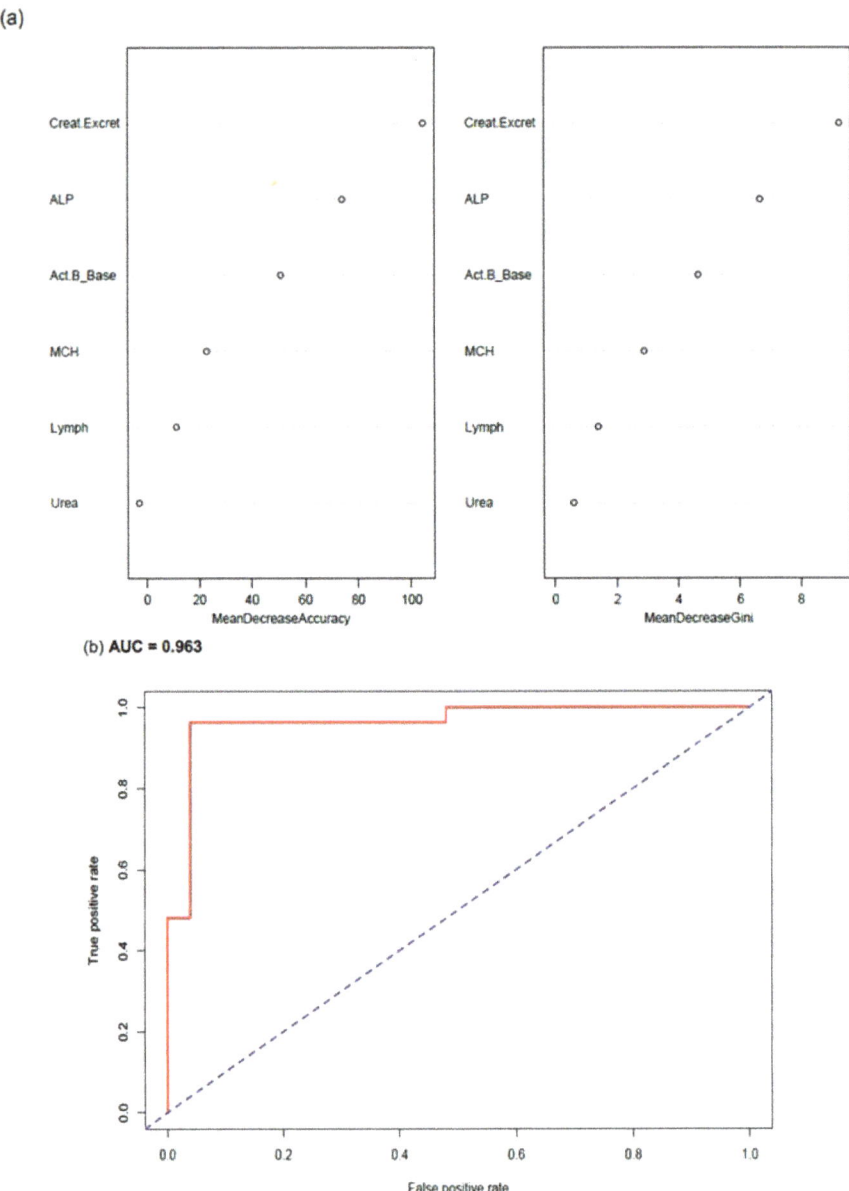

Figure 4. (**a**) Random Forest Analysis (RFA) and (**b**) Receiver Operating Characteristic (ROC) investigations on the prediction of Weighted Standing Time (WST) using only correctly predicted cases from the WST classes 0 versus 1, and the relative importance of activin B and pathology markers in separating the two WST classes of ME/CFS severity. Correct case prediction was performed via RF. AUC—area under curve (accuracy calculation from true and false positive rates).

The correctly predicted cases across the entire WST scale (Table 1b) were investigated by RFA to elucidate the broad pattern of the designated markers associated with the best accuracy prediction (Figure 5).

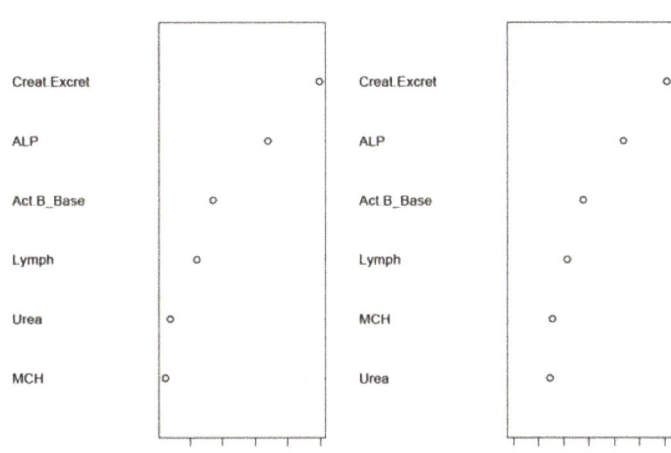

Figure 5. Relative predictor variable importance as determined by Random Forest Analysis (RFA) using only cases that were correctly predicted for each specific WST class (Table 1b) of ME/CFS severity. Correct case prediction by WST class was achieved by RFA.

Similar to the ranking of markers for WST classes 0 versus 1 (Figures 3 and 4), the urinary creatinine excretion rate, ALP and activin B were the top-ranked predictors of all the WST classes (Figure 5), which stratifies ME/CFS severity as according to orthostatic intolerance testing performance. While the cases were correctly predicted, WST class 0 recorded an (OOB) error rate of 8.7%, while class 2 recorded a 17% error rate. However, class 1 (Moderate severity) was perfectly predicted (Figure 5), suggesting again that the marker set including activin B is best for predicting symptom severity ranging from healthy, through mild, to moderate ME/CFS. The extent of the error rate in the severe cases indicates wider variation in these ME/CFS cases. Future studies involving larger participant samples will assist in determining predictive parameters with greater accuracy.

3.6. New Reference Intervals for Serum and Urine Markers Based on Correct Random Forest Prediction

To provide simpler and accurate guidance to clinicians supporting ME/CFS patients, reference intervals were calculated based on cases correctly predicted by RFA. The reference intervals were calculated using the median and 25–75% IQRs.

New reference intervals based on correctly predicted cases for each analyte of interest were calculated based on the following criteria: (1) comparison of the ME/CFS cohort with the healthy control group; (2) calculation of reference intervals following the WST criteria of categories 0 (healthy controls plus mild ME/CFS), 1 (moderate symptoms), and 2 (severe symptoms). The full WST classification definitions are summarised in Table 1.

Tables 5 and 6 show the medians and 25–75th IQR for the ME/CFS predictors correctly detected by RFA (namely, MCH, lymphocyte count, serum urea, ALP, 24-h urinary creatinine excretion rate and activin B), using criteria 1 (Table 5) and 2 (Table 6).

Table 5. Median and 25–75 IQR calculated from ME/CFS or healthy control cases correctly predicted by Random Forest Analysis (RFA). ME/CFS cases ranged from mild to severe symptoms, as determined by the International Consensus Criteria [12] and the standing test.

Blood/Serum/Urine Marker	Median (25–75%)		p-Value *
	ME/CFS (n = 42)	Healthy Control (n = 11)	
MCH (pg)	29.6 (28.5–30.38)	30.8 (29.75–31.45)	0.44
Lymphocytes (×10^9/L)	2.0 (1.48–2.23)	1.9 (1.5–2.6)	0.50
Serum Urea (mmol/L)	5.2 (3.9–5.75)	5.4 (4.65–6.35)	0.02
ALP (U/L)	78.5 (66.75–85.25)	60.0 (50.5–74.0)	0.17
Urinary Creatinine Excretion Rate (mmol/24 h)	10.5 (8.03–10.88)	12.7 (12.12–15.3)	<0.001
Activin B (pg/mL)	82.0 (71.26–104.86)	119.58 (89.49–167.37)	0.002

* Statistical significance $p < 0.05$. IQR (Inter-Quartile Range).

Table 6. Median and 25–75 IQR calculated from a combined class of healthy control and mild ME/CFS cases (WST 0), moderate (WST 1) and severe (WST 2) symptoms correctly predicted by Random Forest Analysis (RFA). ME/CFS was diagnosed via the International Consensus Criteria [12], and WST class calculated from standing test results.

Blood/Serum/Urine Marker	Weighted Standing Time Median (25th–75th)			p-Value *
	WST 0 (n = 23)	WST 1 (n = 23)	WST 2 (n = 12)	
MCH (pg)	30.8 (29.8–31.5)	29.5 (28.6–30.3)	30.95 (30.2–32.25)	(a) 0.006 (b) 0.811
Lymphocytes (×10^9/L)	1.9 (1.5–2.3)	1.9 (1.4–2.1)	2.5 (2.1–3.0)	(a) 0.004 (b) 0.094
Serum Urea (mmol/L)	5.4 (4.6–6.4)	5.4 (3.9–5.9)	4.2 (3.83–4.58)	(a) 0.012 (b) 0.010
ALP (U/L)	60.0 (52.0–74.0)	79.0 (67.0–86.0)	50.5 (34.75–72.5)	(a) <0.001 (b) 0.840
Urinary Creatinine Excretion Rate (mmol/24 h)	13.1 (12.12–15.6)	10.50 (7.5–11.4)	10.45 (9.7–11.23)	(a) <0.001 (b) 0.001
Activin B (pg/mL)	130.36 (97.03–171.45)	81.48 (71.53–106.47)	93.86 (76.46–132.01)	(a) 0.004 (b) 0.013

* p-value set at $p < 0.05$ (Bonferroni correction not required for Kruskal–Wallis tests). p-values (a) Kruskal Wallis test (b) Jonckheere–Terpstra Test. IQR (Inter-Quartile Range).

The small sample sizes led to most markers having a significant overlap of ranges, and therefore not producing distinctive reference intervals. There were some exceptions, namely, for ME/CFS urinary creatinine excretion rate, a 25–75 IQR of 8.03–10.88 mmol/24 h (median—10.5), and 12.12–15.3 mmol/24 h (median—12.7) for healthy controls (Table 5).

For the WST comparison (Table 6), 25–75 IQR overlap was not found between classes for activin B, with separation of confidence intervals observed for MCH and urinary creatine excretion rate (between class 0 and class 1, as well as classes 0 and 2). There was a marginal separation of 25–75 IQR observed for serum urea classes 0 and 2. Using WST data for between class prediction and ROC analyses, the correctly predicted cases (by RFA) for classes 0 and 1 (Figure 4) emphasised the powerful role of 24-h urinary creatinine excretion rate as a potential diagnostic marker; it was the only marker analysed that showed a clear differentiation between class 0 in comparison to class 1 25–75 IQR intervals (results not shown).

The calculation of reference intervals specific to varying levels of ME/CFS severity, as quantitated by WST, was achieved (Tables 5 and 6). With access to larger sample sizes, via large multi-centre studies and/or databases, the capacity to develop novel diagnostic guidelines using pathology results specific for ME/CFS, with and without activin B, will be possible.

Two multi-category, non-parametric statistical tests were used to assess significance for each predictor variable, the Kruskal Wallis (KW) and Jonckheere–Terpstra (J-T) Tests (Table 6). The methods are different in how they estimate significance across three or more classes, with the J-T test designed for investigations of ordered (ordinal) variables. While all variables were clearly significant (≤0.012) by the KW test, only serum urea, 24-h urinary creatinine excretion rate and activin B demonstrated significance for both tests, suggesting enhanced statistical robustness for these markers in terms of variation across the three WST classes.

4. Discussion

As demonstrated previously by us [8,18] and others [26], the results of pathology testing are not remarkable for ME/CFS patients, and often there are no statistically significant differences in the pathology results for ME/CFS when compared to healthy control subjects, although a recent study has identified the pathology test for creatine kinase (CK) as a significant marker to separate ME/CFS from control samples [27]. These difficulties in detecting quantitative markers for ME/CFS diagnosis have stimulated many investigations over the past 30 years, and with research consistently suggesting immune system involvement or dysfunction [28], cytokine studies have featured prominently in these attempts at biomarker development [1–7]. The search for a cytokine biomarker has been fraught with frustration, for example, the promise of a TGF-β marker was stymied by the realisation that sample preparation may explain serum concentration variation [7]. To this literature on putative ME/CFS serum biomarkers, we added activin B, which is useful in isolation, but also as a ratio with activin A or follistatin [8] and maintains statistical significance across WST classes [18].

The research presented here is a validation study on the potential of activin B as a reliable serum marker for ME/CFS, which would be a major advance in this field in light of the history of biomarker development. As reported, serum activin B showed statistical significance in separating ME/CFS participants from healthy controls, and additionally, demonstrated a capacity to differentiate WST classes in combination with select pathology markers. However, for this new research population, the trend was reversed, with healthy control participants showing a significantly increased median compared to the ME/CFS cohort. A cohort of existing CFS Discovery patients were recruited as research participants for this study, and issues associated with small to medium samples sizes may have contributed to these findings. The re-calibration of the activin B assay, due to sensitivity variation across the range of detection, improved the accuracy of the assay at lower serum concentrations, thus enhancing activin B detection capacity and broadening the reference interval range, which may explain the differences in activin B results found for this study when compared to the previous results [8].

Exploratory random forest analysis (RFA) was performed on the same data, with subsequent analyses focussed on WST data only (see Table 1b). The standard RFA of WST data (5000 trees per analysis, four predictor variables tested per node) resulted in (OOB) error rates of 38.14%. Activin B was also investigated as a member of a six-marker profile that included 24-h urinary creatinine excretion rate, mean corpuscular haemoglobin (MCH), alkaline phosphatase (ALP), serum urea, and total lymphocyte count. RFA, with or without activin B, showed an identical overall prediction error rate (OOB), but with the addition of activin B to the marker profile, a reduction in WST 2 (severe) class prediction error rate was identified, at the expense of an error rate increase for WST 0 (WST 1 error rate remained stable). For this RFA, urinary creatinine, ALP and activin B were the top predictors of WST class. The capacity of activin B to enhance discrimination between WST classes was also a feature identified by RFA.

Single decision trees confirmed the primacy of 24-h urinary creatinine clearance as a ME/CFS predictor, with a calculated decision threshold of 11.96 mmol/L separating class 0 (accuracy 83.3%) from classes 1 and 2, while ALP separated classes 1 and 2 at 62.5 U/L (accuracies of 86.4% and 75% respectively). Caution must be exercised when interpreting these results, since the final accuracy scores were often calculated from ≤20 cases.

As an extension of RFA, the panel of six predictive markers was assessed by receiver operating characteristic (ROC) curves to investigate the impact of test profile sensitivity and specificity (false negative, false positive rates). Pairwise WST classes were analysed per ROC, both for the entire data set, and for the correctly predicted cases for each WST class (0, 1, 2). Activin B remained in the top three in terms of predictor importance, with the model producing an AUC of 0.76 for all cases and an AUC of 0.963 for models comprising only correctly predicted outcomes. The correctly predicted cases from each WST class were subsequently used to calculate new reference intervals for each of the six RFA predictors (Figure 2).

Due to the broad reference intervals calculated as medians and 25th–75th IQRs, distinct separation between WST classes was not common, but did feature for 24-h urinary creatinine clearance and some class comparisons for activin B. As stated earlier, larger participant cohorts are required for validation, and the calculation of accurate reference intervals via the method presented here.

In tandem with research on ME/CFS immunology, pathology and cytokine biology, metabolomics is yielding valuable insights into ME/CFS aetiology [29,30], which in turn crosses into mitochondrial function [31]. New and sophisticated evidence of mitochondrial dysfunction in ME/CFS patients has emerged recently from patients involved as research participants in this project, with blast lymphocytes grown from blood samples collected at CFS Discovery and analysed via *Seahorse* technology [32].

Potential exists to meld metabolomics with immunity, and mTOR (mammalian targets of rapamycin and TORC subunits), which has a role in amino acid transport and protein synthesis [33], may be central to this link, particularly in the context of muscle growth [34,35]. Muscle pain and weakness are often reported as leading ME/CFS symptoms [12,18]. TGF-β and activin proteins involve mTOR interaction, including for natural killer (NK) cells [36], which are regularly noted as deficient in ME/CFS patients [37], as well as for cartilage and bone biology [38]. Separating the specific biology of activin B from the well-studied roles of activin A has shown insights in relation to SMAD signalling [10,39,40], which will further illuminate activin B utility in the context of ME/CFS.

The centrality of NK cells to ME/CFS has been challenged recently by a comprehensive study involving more than 300 total participants, which included healthy and fatigue controls, as well as participants with varying levels of ME/CFS symptom severity [41]. NK cell numbers and function, as reflected by subtype proportions or responsiveness post in vitro stimulation, were not different between the control and ME/CFS cohorts. Instead, $CD8^+$ T-cell proportions were altered, and mucosal associated invariant T cells (MAIT) increased for ME/CFS.

Future investigations will present results from the interrogation of databases that contain activin, pathology, mitochondrial and metabolomics results, and thereafter assist in the identification of additional immune-metabolomic biomarker patterns. Such results will thereafter contribute to the elucidation of disease mechanism via the unravelling of impaired metabolomic pathways, and understanding of the subsequent impact on immune function, muscle physiology and neurophysiology for ME/CFS patients.

In conclusion, activin B retained the capacity to separate ME/CFS cases from healthy controls (Table 2), but as an inverse relationship compared to the situation reported previously [8], with healthy controls having a higher median. The potential, therefore, to develop activin B as a general serum marker of ME/CFS needs multi-centre studies with large participant cohorts. While the current project recruited 97 participants, these were spread across the spectrum of good health to severe ME/CFS symptoms, hence resulting in small to moderate samples sizes. RFA studies revealed the unexpected role of activin B as a useful supporting marker for the discrimination of mild to moderate ME/CFS symptoms, as reflected by WST class, while severe cases were more difficult to predict via multi-marker RFA and the other methods developed to predict ME/CFS.

Supplementary Materials: The following are available online at http://www.mdpi.com/2075-4418/9/3/79/s1.

Author Contributions: Study conceptualization involved, B.A.L., B.K. and D.d.K.; Methodology, B.A.L., E.P., S.H., M.H. and D.P.L.; Validation, E.P., B.A.L., A.M.R. and S.H.; Formal analysis, B.A.L., M.H. and A.M.R.; Investigation, All authors.; Resources, E.P., D.P.L., S.H., B.K., M.H. and D.d.K.; Data curation, B.A.L.; Writing—original draft preparation, B.A.L., B.K. and D.d.K.; Writing—review and editing, All authors; Visualization, B.A.L. and A.M.R.; Supervision, B.A.L., B.K. and D.d.K.; Project administration, B.A.L., M.H. and B.K.; Funding acquisition, B.A.L., B.K. and D.d.K.

Funding: This research was funded by the Judith. J. Mason and Harold S. Williams Memorial Foundation (The Mason Foundation), grant number CT23141–23142.

Acknowledgments: The authors thank The Mason Foundation (Australia) for funding this project. Many thanks also to the staff at CFS Discovery (Donvale), and particularly to the patients and other volunteers for contributing to research as study participants. The authors also acknowledge the valuable role of Australian Clinical Laboratories (ACL – Adelaide) for the provision of pathology services. Results from this study were presented at the Emerge Australia International Research Symposium, "ME/CFS—The Biomedical Basis, Diagnosis, Treatment and Management" (12–15 March 2019, Geelong, Australia).

Conflicts of Interest: Donald P. Lewis (retired) was the Director and senior clinician at CFS Discovery, Donvale, where the research participants were recruited and assessed for this project. Edwina Privitera was an employee of CFS Discovery. Badia Kita is an employee of Paranta Bioscience, with David de Kretser and Mark Hedger also associated with this company. Paranta Bioscience has an interest in the commercial development of activin proteins. The funders had no role in the design of the study; in the collection, analyses, or interpretation of data; in the writing of the manuscript, or in the decision to publish the results.

References

1. Chao, C.C.; Janoff, E.N.; Hu, S.; Thomas, K.; Gallagher, M.; Tsang, M.; Peterson, P.K. Altered cytokine release in peripheral blood mononuclear cell cultures from patients with the chronic fatigue syndrome. *Cytokine* **1991**, *3*, 292–298. [CrossRef]
2. Bennett, A.L.; Chao, C.C.; Hu, S.; Buchwald, D.; Fagioli, L.R.; Schur, P.H.; Peterson, P.K.; Komaroff, A.L. Elevation of bioactive transforming growth factor-beta in serum from patients with chronic fatigue syndrome. *J. Clin. Immunol.* **1997**, *17*, 160–166. [CrossRef] [PubMed]
3. Blundell, S.; Ray, K.K.; Buckland, M.; White, P.D. Chronic fatigue syndrome and circulating cytokines: A systematic review. *Brain Behav. Immun.* **2015**, *50*, 186–195. [CrossRef] [PubMed]
4. Peterson, D.; Brenu, E.W.; Gottschalk, G.; Ramos, S.; Nguyen, T.; Staines, D.; Marshall-Gradisnik, S. Cytokines in the cerebrospinal fluids of patients with chronic fatigue syndrome/myalgic encephalomyelitis. *Mediat. Inflamm.* **2015**, *2015*, 929720. [CrossRef] [PubMed]
5. Clark, L.V.; Buckland, M.; Murphy, G.; Taylor, N.; Vleck, V.; Mein, C.; Wozniak, E.; Smuk, M.; White, P.D. Cytokine responses to exercise and activity in patients with chronic fatigue syndrome: Case-control study. *Clin. Exp. Immunol.* **2017**, *190*, 360–371. [CrossRef] [PubMed]
6. Montoya, J.G.; Holmes, T.H.; Anderson, J.N.; Maecker, H.T.; Rosenberg-Hasson, Y.; Valencia, I.J.; Chu, L.; Younger, J.W.; Tato, C.M.; Davis, M.M. Cytokine signature associated with disease severity in chronic fatigue syndrome patients. *Proc. Natl. Acad. Sci. USA* **2017**, *114*, e7150–e7158. [CrossRef]
7. Roerink, M.E.; Van Der Schaaf, M.E.; Hawinkels, L.J.; Raijmakers, R.P.; Knoop, H.; Van Der Meer, J.W. Pitfalls in cytokine measurements—Plasma TGF-beta1 in chronic fatigue syndrome. *Neth. J. Med.* **2018**, *76*, 310–313.
8. Lidbury, B.A.; Kita, B.; Lewis, D.P.; Hayward, S.; Ludlow, H.; Hedger, M.P.; De Kretser, D.M. Activin B is a novel biomarker for chronic fatigue syndrome/myalgic encephalomyelitis (CFS/ME) diagnosis: A cross sectional study. *J. Transl. Med.* **2017**, *15*, 60. [CrossRef]
9. Hedger, M.P.; De Kretser, D.M. The activins and their binding protein, follistatin-Diagnostic and therapeutic targets in inflammatory disease and fibrosis. *Cytokine Growth Factor Rev.* **2013**, *24*, 285–295. [CrossRef]
10. Besson-Fournier, C.; Latour, C.; Kautz, L.; Bertrand, J.; Ganz, T.; Roth, M.P.; Coppin, H. Induction of activin B by inflammatory stimuli up-regulates expression of the iron-regulatory peptide hepcidin through Smad1/5/8 signaling. *Blood* **2012**, *120*, 431–439. [CrossRef]
11. De Kretser, D.M.; Bensley, J.G.; Phillips, D.J.; Levvey, B.J.; Snell, G.I.; Lin, E.; Hedger, M.P.; O'Hehir, R.E. Substantial increases occur in serum activins and follistatin during lung transplantation. *PLoS ONE* **2016**, *11*, e0140948. [CrossRef] [PubMed]
12. Carruthers, B.M.; Van De Sande, M.I.; De Meirleir, K.L.; Klimas, N.G.; Broderick, G.; Mitchell, T.; Staines, D.; Powles, A.P.; Speight, N.; Vallings, R.; et al. Myalgic encephalomyelitis: International Consensus Criteria. *J. Intern. Med.* **2011**, *270*, 327–338. [CrossRef] [PubMed]
13. Reynolds, G.K.; Lewis, D.P.; Richardson, A.M.; Lidbury, B.A. Comorbidity of postural orthostatic tachycardia syndrome and chronic fatigue syndrome in an Australian cohort. *J. Intern. Med.* **2014**, *275*, 409–417. [CrossRef] [PubMed]
14. Johns, M.W. A new method for measuring daytime sleepiness: The Epworth Sleepiness Scale. *Sleep* **1991**, *14*, 50–55. [CrossRef] [PubMed]

15. Lovibond, S.H.; Lovibond, P.F. *Manual for the Depression Anxiety Stress Scales*, 2nd ed.; Psychology Foundation: Sydney, Australia, 1995.
16. Depression Anxiety Stress Scales (DASS). Psychology Foundation of Australia. Available online: http://www2.psy.unsw.edu.au/dass/ (accessed on 19 October 2018).
17. Lewis, I.; Pairman, J.; Spickett, G.; Newton, J.L. Clinical characteristics of a novel subgroup of chronic fatigue syndrome patients with postural orthostatic tachycardia syndrome. *J. Intern. Med.* **2013**, *273*, 501–510. [CrossRef] [PubMed]
18. Richardson, A.M.; Lewis, D.P.; Kita, B.; Ludlow, H.; Groome, N.P.; Hedger, M.P.; De Kretser, D.M.; Lidbury, B.A. Weighting of orthostatic intolerance time measurements with standing difficulty score stratifies ME/CFS symptom severity and analyte detection. *J. Transl. Med.* **2018**, *16*, 97. [CrossRef] [PubMed]
19. Liaw, A.; Wiener, M. Classification and Regression by randomForest. *R News* **2002**, *2*, 18–22.
20. Therneau, T.; Atkinson, B. Rpart: Recursive Partitioning and Regression Trees, R package version 4.1-13. 2018. Available online: https://CRAN.R-project.org/package=rpart (accessed on 20 October 2018).
21. Kuhn, M.; Wing, J.; Weston, S.; Williams, A.; Keefer, C.; Engelhardt, A.; Cooper, T.; Mayer, Z.; Kenkel, B.; The R Core Team; et al. Caret: Classification and Regression Training, R package version 6.0-80. 2018; Available online: https://CRAN.R-project.org/package=caret (accessed on 20 October 2018).
22. Brownlee, J. How to Build an Ensemble of Machine Learning Algorithms in R (ready to use boosting, bagging and stacking). Available online: https://machinelearningmastery.com/machine-learning-ensembles-with-r/ (accessed on 20 October 2018).
23. Sing, T.; Sander, O.; Beerenwinkel, N.; Lengauer, T. ROCR: Visualizing classifier performance in R. *Bioinformatics* **2005**, *21*, 7881. Available online: http://rocr.bioinf.mpi-sb.mpg.de (accessed on 20 October 2018). [CrossRef] [PubMed]
24. Ludlow, H.; Phillips, D.J.; Myers, M.; McLachlan, R.I.; De Kretser, D.M.; Allan, C.A.; Anderson, R.A.; Groome, N.P.; Hyvönen, M.; Colin Duncan, W.; et al. A new 'total' activin B enzyme-linked immunosorbent assay (ELISA): Development and validation for human samples. *Clin. Endocrinol.* **2009**, *71*, 867–873. [CrossRef]
25. De Kretser, D.M.; Bensley, J.G.; Pettilä, V.; Linko, R.; Hedger, M.P.; Hayward, S.; Allan, C.A.; McLachlan, R.I.; Ludlow, H.; Phillips, D.J. Serum activin A and B levels predict outcomes in patients with acute respiratory failure: A prospective cohort study. *Crit. Care* **2013**, *17*, R263. [CrossRef]
26. Niblett, S.H.; King, K.E.; Dunstan, R.H.; Clifton-Bligh, P.; Hoskin, L.A.; Roberts, T.K.; Fulcher, G.R.; McGregor, N.R.; Dunsmore, J.C.; Butt, H.L.; et al. Hematologic and urinary excretion anomalies in patients with chronic fatigue syndrome. *Exp. Biol. Med.* **2007**, *232*, 1041–1049. [CrossRef] [PubMed]
27. Nacul, L.; de Barros, B.; Kingdon, C.C.; Cliff, J.M.; Clark, T.G.; Mudie, K.; Dockrell, H.M.; Lacerda, E.M. Evidence of Clinical Pathology Abnormalities in People with Myalgic Encephalomyelitis/Chronic Fatigue Syndrome (ME/CFS) from an Analytic Cross-Sectional Study. *Diagnostics* **2019**, *9*, 41. [CrossRef] [PubMed]
28. Sotzny, F.; Blanco, J.; Capelli, E.; Castro-Marrero, J.; Steiner, S.; Murovska, M.; Scheibenbogen, C. Myalgic Encephalomyelitis/Chronic Fatigue Syndrome—Evidence for an autoimmune disease. *Autoimmun. Rev.* **2018**, *17*, 601–609. [CrossRef] [PubMed]
29. Armstrong, C.W.; McGregor, N.R.; Sheedy, J.R.; Buttfield, I.; Butt, H.L.; Gooley, P.R. NMR metabolic profiling of serum identifies amino acid disturbances in chronic fatigue syndrome. *Clin. Chim. Acta* **2012**, *413*, 1525–1531. [CrossRef] [PubMed]
30. Armstrong, C.W.; McGregor, N.R.; Butt, H.L.; Gooley, P.R. Metabolism in chronic fatigue syndrome. *Adv. Clin. Chem.* **2014**, *66*, 121–172.
31. Booth, N.E.; Myhill, S.; McLaren-Howard, J. Mitochondrial dysfunction and the pathophysiology of Myalgic Encephalomyelitis/Chronic Fatigue Syndrome (ME/CFS). *Int. J. Clin. Exp. Med.* **2012**, *5*, 208–220. [PubMed]
32. Missailidis, D.; Annesley, S.; Fisher, P. Unpublished results (manuscript under review). 2019.
33. Freitag, J.; Berod, L.; Kamradt, T.; Sparwasser, T. Immunometabolism and autoimmunity. *Immunol. Cell Biol.* **2016**, *94*, 925–934. [CrossRef]
34. Chen, J.L.; Walton, K.L.; Winbanks, C.E.; Murphy, K.T.; Thomson, R.E.; Makanji, Y.; Qian, H.; Lynch, G.S.; Harrison, C.A.; Gregorevic, P. Elevated expression of activins promotes muscle wasting and cachexia. *FASEB J.* **2014**, *28*, 1711–1723. [CrossRef]

35. Bodine, S.C.; Stitt, T.N.; Gonzalez, M.; Kline, W.O.; Stover, G.L.; Bauerlein, R.; Zlotchenko, E.; Scrimgeour, A.; Lawrence, J.C.; Glass, D.J.; et al. Akt/mTOR pathway is a crucial regulator of skeletal muscle hypertrophy and can prevent muscle atrophy in vivo. *Nat. Cell Biol.* **2001**, *3*, 1014–1019. [CrossRef]
36. Viel, S.; Marçais, A.; Guimaraes, F.S.; Loftus, R.; Rabilloud, J.; Grau, M.; Degouve, S.; Djebali, S.; Sanlaville, A.; Charrier, E.; et al. TGF-beta inhibits the activation and functions of NK cells by repressing the mTOR pathway. *Sci. Signal* **2016**, *9*, ra19. [CrossRef]
37. Brenu, E.W.; Van Driel, M.L.; Staines, D.R.; Ashton, K.J.; Hardcastle, S.L.; Keane, J.; Tajouri, L.; Peterson, D.; Ramos, S.B.; Marshall-Gradisnik, S.M. Longitudinal investigation of natural killer cells and cytokines in chronic fatigue syndrome/myalgic encephalomyelitis. *J. Transl. Med.* **2012**, *10*, 88. [CrossRef] [PubMed]
38. Hino, K.; Horigome, K.; Nishio, M.; Komura, S.; Nagata, S.; Zhao, C.; Jin, Y.; Kawakami, K.; Yamada, Y.; Ohta, A.; et al. Activin-A enhances mTOR signalling to promote aberrant chondrogenesis in fibrodysplasia ossificans progressiva. *J. Clin. Investig.* **2017**, *127*, 3339–3352. [CrossRef] [PubMed]
39. Canali, S.; Core, A.B.; Zumbrennen-Bullough, K.B.; Merkulova, M.; Wang, C.Y.; Schneyer, A.L.; Pietrangelo, A.; Babitt, J.L. Activin B Induces Noncanonical SMAD1/5/8 Signaling via BMP Type I Receptors in Hepatocytes: Evidence for a Role in Hepcidin Induction by Inflammation in Male Mice. *Endocrinology* **2016**, *157*, 1146–1162. [CrossRef] [PubMed]
40. Xiong, S.; Klausen, C.; Cheng, J.C.; Zhu, H.; Leung, P.C. Activin B induces human endometrial cancer cell adhesion, migration and invasion by up-regulating integrin β3 via SMAD2/3 signalling. *Oncotarget* **2015**, *6*, 31659–31673. [CrossRef] [PubMed]
41. Cliff, J.M.; King, E.C.; Lee, J.S.; Sepúlveda, N.; Wolf, A.S.; Kingdon, C.; Bowman, E.; Dockrell, H.M.; Nacul, L.C.; Lacerda, E.; et al. Cellular Immune Function in Myalgic Encephalomyelitis/Chronic Fatigue Syndrome (ME/CFS). *Front. Immunol.* **2019**, *10*, 796. [CrossRef] [PubMed]

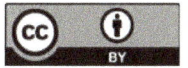 © 2019 by the authors. Licensee MDPI, Basel, Switzerland. This article is an open access article distributed under the terms and conditions of the Creative Commons Attribution (CC BY) license (http://creativecommons.org/licenses/by/4.0/).

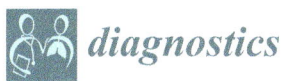

Article

Post-Exertional Malaise Is Associated with Hypermetabolism, Hypoacetylation and Purine Metabolism Deregulation in ME/CFS Cases

Neil R. McGregor [1,*], Christopher W. Armstrong [2], Donald P. Lewis [3] and Paul R. Gooley [2]

1 Faculty of Medicine, Dentistry and Health Sciences, University of Melbourne, Parkville VIC 3010, Australia
2 Department of Biochemistry and Molecular Biology, Bio21 Molecular Science and Biochemistry Institute, 30 Flemington Road, Parkville VIC 3010, Australia
3 CFS Discovery, Donvale Medical Centre, Donvale VIC 3111, Australia
* Correspondence: neilm@unimelb.edu.au; Tel.: +61-041-246-9832

Received: 17 June 2019; Accepted: 2 July 2019; Published: 4 July 2019

Abstract: Post-exertional malaise (PEM) is a cardinal predictive symptom in the definition of Myalgic Encephalomyelitis/Chronic Fatigue Syndrome (ME/CFS). If the cases overexert themselves they have what is termed "payback" resulting in a worsening of symptoms or relapse which can last for days, weeks or even months. The aim was to assess the changes in biochemistry associated with the cases self-reported PEM scores over a 7-day period and the frequency of reporting over a 12-month period. Forty-seven ME/CFS cases and age/sex-matched controls had a clinical examination, completed questionnaires; were subjected to standard serum biochemistry; had their serum and urine metabolomes analyzed in an observational study. Thirty-five of the 46 ME/CFS cases reported PEM in the last 7-days and these were allocated to the PEM group. The principal biochemical change related to the 7-day severity of PEM was the fall in the purine metabolite, hypoxanthine. This decrease correlated with alterations in the glucose:lactate ratio highly suggestive of a glycolytic anomaly. Increased excretion of urine metabolites within the 7-day response period indicated a hypermetabolic event was occurring. Increases in urine excretion of methylhistidine (muscle protein degradation), mannitol (intestinal barrier deregulation) and acetate were noted with the hypermetabolic event. These data indicate hypoacetylation was occurring, which may also be related to deregulation of multiple cytoplasmic enzymes and DNA histone regulation. These findings suggest the primary events associated with PEM were due to hypoacetylation and metabolite loss during the acute PEM response.

Keywords: fatigue syndrome; chronic; exercise; hypoacetylation; methylhistidine; histone deacetylation

1. Introduction

Myalgic Encephalomyelitis/Chronic Fatigue Syndrome (ME/CFS) is a medically unexplained condition which occurs predominantly in females. It is characterized by persistent or relapsing fatigue and altered responses to exercise and alterations in normal sleep structure. Post-exertional malaise (PEM) is 10.4-fold more frequent in ME/CFS cases compared with controls [1]. However, very little is known about the underlying pathophysiology of PEM.

ME/CFS females were reported to have biochemical changes consistent with the deregulation of glycolysis and urea cycle activity [2], which were indicated by increases in the fasted first morning serum metabolome glucose and falls in lactate and acetate. The deregulation of glycolysis at pyruvate dehydrogenase (EC 1.2.4.1), has been confirmed by other researchers [3]. This deregulation of glycolysis results in falls of acetate and activation of histone deacetylation [4,5] as well as deregulation of acetylation of cytoplasmic and mitochondrial enzymes. Importantly, histone deacetylase 2 (HDAC2) was ~four fold higher and HDAC3 was ~two-fold higher, in ME/CFS cases compared with controls [6]. In further support, a study of gene upregulation in ME/CFS cases, following an exercise test, revealed two histone genes were upregulated [7]. Analysis of HDAC binding sites within the genes of that study revealed that 19 of the 20 upregulated genes had binding sites for HDAC1 and HDAC2 but also members of the SMAD transcription factor family that convey the signal from the transforming growth factor beta (TGF-β) receptor, namely SMAD1, SMAD4, and SMAD5 [8,9] (Table S1). The Whistler et al. study [7] also supports the hypothesis that acetylation changes may occur, when ME/CFS cases have PEM. Anomalies in TGF-β have also been identified in some ME/CFS studies but not all [10,11]. However, none of these were assessed against PEM activity. These data indicate that the change in glycolysis in ME/CFS cases may be related to either or combined effects of at least: (1) histone deacetylation; (2) a chronic reduction in acetate production via glycolysis; (3) deregulation of cytoplasmic and mitochondrial enzyme acetylation.

Reductions in the purine metabolite, hypoxanthine, were also found in the serum metabolomes of the females in first morning fasted samples [2] and potentially indicated reductions in the ability to produce ATP. During exercise, the release of hypoxanthine from muscle occurs as part of a hypermetabolic event when the levels of mitochondrial/cytoplasmic ATP fall. The hypermetabolic event relates to the release of metabolites from muscle associated with inhibition of protein synthesis within muscle once exercise starts. This same event occurs in lymphocytes when glycolysis is inhibited [12,13]. Whilst multiple immune issues have been detected in ME/CFS cases, the underlying mechanism behind the changes have not been identified [14]. Activation of glycolysis and histone acetylation are essential steps in immune activation [15], in particular T-cells and NK-cells [16]. An interesting study of lymphocytes showed that when the ATP levels fell after inhibition of glycolysis and adenosine degradation products increased, the incorporation of leucine into protein was also dramatically inhibited [12]. Thus, the ME/CFS case immune system issues may be a result of glycolytic and acetylation dysregulation, resulting in a reduced ability to translate DNA into proteins and hence protein synthesis. Evidence also indicates a switch toward utilization of branched-chain amino acids as an energy source, especially during exhaustive events [17].

Acetate is associated with control of multiple enzymes within the cell [18], which could be critically important in the biochemical changes in ME/CFS. A total of 1750 cellular proteins have been identified to have the characteristics to bind acetate and alter the protein function, these include DNA replication (52 proteins), DNA repair (72 proteins), cell cycle switching (132 proteins), nucleotide exchange factors (55 proteins), and acetylation and deacetylation (21 proteins) [18]. The biochemistry of these acetate regulated events may be secondary to the fall in acetate but are likely to have profound effects upon cellular function in ME/CFS cases.

The objective of this paper was to assess PEM 7-day severity and 12-month frequency symptoms scores and related biochemistry (blood and urine) in ME/CFS cases and controls. Associations of the PEM scores were examined using standard serum biochemistry, a 24-hour urine assessment and a blood and urine metabolome.

2. Methods

Forty-six cases with ME/CFS and 26 fatigue-free, age and sex-matched healthy individuals were recruited. Obtaining age and sex-matched controls was undertaken by placing advertisements on University billboards and selecting individuals of the same sex and age (±5 years) who were then assessed using the same clinical examinations. The ME/CFS group comprised cases that were currently symptomatic and diagnosed as having ME/CFS in accordance with the Canadian guidelines and its exclusionary criteria [19]. A Depression Anxiety Stress assessment (DASS) [20] was used to assess their psychiatric comorbidity. Only those ME/CFS subjects who complied with the criteria were included in the study. All subjects were asked to list their drugs and oral supplements. None of the participants were related to one another nor did they ever live together. All subjects signed consent forms. This study was approved by the University of Melbourne human research ethics committee (HREC# 0723086, 2010) and the first specimens were collected on 23 September 2010.

2.1. Clinical Measures

The subjects had a full clinical examination and were questioned about their illness, onset, and family histories to determine whether they fulfilled criteria for the Canadian ME/CFS guidelines. All subjects completed several questionnaires, including a large symptom questionnaire developed for chronic pain research [21]. It asked subjects to score how severe a symptom was in the last seven days (0–4 scalar response) and how frequently the symptom occurred over the last 12-month period (0–4 scalar response), as previously published [22]. The 7-day severity and 12-month frequency scores, designed to differentiate between acute and chronic responses, have been assessed against the biochemistry and found to differentiate between an acute response and a chronic response [22]. These questionnaires were checked for completeness by the reception staff and the medical clinician (DL). The medical clinician questioned the subjects about their responses to ensure accuracy.

2.2. Biochemistry Assessments

The sample collection and processing has previously been published [2] and are provided here in summary. Subjects had a phlebotomy for either standard serum biochemistry, which was performed at a commercial (National Association of Testing Authorities (NATA) accredited) laboratory; or a metabolome. A second urine sample was collected upon rising by each subject at their home and stored at 4 °C. Within 6 h, a blood sample was taken by venipuncture into BD Vacutainer®blood collection tubes (Beckton Dickinson, Mississauga, ON, Canada). All samples were stored at −80 °C prior to performing an NMR analysis as previously described [2] using a liquid-liquid extraction technique [23], data were acquired on an 800 MHz Bruker Avance II NMR spectrometer (Bruker, Billerica, MA, USA); metabolites were identified and quantitated with the compound libraries in the Chenomx software (v6.1, Chenomx, Edmonton, AB, Canada). Twenty-nine metabolites per blood serum sample and thirty metabolites per urine sample were identified.

2.3. Data Analysis

The metabolome data were prepared as raw data (μM) and as relatively distributed data (%) by dividing each metabolite concentration by the total concentration of metabolites quantified in each sample. The parametric data prior to statistical analysis was assessed for normality and log converted if not normally distributed. All percentage data were arcsine converted for analysis. The dataset was evaluated using Statistica for Windows Ver. 12.0 (TIBCO Software, Palo Alto, CA, USA) using statistical calculations, including t-tests and Pearson correlation coefficients, ANOVA and multivariate analysis. The nonparametric data were assessed using Spearman rank correlations, Mann-Whitney U-tests or Kruskal-Wallis ANOVA. Small sample frequency data were analyzed with Fisher exact Chi-square analysis (χ^2). Multiplicity (Bonferroni) correction was carried out on the data based upon the number of variables assessed in each statistical test.

3. Results

3.1. Demographics

To examine the PEM biochemistry, we chose to divide the ME/CFS group on presence/absence of significant PEM responses in the last 7 days (PEM, NoPEM meaning those without current symptoms, Controls (C)). Table 1 shows the subject demographics for the ME/CFS cases divided on the basis of the presence or absence of significant PEM and the control group. No differences were found for sudden versus gradual onset or triggers at onset, such as infections (significance $p < 0.01$). Table 1 also shows the ME/CFS-defined symptom clusters across the three groups (control, ME/CFS: NoPEM, PEM). Apart from the PEM scores, there were no differences in symptom profiles between the NoPEM and PEM groups. Both groups presented higher scores compared with controls.

Table 1. Subject demographics, post-exertional malaise (PEM) scores within the ME/CFS cases divided on the basis of PEM 7-day severity scores compared with controls. The symptom scores are given as the median and the 10–90% percentile distribution.

	Control	ME/CFS NoPEM	ME/CFS PEM
Number	25	11	35
Age	33.6 ± 7.8 *	30.9 ± 9.6	42.1 ± 16.3
%Females	96%	100%	80%
Duration (years)	-	8.7 ± 5.4	12.1 ± 9.7
Age at Onset	-	22.8 ± 6.8	30 ± 13.9
Systolic BP	-	116 ± 12	129 ± 17
Diastolic BP	-	79 ± 7	83 ± 9
Pulse rate	-	78 ± 11	73 ± 13
BMI x ± SD	23.1 ± 2.6	22.7 ± 3.6	24.9 ± 6.1
DASS Depression	0	11.2 ± 10.7	11.1 ± 11.1
DASS Anxiety	0.5 ± 0.6	13.3 ± 8.3	9.8 ± 7.8
DASS Stress	3.5 ± 3.6 *	20.7 ± 9.4 *	12.9 ± 8.7
PEM 7D	0.1 ± 0.4 **	1.3 ± 0.65 **	3.7 ± 0.5 **,‡
12F	0.1 ± 0.4 **	2.8 ± 1.2 **	3.5 ± 0.6 **,†
Fatigue 7D	0.7 ± 0.8 **	3.2 ± 0.9 **	3.7 ± 0.6 **
12F	1.1 ± 0.8 **	3.8 ± 0.6 **	3.8 ± 0.4 **
Sleep Disturbance 7D	1.6 ± 2.6 **	10.9 ± 2.5 **	10.5 ± 3.2 **
12F	2.6 ± 2.3 **	12.3 ± 2.7 **	11.1 ± 2.8 **
Cognition scores 7D	2.3 ± 2.9 **	16.1 ± 5.8 **	17.3 ± 6.5 **
12F	3.6 ± 3.7 **	18.8 ± 5.6 **	18.3 ± 5.9 **
Body Pain 7D	1.3 ± 1.3 **	6.3 ± 2.1 **	6.3 ± 2.2 **
Distribution 12F	2.6 ± 1.3 **	7.1 ± 1.5 **	6.9 ± 2.1 **

Statistical methods: ANOVA and post-hoc Tukey Honest Significance (THS) analysis. Multiplicity (Bonferroni) correction: Data only included if one measure reached $p < 0.01$. PEM = PEM group. NoPEM = those with very low or absent PEM scores. BMI = body mass index, 7D = 7-Day severity score, 12F = 12-month frequency score. In control column * = $p < 0.01$ or ** = $p < 0.001$ for the ANOVA. In the ME/CFS NoPEM or PEM columns * = $p < 0.01$ or ** = $p < 0.001$ for post hoc analysis vs. controls. In the ME/CFS NoPEM or PEM columns † = $p < 0.01$ or ‡ = $p < 0.001$ for post hoc analysis of NoPEM vs. PEM.

3.2. Biochemistry

Table 2 shows a summary of the statistically significant metabolome measures between the groups. The ME/CFS groups had significant reductions in serum hypoxanthine (NoPEM 4.4-fold lower, PEM 2.4-fold lower versus controls), serum lactate (NoPEM 1.9-fold lower, PEM 1.6-fold lower versus controls), phenylalanine (Both NoPEM and PEM 1.3-fold lower versus controls). Glucose was increased in the ME/CFS cases (both NoPEM and PEM 1.2-fold higher versus controls). In the urine the fall in acetate was greatest (NoPEM 2.5-fold lower, PEM 1.5-fold lower versus controls) and this was statistically different between the NoPEM and PEM subgroups ($p < 0.01$). The excretion of methylhistidine was higher in the PEM subgroup (1.6 fold) and control (1.3 fold) groups, respectively, compared with the NoPEM subgroup. In the fecal metabolome, the % butyrate was increased in the NoPEM group compared with both the PEM and control groups. (Figure S1 shows the group canonical plots of separations using different analyses).

Table 3 is a summary of the correlation analysis of the PEM scores across the whole group and within the ME/CFS group. In the whole group analysis, the 7-day severity PEM score and 12-month frequency PEM scores were positively correlated with serum glucose and negatively correlated with hypoxanthine, phenylalanine, lactate and threonine. No significant correlates were noted within the

ME/CFS group. The absolute urine levels showed a significant correlation between the 7-day PEM score along with mannitol, serine, acetate, methylhistidine and glucose. The 12-month frequency of PEM correlated with a fall in acetate alone. The urine percentage data showed falls in urea, pyruvate and acetate with both the 7-day severity and 12-month frequency scores. The only fecal component to reach statistical significance was the percentage uracil. These data show a significant renal concentrating issue is occurring in the ME/CFS group during a PEM event and this was principally related to falls in urea and acetate. To check this, we calculated the serum to urine ratios of multiple metabolites. The 7-day severity of PEM correlated with the following ratios: serum acetate:urine acetate ratio ($r = -0.44$, $p < 0.002$), serum tyrosine:urine tyrosine ratio ($r = -0.40$, $p < 0.006$), serum serine:urine serine ratio ($r = -0.39$, $p < 0.008$), serum creatine:urine creatine ratio ($r = -0.38$, $p < 0.009$), and the serum leucine:urine leucine ratio ($r = -0.37$, $p < 0.01$). Thus, the 7-day severity of PEM was associated with an increased urinary excretion of metabolites within the ME/CFS group and this was associated with a reduction in multiple serum metabolites including the important protein synthesis regulating amino acid, leucine.

Table 2. Summary of ANOVA assessment of the changes in the serum, urine and fecal metabolomes.

	Control Mean (SD)	ME/CFS NoPEM Mean (SD)	ME/CFS PEM Mean (SD)
Serum			
Hypoxanthine (µM)	15.7 ± 12.2 **	3.6 ± 1.4 **	6.6 ± 8.2 **
Lactate (µM)	637 ± 335 **	339 ± 68 *	399 ± 240 **
Phenylalanine (µM)	18.4 ± 3.1 **	15.5 ± 2.2	15.1 ± 3.5 **
Glucose (µM)	971 ± 233 *	1266 ± 249 *	1189 ± 318 *
Hypoxanthine %	0.55 ± 0.39 **	0.14 ± 0.05 **	0.24 ± 0.25 **
Lactate %	22.7 ± 10.5 **	12.9 ± 2.0 *	14.7 ± 6.5 **
Phenylalanine %	0.68 ± 0.09 **	0.60 ± 0.10	0.58 ± 0.10 **
Glucose %	36.2 ± 9.5 **	48.1 ± 5.3 **	45.4 ± 7.5 **
Urine			
Acetate (µM)	91.9 ± 60.3 **	37.0 ± 14.9 **	63.3 ± 31.8 †
Formate (µM)	81.1 ± 56.1 *	27.1 ± 15.2 **	43.0 ± 30.3 *
Urea (µM)	7969 ± 3050 *	4868 ± 2678 **	5821 ± 2425
Mannitol (µM)	312 ± 198 *	96 ± 57 **	258 ± 344 *
Serine (µM)	383 ± 198 *	178 ± 108 **	313 ± 193
Pyruvate (µM)	22.2 ± 10.7 *	11.3 ± 6.4 **	18.4 ± 12.6
Hippurate (µM)	632 ± 424 *	297 ± 253 *	666 ± 612
Methylhistidine (µM)	278 ± 192 *	230 ± 418 *	358 ± 373 †
Pyruvate %	0.36 ± 0.08 **	0.26 ± 0.11 *	0.27 ± 0.09 **
Urea %	4.7 ± 3.4 **	3.8 ± 5.3	5.6 ± 5.1 **
Serine %	6.1 ± 1.6 *	4.2 ± 0.9 *	4.8 ± 1.9 *
Creatinine %	19.7 ± 10.3 *	33.4 ± 9.2 *	25.7 ± 11.5
Acetate %	1.53 ± 0.67 *	0.94 ± 0.26 *	1.08 ± 0.61 *
Allantoin %	0.53 ± 0.28 *	0.96 ± 0.33 *	0.78 ± 0.53
Tryptophan %	0.49 ± 0.16 *	0.49 ± 0.35	0.36 ± 0.10 *
Fecal			
Butyrate %	9.8 ± 3.5 *	15.2 ± 4.5 *	11.3 ± 4.4 †
Ratios			
Serum Glucose: Lactate	2.2 ± 1.4 **	3.8 ± 0.7 **	3.6 ± 1.4 **
Urine Glucose: Lactate	5.2 ± 2.3 *	7.8 ± 4.7 *	6.2 ± 1.8
Serum Glucose: Acetate	96.4 ± 53.6 **	150.6 ± 45.8 *	155.2 ± 72.0 **
Urine Glucose: Acetate	1.37 ± 0.61 *	1.91 ± 0.52 *	1.78 ± 0.70
Serum Acetate: Urine Acetate	0.16 ± 0.09 *	0.30 ± 0.18 *	0.18 ± 0.09 †

Statistical method: ANOVA, multiplicity correction $p < 0.01$. In control column * = $p < 0.01$ or ** = $p < 0.001$ for the ANOVA. In the ME/CFS NoPEM or PEM columns * = $p < 0.01$ or ** = $p < 0.001$ for post hoc analysis vs. controls. In the ME/CFS NoPEM or PEM columns † = $p < 0.01$ for post hoc analysis of NoPEM vs. PEM.

Table 3. PEM 7-day severity and 12-month frequency score correlate with biochemistry in the Serum urine and fecal metabolomes.

Serum	7-Day PEM All Subjects	7-Day PEM ME/CFS Subjects	12-Month PEM All Subjects	12-Month PEM ME/CFS Subjects
Phenylalanine	−0.40 **	−0.11	−0.42 **	−0.08
Hypoxanthine	−0.35 *	+0.25	−0.43 **	+0.21
Lactate	−0.33 *	+0.13	−0.37 *	+0.18
Threonine	−0.31 *	−0.13	−0.25	+0.07
Glucose	+0.31 *	−0.09	+0.38 **	+0.02
Urine				
Total Metabolite	+0.10	+0.38 *	−0.02	+0.18
Mannitol	−0.01	+0.43 *	−0.15	+0.20
Serine	−0.07	+0.42 *	−0.22	+0.17
Acetate	−0.18	+0.41 *	−0.32 *	+0.21
p-Methylhistidine	+0.08	+0.40 *	−0.14	−0.02
Glucose	+0.02	+0.37 *	−0.09	+0.23
Urine %				
Urea%	−0.42 **	−0.24	−0.37 **	−0.04
Pyruvate%	−0.35 *	+0.06	−0.37 **	0.13
Tryptophan%	−0.32 *	−0.28	−0.20	0.06
Malonate%	−0.32 *	−0.37 *	−0.18	0.05
Acetate%	−0.30 *	+0.06	−0.35 *	−0.01
Fecal %				
Uracil	+0.04	+0.46 **	−0.09	0.27

Statistical method: Spearman Rank correlation. Multiplicity correction $p < 0.01$, * = $p < 0.01$ or ** = $p < 0.001$.

The serum glucose:lactate ratio is very similar to the changes in the urine glucose:lactate ratio, which is consistent with the change seen in the serum acetate: urine acetate ratio. This suggests that the serum and urine changes are very similar. Thus, the available acetate in serum appears to be significantly reduced and is lowest in the NoPEM cases.

3.3. Purine Metabolism Changes

As serum hypoxanthine was the prime predictive variable for alterations in the PEM scores, we assessed the relationships between serum Hypoxanthine and the purine related metabolites (Table 4). Serum and urine hypoxanthines were lower in the PEM subgroups versus the controls. Whilst there was no difference in the serum urate levels, the marker of purine degradation in the liver, the serum hypoxanthine: urate ratio was lower in the ME/CFS group. The ratio in the NoPEM subgroup was 5.4-fold lower whilst in the PEM group the ratio was 3.5-fold lower. The hypoxanthine:urate ratio was negatively correlated with serum glucose ($r = −0.48$, $p < 0.001$) and positively correlated with serum lactate ($r = 0.77$, $p < 0.001$), the purine ring precursor amino acids ($r = 0.54$, $p < 0.001$), acetate ($r = 0.49$, $p < 0.001$), and the total serum amino acids ($r = 0.38$, $p < 0.006$). The correlation between serum hypoxanthine and the purine ring precursors, indicative of purine synthesis, was not different between the ME/CFS cases and the controls (ME/CFS $r = 0.66$, $p < 0.001$, control $r = 0.61$, $p < 0.001$). However, the ratio was significantly lower in the ME/CFS group (Table 4 and Figure S2) and the purine ring precursor amino acids correlated positively with serum acetate ($r = 0.52$, $p < 0.001$). Thus, the synthesis and possibly the salvage of hypoxanthine were reduced whilst purine degradation was in the normal range. The levels of hypoxanthine in the serum were associated with the availability of the purine ring precursors, the glucose: lactate ratio and acetate. This suggests that acetylation is a major factor in the change in the purine metabolism deregulation in ME/CFS. Thus, the increase in urine metabolite loss during exercise events in ME/CFS cases results in a loss of purine ring precursors and a fall in acetate and hypoxanthine.

Table 4. Assessment of Purine metabolite changes in serum and urine in the PEM, NoPEM and control subjects.

Metabolite	Control	NoPEM	PEM
Serum Hypoxanthine	15.7 ± 12.2 **	3.6 ± 1.4 **	6.6 ± 8.2 **
% Serum Hypoxanthine	0.55 ± 0.39% **	0.14 ± 0.05% **	0.24 ± 0.25% **
Urine Hypoxanthine	14.9 ± 6.7 *	7.6 ± 4.0*	14.3 ± 11.3
%Urine Hypoxanthine	0.26 ± 0.13% *	0.17 ± 0.04%	0.21 ± 0.10%
Urine Allantoin	32.8 ± 19.0	36.0 ± 13.5	43.7 ± 25.1
% Urine Allantoin	0.53 ± 0.28% *	0.96 ± 0.33% *	0.78 ± 0.53%
Serum Urate	0.28 ± 0.03	0.28 ± 0.06	0.29 ± 0.09
Serum Purine Ring Precursors	138.6 ± 32.8	117.9 ± 23.9	130.2 ± 29.8
Ratios			
Serum Hypoxanthine: Urine Hypoxanthine	1.3 ± 1.6	0.7 ± 0.6	0.9 ± 1.4
Serum Hypoxanthine: Urate	74.2 ± 65.3 **	13.6 ± 6.2 **	21.6 ± 26.3 **
Serum Hypoxanthine: Urine Allantoin	0.75 ± 1.26	0.11 ± 0.05	0.34 ± 0.09
Urine Allantoin: Serum Urate	135.5 ± 71.7	134.2 ± 57.1	162.5 ± 96.2

Statistical method: ANOVA. In control column * = $p < 0.05$ or ** = $p < 0.001$ for the ANOVA. In the ME/CFS NoPEM or PEM columns * = $p < 0.05$ or ** = $p < 0.001$ for post hoc analysis vs. controls.

4. Discussion

This paper has identified that the post-exertional malaise experienced by an Australian Anglo-Celtic cohort of ME/CFS cases is associated with a deregulation of purine metabolism and low acetate levels. This deregulation of purine metabolism is associated with a change in glycolytic activity and a switch to urea cycle creatine phosphate energy usage [2]. This has the effect of reducing the availability of acetate and upregulating histone deacetylase activity [4]. A four- and two-fold increase in HDAC2 and HDAC3, respectively, have been confirmed in ME/CFS cases [6] and a very high level of HDAC1 and HDAC2 binding sites occur within the genes upregulated in ME/CFS cases following exercise (see Table S1) [7]. The enzyme hypoxanthine phosphoribosyltransferase (EC 2.4.2.8) is an important enzyme in the salvage of the purines, adenosine and guanine [24]. Its gene (*HPRT1*) is on the X chromosome and has an unusual regulatory issue. Acetylation and methylation of one X chromosome silence its activity in females, which results in a single X chromosome being active for transcription, as in males [25,26]. This potentially poses a significant issue if there is a loss of silencing of the second X chromosome. This study has too few males to properly assess this potential issue. Deregulation of X chromosome silencing may be related to the fall in hypoxanthine salvage and the more severe illness in females compared with males [1]. Studies are warranted to investigate this interesting possibility.

There is increased urine excretion of metabolites associated with the 7-day PEM scores, in-particular, mannitol, methylhistidine, acetate, and glucose. This increased metabolite excretion correlates with the ME/CFS case reported 7-day severity of PEM symptoms. Relative abundance assessment shows that the efflux of metabolites is associated with reductions in urine urea, pyruvate and acetate suggesting an energy and renal concentrating issue, possibly associated with hypoacetylation, is most likely occurring at the time of the metabolite loss. In diabetic nephropathy, the renal tubular cells upregulate glycolysis and lactate production [27]. This may also be the case in this study as the excretion of glucose ($r = +0.37$, $p < 0.01$) and acetate ($r = +0.41$, $p < 0.01$) were positively correlated with the 7-day PEM severity. Importantly, acetate was negatively correlated with the 12-month frequency of PEM events ($r = −0.32$, $p < 0.01$). This change in renal acetate retention is also supported by the negative correlation between the 7-day PEM score and the serum acetate:urine acetate ratio ($r = -0.44$, $p < 0.002$). Thus, the greater the frequency of PEM events the greater the loss of acetate. Renal glomerular podocytes are damaged by increases in blood glucose in diabetic patients and this has been linked to deacetylation of Nephrin and microRNA activity [28]. In this study, the reduction in serum acetate levels appears to result in a conditional renal hypoacetylation event which will allow increased metabolite loss from the kidney. Renal changes in diabetes nephropathy are also associated with down-regulation of bone morphogenic protein (BMP) receptor function and TGF-β mediated transcription factor production and supply of BMP-7 restores function [29,30]. Whilst the renal changes are very similar to the renal changes seen in central diabetes insipidus, protein-calorie restriction and infection/inflammatory mediated events, no subjects had diabetes insipidus or were protein calorie restricted, and all had average BMI's. These renal changes provide additional support for either an inflammatory origin or a possibly an energy/acetylation or even a transcription factor problem. Importantly, multiple studies have found that the level of serum cytokines are not significantly different between ME/CFS and controls and do not correlate with symptom expression [31]. Therefore, studies to assess the activities of HDAC and BMP transcription factors in MEC/CFS cases are warranted.

The change in renal metabolite loss is associated with increased mannitol excretion, which suggests a gastrointestinal barrier issue may also be occurring. NoPEM ME/CFS cases had a 3.2-fold lower urinary mannitol, not unlike that seen in multiple sclerosis patients [32]. However, the level of urinary mannitol increased with the 7-day PEM scores ($r = +0.38$, $p < 0.01$). This increase in mannitol indicates a potential intestinal barrier change, which is consistent with the finding of bacteremia following exercise in ME/CFS cases [33]. The presence of bacteremia is supported by the correlation between fecal uracil and the 7-day PEM score ($r = +0.46$, $p < 0.001$). The increase in fecal uracil was also correlated with the serum hypoxanthine level in the PEM group ($r = +0.39$, $p < 0.03$) showing that they rose together as part of the PEM-associated hypermetabolic event. Uracil is a breakdown product of RNA but may also be of bacterial origin. Whether this indicates a breakdown in enterocytes or an alteration in the fecal flora or their metabotoxins/toxins is not known. Further investigation of these changes is warranted.

A 1.6-fold increase in urinary excretion of methylhistidine within the PEM subgroup was also seen compared with the NoPEM subgroup. Methylhistidine is a breakdown product of muscle contractile proteins, following a short term bout of resistance exercise [34]. Muscle protein synthesis is controlled by the available leucine and phenylalanine [35] and by BMP protein receptor activity [36]. In this study urinary methylhistidine positively correlated with urinary creatine ($r = +0.63$, $p < 0.001$), leucine ($r = +0.59$, $p < 0.001$), phenylalanine ($r = +0.40$, $p < 0.001$) and acetate ($r = +0.47$, $p < 0.001$) across all groups. A reduction in available acetate during exercise is associated with a reduction in phosphocreatine degradation and hence is associated with increased phosphocreatine and mitochondrial energy provision [37], which is consistent with the glycolysis/urea cycle energy switch identified in this ME/CFS cohort [2]. Interestingly, 3-methylhistidine in the nonacetylated form is excreted in greater amounts when rats are exposed to bacterial lipopolysaccharides [38]. It is likely that the increased 3-methylhistidine excretion observed during the 7-day PEM response is the result of the reduced energy provision and the fall in amino acids, which may be acetylation mediated. However, the response could also be exacerbated by the gastrointestinal barrier anomalies suggested by the increased bacteremia identified in ME/CFS cases [33]. Alternatively, an anomaly in BMP regulation may also be involved in the increased 3-methylhistidine excretion. Thus, a combination of at least three different events may contribute to the increased 3-methylhistidine excretion and this may be reflected in different genetic susceptibilities within different subjects.

The findings that the PEM is associated with a loss of metabolites, reduction in acetylation, deregulation of purine metabolism, increased contractile protein breakdown and bacteremia associated with exercise suggest that treatments such as graded exercise may be more detrimental than beneficial as claimed in some studies [39,40]. Until such time as these biological changes can be further investigated, the use of graded exercise as a therapy for those with severe forms of ME/CFS should be considered potentially harmful. In support of this, the use of graded exercise therapy has caused significant protest by ME/CFS sufferers as they see it as harmful [41,42].

This study was designed to investigate metabolic changes in ME/CFS subjects using a discovery hypothesis and not a specific hypothesis-driven method to assess specific biochemical events. This study with these limitations has resulted in the development of a hypothesis which now requires to be assessed by a typical hypothesis-driven process. Whilst the study size is small it reproduced the earlier findings but should be reproduced with a larger sample or multi-centers to reconfirm the findings. The use of self-reported symptoms may introduce a recall bias within the subjects and in a larger study, each of the variables found to be associated with the symptom severity and distribution need to be evaluated by other methods. Studies investigating acetylation and its related DNA transcription changes and the alteration in cytosol enzyme activity should allow the development of the understanding of the mechanisms of PEM development and the development of appropriate therapies based upon the underlying biochemistry.

5. Conclusions

This study revealed that post-exertional malaise is associated with changes in glycolysis and acetylation in ME/CFS cases. These changes are consistent with a hypoacetylation state and are likely to significantly alter histone acetylation and the actions of acetylation and deacetylation in controlling cellular enzymatic events. Well-designed studies evaluating these important factors are warranted.

Supplementary Materials: The following are available online at http://www.mdpi.com/2075-4418/9/3/70/s1.

Author Contributions: Conceptualization, investigation, curation of the data and review of the manuscript involved all authors; The methodology and validation of the data was undertaken at the Bio21 Institute, University of Melbourne by C.W.A. and P.R.G.; The resources to obtain and process the data were provided by D.P.L. at CFS discovery and at the Bio21 Institute by P.R.G.; Data analysis and writing the original draft was performed by N.R.M.; The project was administered by P.R.G. and the funding acquired by P.R.G. and/or C.W.A.

Funding: This research was funded by the Judith Jane Mason and Harold Stannett Williams memorial foundation (The Mason Foundation) (MAS2017F046 in addition to funding without reference numbers in 2009, 2010, 2012 and 2015), philanthropic donations by Mr Douglas Stutt, the Field family and the Blake Beckett trust, and equipment grants from the Rowen White Foundation and the State of Victoria.

Acknowledgments: The authors of this work would like to thank the nursing and administrative staff at the CFS Discovery clinic for their important help throughout this study.

Conflicts of Interest: There are no conflicts of interest.

Abbreviations

BMP	Bone Morphogenic Protein
HDAC	Histone Deacetylase
ME/CFS	FS Myalgic encephalomyelitis/Chronic Fatigue Syndrome
PEM	Post-Exertional Malaise
SMAD	Transforming Growth Factor-Beta Signaling Proteins
TGF-β	Transforming Growth Factor-Beta
TCA	tricarboxylic acid cycle

References

1. Brown, A.; Jason, L.A. Meta-analysis investigating post-exertional malaise between patients and controls. *J. Health Psychol.* **2018**. [CrossRef] [PubMed]
2. Armstrong, C.W.; McGregor, N.R.; Lewis, D.P.; Butt, H.L.; Gooley, P.R. Metabolic profiling reveals anomalous energy metabolism and oxidative stress pathways in chronic fatigue syndrome patients. *Metabolomics* **2015**, *11*, 1626–1639. [CrossRef]
3. Fluge, O.; Mella, O.; Bruland, O.; Risa, K.; Dyrstad, S.E.; Alme, K.; Rekeland, I.G.; Sapkota, D.; Rosland, G.V.; Fossa, A.; et al. Metabolic profiling indicates impaired pyruvate dehydrogenase function in myalgic encephalopathy/chronic fatigue syndrome. *JCI Insight* **2016**, *1*, e89376. [CrossRef] [PubMed]

4. Liu, X.S.; Little, J.B.; Yuan, Z.M. Glycolytic metabolism influences global chromatin structure. *Oncotarget* **2015**, *6*, 4214–4225. [CrossRef] [PubMed]
5. Chano, T.; Avnet, S.; Kusuzaki, K.; Bonuccelli, G.; Sonveaux, P.; Rotili, D.; Mai, A.; Baldini, N. Tumour-specific metabolic adaptation to acidosis is coupled to epigenetic stability in osteosarcoma cells. *Am. J. Cancer Res.* **2016**, *6*, 859–875. [PubMed]
6. Jason, L.; Sorenson, M.; Sebally, K.; Alkazemi, D.; Lerch, A.; Porter, N.; Kubow, S. Increased HDAC in association with decreased plasma cortisol in older adults with chronic fatigue syndrome. *Brain Behav. Immun.* **2011**, *25*, 1544–1547. [CrossRef]
7. Whistler, T.; Jones, J.F.; Unger, E.R.; Vernon, S.D. Exercise responsive genes measured in peripheral blood of women with chronic fatigue syndrome and matched control subjects. *BMC Physiol.* **2005**, *5*, 5. [CrossRef]
8. Boeuf, S.; Bovee, J.V.; Lehner, B.; van den Akker, B.; van Ruler, M.; Cleton-Jansen, A.M.; Richter, W. BMP and TGFbeta pathways in human central chondrosarcoma: Enhanced endoglin and Smad 1 signaling in high grade tumors. *BMC Cancer* **2012**, *12*, 488. [CrossRef]
9. Hu, W.; Zhang, Y.; Wang, L.; Lau, C.W.; Xu, J.; Luo, J.Y.; Gou, L.; Yao, X.; Chen, Z.Y.; Ma, R.C.; et al. Bone Morphogenic Protein 4-Smad-Induced Upregulation of Platelet-Derived Growth Factor AA Impairs Endothelial Function. *Arter. Thromb Vasc. Biol.* **2016**, *36*, 553–560. [CrossRef]
10. Montoya, J.G.; Holmes, T.H.; Anderson, J.N.; Maecker, H.T.; Rosenberg-Hasson, Y.; Valencia, I.J.; Chu, L.; Younger, J.W.; Tato, C.M.; Davis, M.M. Cytokine signature associated with disease severity in chronic fatigue syndrome patients. *Proc. Natl. Acad Sci. USA* **2017**, *114*, E7150–E7158. [CrossRef]
11. Wyller, V.B.; Nguyen, C.B.; Ludviksen, J.A.; Mollnes, T.E. Transforming growth factor beta (TGF-beta) in adolescent chronic fatigue syndrome. *J. Transl. Med.* **2017**, *15*, 245. [CrossRef] [PubMed]
12. Matsumoto, S.S.; Raivio, K.O.; Seegmiller, J.E. Adenine nucleotide degradation during energy depletion in human lymphoblasts. Adenosine accumulation and adenylate energy charge correlation. *J. Biol. Chem.* **1979**, *254*, 8956–8962. [PubMed]
13. Matsumoto, S.S.; Raivio, K.O.; Willis, R.C.; Seegmiller, J.E. Interactions between energy metabolism and adenine nucleotide metabolism in human lymphoblasts. *Adv. Exp. Med. Biol.* **1979**, *122B*, 277–282. [PubMed]
14. Mensah, F.K.F.; Bansal, A.S.; Ford, B.; Cambridge, G. Chronic fatigue syndrome and the immune system: Where are we now? *Neurophysiol. Clin.* **2017**, *47*, 131–138. [CrossRef] [PubMed]
15. Poznanski, S.M.; Barra, N.G.; Ashkar, A.A.; Schertzer, J.D. Immunometabolism of T cells and NK cells: Metabolic control of effector and regulatory function. *Inflamm. Res.* **2018**, *67*, 813–828. [CrossRef]
16. Cheng, S.C.; Quintin, J.; Cramer, R.A.; Shepardson, K.M.; Saeed, S.; Kumar, V.; Giamarellos-Bourboulis, E.J.; Martens, J.H.; Rao, N.A.; Aghajanirefah, A.; et al. mTOR- and HIF-1alpha-mediated aerobic glycolysis as metabolic basis for trained immunity. *Science* **2014**, *345*, 1250684. [CrossRef] [PubMed]
17. Georgiades, E.; Behan, W.M.; Kilduff, L.P.; Hadjicharalambous, M.; Mackie, E.E.; Wilson, J.; Ward, S.A.; Pitsiladis, Y.P. Chronic fatigue syndrome: New evidence for a central fatigue disorder. *Clin. Sci. (Lond.)* **2003**, *105*, 213–218. [CrossRef]
18. Choudhary, C.; Kumar, C.; Gnad, F.; Nielsen, M.L.; Rehman, M.; Walther, T.C.; Olsen, J.V.; Mann, M. Lysine acetylation targets protein complexes and co-regulates major cellular functions. *Science* **2009**, *325*, 834–840. [CrossRef]
19. Carruthers, B.M.; van de Sande, M.I.; De Meirleir, K.L.; Klimas, N.G.; Broderick, G.; Mitchell, T.; Staines, D.; Powles, A.C.; Speight, N.; Vallings, R.; et al. Myalgic encephalomyelitis: International Consensus Criteria. *J. Intern. Med.* **2011**, *270*, 327–338. [CrossRef]
20. Crawford, J.R.; Henry, J.D. The Depression Anxiety Stress Scales (DASS): Normative data and latent structure in a large non-clinical sample. *Br. J. Clin. Psychol.* **2003**, *42*, 111–131. [CrossRef]
21. McGregor, N.R. An Investigation of the Association between Toxin Producing Staphylococcus, Biochemical Changes and Jaw Muscle Pain. Ph.D. Thesis, University of Sydney, Sydney, NSW, Australia, 2000.
22. McGregor, N.R.; Armstrong, C.W.; Lewis, D.P.; Butt, H.L.; Gooley, P.R. Widespread pain and altered renal function in ME/CFS patients. *Fatigue Biomed. Health Behav.* **2016**, *4*, 12. [CrossRef]
23. Sheedy, J.R.; Ebeling, P.R.; Gooley, P.R.; McConville, M.J. A sample preparation protocol for 1H nuclear magnetic resonance studies of water-soluble metabolites in blood and urine. *Anal. Biochem.* **2010**, *398*, 263–265. [CrossRef] [PubMed]
24. Townsend, M.H.; Robison, R.A.; O'Neill, K.L. A review of HPRT and its emerging role in cancer. *Med. Oncol.* **2018**, *35*, 89. [CrossRef] [PubMed]

25. Goto, Y.; Gomez, M.; Brockdorff, N.; Feil, R. Differential patterns of histone methylation and acetylation distinguish active and repressed alleles at X-linked genes. *Cytogenet Genome Res.* **2002**, *99*, 66–74. [CrossRef] [PubMed]
26. Keohane, A.M.; O'Neill, L.P.; Belyaev, N.D.; Lavender, J.S.; Turner, B.M. X-Inactivation and histone H4 acetylation in embryonic stem cells. *Dev. Biol.* **1996**, *180*, 618–630. [CrossRef] [PubMed]
27. Sas, K.M.; Kayampilly, P.; Byun, J.; Nair, V.; Hinder, L.M.; Hur, J.; Zhang, H.; Lin, C.; Qi, N.R.; Michailidis, G.; et al. Tissue-specific metabolic reprogramming drives nutrient flux in diabetic complications. *JCI Insight* **2016**, *1*, e86976. [CrossRef]
28. Lin, C.L.; Lee, P.H.; Hsu, Y.C.; Lei, C.C.; Ko, J.Y.; Chuang, P.C.; Huang, Y.T.; Wang, S.Y.; Wu, S.L.; Chen, Y.S.; et al. MicroRNA-29a promotion of nephrin acetylation ameliorates hyperglycemia-induced podocyte dysfunction. *J. Am. Soc. Nephrol.* **2014**, *25*, 1698–1709. [CrossRef]
29. Wang, S.; de Caestecker, M.; Kopp, J.; Mitu, G.; Lapage, J.; Hirschberg, R. Renal bone morphogenetic protein-7 protects against diabetic nephropathy. *J. Am. Soc. Nephrol.* **2006**, *17*, 2504–2512. [CrossRef]
30. Wang, Y.; Xiao, Y.; Li, S.; Shi, L.; Liu, L.; Zhang, Y.; Shi, M.; Guo, B. BMP-7 enhances SnoN mRNA expression in renal tubular epithelial cells under high-glucose conditions. *Mol. Med. Rep.* **2017**, *16*, 3308–3314. [CrossRef]
31. Vollmer-Conna, U.; Cameron, B.; Hadzi-Pavlovic, D.; Singletary, K.; Davenport, T.; Vernon, S.; Reeves, W.C.; Hickie, I.; Wakefield, D.; Lloyd, A.R.; et al. Postinfective fatigue syndrome is not associated with altered cytokine production. *Clin. Infect. Dis.* **2007**, *45*, 732–735. [CrossRef]
32. Buscarinu, M.C.; Cerasoli, B.; Annibali, V.; Policano, C.; Lionetto, L.; Capi, M.; Mechelli, R.; Romano, S.; Fornasiero, A.; Mattei, G.; et al. Altered intestinal permeability in patients with relapsing-remitting multiple sclerosis: A pilot study. *Mult. Scler.* **2017**, *23*, 442–446. [CrossRef] [PubMed]
33. Shukla, S.K.; Cook, D.; Meyer, J.; Vernon, S.D.; Le, T.; Clevidence, D.; Robertson, C.E.; Schrodi, S.J.; Yale, S.; Frank, D.N. Changes in Gut and Plasma Microbiome following Exercise Challenge in Myalgic Encephalomyelitis/Chronic Fatigue Syndrome (ME/CFS). *PLoS ONE* **2015**, *10*, e0145453. [CrossRef] [PubMed]
34. Bird, S.P.; Tarpenning, K.M.; Marino, F.E. Liquid carbohydrate/essential amino acid ingestion during a short-term bout of resistance exercise suppresses myofibrillar protein degradation. *Metabolism* **2006**, *55*, 570–577. [CrossRef] [PubMed]
35. Borsheim, E.; Tipton, K.D.; Wolf, S.E.; Wolfe, R.R. Essential amino acids and muscle protein recovery from resistance exercise. *Am. J. Physiol. Endocrinol. Metab.* **2002**, *283*, E648–E657. [CrossRef] [PubMed]
36. Chen, J.L.; Walton, K.L.; Hagg, A.; Colgan, T.D.; Johnson, K.; Qian, H.; Gregorevic, P.; Harrison, C.A. Specific targeting of TGF-beta family ligands demonstrates distinct roles in the regulation of muscle mass in health and disease. *Proc. Natl. Acad Sci. USA* **2017**, *114*, E5266–E5275. [CrossRef]
37. Timmons, J.A.; Gustafsson, T.; Sundberg, C.J.; Jansson, E.; Greenhaff, P.L. Muscle acetyl group availability is a major determinant of oxygen deficit in humans during submaximal exercise. *Am. J. Physiol.* **1998**, *274*, E377–E380. [CrossRef] [PubMed]
38. Nakhooda, A.F.; Wei, C.N.; Marliss, E.B. Muscle protein catabolism in diabetes: 3-methylhistidine excretion in the spontaneously diabetic "BB" rat. *Metabolism* **1980**, *29*, 1272–1277. [CrossRef]
39. White, P.D.; Goldsmith, K.; Johnson, A.L.; Chalder, T.; Sharpe, M. Recovery from chronic fatigue syndrome after treatments given in the PACE trial. *Psychol. Med.* **2013**, *43*, 2227–2235. [CrossRef]
40. White, P.D.; Goldsmith, K.A.; Johnson, A.L.; Potts, L.; Walwyn, R.; DeCesare, J.C.; Baber, H.L.; Burgess, M.; Clark, L.V.; Cox, D.L.; et al. Comparison of adaptive pacing therapy, cognitive behaviour therapy, graded exercise therapy, and specialist medical care for chronic fatigue syndrome (PACE): A randomised trial. *Lancet* **2011**, *377*, 823–836. [CrossRef]
41. Kindlon, T. Do graded activity therapies cause harm in chronic fatigue syndrome? *J. Health Psychol.* **2017**, *22*, 1146–1154. [CrossRef]
42. Geraghty, K.J.; Blease, C. Myalgic encephalomyelitis/chronic fatigue syndrome and the biopsychosocial model: A review of patient harm and distress in the medical encounter. *Disabil. Rehabil.* **2018**, 1–10. [CrossRef] [PubMed]

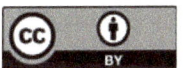

© 2019 by the authors. Licensee MDPI, Basel, Switzerland. This article is an open access article distributed under the terms and conditions of the Creative Commons Attribution (CC BY) license (http://creativecommons.org/licenses/by/4.0/).

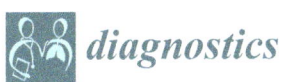

Article

The IDO Metabolic Trap Hypothesis for the Etiology of ME/CFS

Alex A. Kashi [1], Ronald W. Davis [1,2] and Robert D. Phair [3,*]

1. Stanford Genome Technology Center, Stanford University, Palo Alto, CA 94304, USA
2. Departments of Biochemistry and Genetics, Stanford University, Stanford, CA 94305, USA
3. Integrative Bioinformatics Inc., Mountain View, CA 94041, USA
* Correspondence: rphair@integrativebioinformatics.com

Received: 24 May 2019; Accepted: 24 July 2019; Published: 26 July 2019

Abstract: Myalgic encephalomyelitis/chronic fatigue syndrome (ME/CFS) is a debilitating noncommunicable disease brandishing an enormous worldwide disease burden with some evidence of inherited genetic risk. Absence of measurable changes in patients' standard blood work has necessitated ad hoc symptom-driven therapies and a dearth of mechanistic hypotheses regarding its etiology and possible cure. A new hypothesis, the indolamine-2,3-dioxygenase (IDO) metabolic trap, was developed and formulated as a mathematical model. The historical occurrence of ME/CFS outbreaks is a singular feature of the disease and implies that any predisposing genetic mutation must be common. A database search for common damaging mutations in human enzymes produces 208 hits, including IDO2 with four such mutations. Non-functional IDO2, combined with well-established substrate inhibition of IDO1 and kinetic asymmetry of the large neutral amino acid transporter, LAT1, yielded a mathematical model of tryptophan metabolism that displays both physiological and pathological steady-states. Escape from the pathological one requires an exogenous perturbation. This model also identifies a critical point in cytosolic tryptophan abundance beyond which descent into the pathological steady-state is inevitable. If, however, means can be discovered to return cytosolic tryptophan below the critical point, return to the normal physiological steady-state is assured. Testing this hypothesis for any cell type requires only labelled tryptophan, a means to measure cytosolic tryptophan and kynurenine, and the standard tools of tracer kinetics.

Keywords: tryptophan metabolism; indoleamine-2,3-dioxygenase; bistability; kynurenine pathway; substrate inhibition; myalgic encephalomyelitis; chronic fatigue syndrome; mathematical model; critical point

---

1. Introduction

Diagnostic measurements for a given disease are most definitive, most specific, and most useful when the measurements are closely related to the molecular basis of the disease. Compare, for example, the ancient diagnosis of diabetes based on excessive urine output versus a diagnosis based on the measurement of plasma glucose and plasma insulin. For a disease like myalgic encephalomyelitis/chronic fatigue syndrome (ME/CFS), whose mechanistic basis is unknown, a specific diagnostic is difficult to identify. Medicine thus resorts to complex pattern recognition in lists of symptoms [1,2], statistical principal component analysis [3–6], advanced physical measurements of yet unproven specificity [7], and even, when just a few thousand critical cells are dysfunctional and standard blood measurements are therefore unremarkable, the unhelpful assertion that patient is "not ill". Here, we aim to advance the search for underlying mechanisms by proposing a new class of theoretical models for ME/CFS and demonstrating that one specific member of that class, the IDO metabolic trap, can reproduce important features of the disease and promises to be experimentally testable.

The idea of a metabolic trap arises from the well-established concept of bistability in nonlinear systems. A system, such as a metabolic pathway, is said to be nonlinear if a doubling of its input does not yield a doubling of its output. Saturation of enzymatic catalysis, characterized by the classic Michaelis-Menten equation, is one source of biological nonlinearity. A more important source of biological nonlinearity is feedback control whether it be transcriptional regulation, allosteric control mediated by binding of a specific metabolite, post-translational modification mediated by, for example, a kinase, or physiological regulation mediated by hormones, cytokines, and their receptors. Importantly, some nonlinear systems, unlike all linear systems, can settle into multiple different steady-states, depending on external conditions or perturbations. This is called bistability. If one of those steady-states is pathological, we refer to it as a metabolic trap because organisms are vulnerable to external perturbations that precipitate a shift from normal physiology to pathophysiology, a shift that is not easily reversed. If we now turn to the specific case—the IDO metabolic trap developed here—we find that this new theoretical model rests on three ideas: (1) the potential importance of common damaging mutations, (2) a possibly detrimental aspect of the phenomenon in enzyme kinetics known as substrate inhibition, and (3) the bistable metabolic system that can result.

Genetics must hold clues to ME/CFS because, like other chronic diseases, there is evidence that this disease can run in families, but it is clearly not a disease one has at birth. Rather, there appears to be a genetic propensity that lies hidden until a particular collection of triggering circumstances arises in the patient's microbial, dietary, micronutrient, physiological, emotional or physical environment. One clue that distinguishes ME/CFS from most other chronic diseases is its long history epidemics, outbreaks or clusters [8]. Historically, it has been assumed that the effect of common genetic variations on phenotype is small [9]. Outbreaks or epidemics of a noncontagious disease raise the possibility that genetic predisposition to ME/CFS is very common in the population and that the disease has low penetrance only because the initiating triggers are multifactorial, and those pathogenic *combinations* of triggers are, themselves, rare. Outbreaks are then explained by a geographically localized combination of factors superimposed on a genetic predisposition that is common in the population. Thus, it is the existence of ME/CFS outbreaks that pointed to the potential importance of common damaging mutations. This inference from the existence of outbreaks does *not* limit the model to patients who became sick as part of an outbreak.

A second foundational idea for the IDO metabolic trap model is the phenomenon of substrate inhibition. In contrast to the widely understood Michaelis-Menten kinetics, there are enzymes for which velocity decreases, rather than saturates, at substrate concentrations 3- to 10-fold above the substrate's K_M. This unusual behavior has been a part of the enzyme kinetics literature for decades [10–12]. One of the giants of enzyme kinetics, W.W. Cleland, took the position that substrate inhibition was almost always a nonphysiological phenomenon [13]. What he meant by "nonphysiological" was that the phenomenon was most often observed when reactions were run opposite the physiological direction with the normal intracellular products as substrates, and thus were examples of product inhibition. Subsequent experience has shown that at least 80 enzymes demonstrate this behavior [10,14]. A recent review [14] describes several desirable consequences of substrate inhibition such as stabilization of product formation in the context of large swings in the substrate (tyrosine hydroxylase), and allosteric regulation (phosphofructokinase). Nevertheless, tryptophan inhibition of the particular enzyme, human indoleamine-2,3-dioxygenase 1 (IDO1), that is central to the model presented here, has been demonstrated in multiple laboratories over multiple decades [15–18] running in the physiological direction with tryptophan and oxygen as substrates and n-formyl-L-kynurenine as a product. While the phenomenon of IDO1 substrate inhibition is well-established, its mechanism remains a matter of scientific debate [17–19]. The model presented here explores the possibility that substrate inhibition of IDO1 has a dark side and may be involved in the pathogenesis of ME/CFS.

A third concept, bistability as a feature of some enzymatic systems, has been studied extensively. Even 40 years ago an itemization of biological oscillators included hundreds of published papers [20]. Later, an oxidase in vitro was shown to exhibit all three of the major dynamic features of nonlinear systems: bistability, limit cycle oscillations, and chaos [21]. And in recent years, bistability in metabolism is enjoying a resurgence of research interest [22–24]. While the IDO metabolic trap model is focused on metabolic bistability, other research in ME/CFS has sought bistability at cell biological and physiological levels of organization [25,26]. Some ME/CFS patients experience the onset of the disease as a switch being thrown, and researchers with backgrounds in nonlinear system theory are therefore drawn to theories that involve bistability [27].

This paper is largely theoretical. Its aim is to formulate an internally consistent hypothetical mechanistic model of the etiology of ME/CFS and to propose an experiment capable of rejecting or corroborating this model. The IDO metabolic trap model represents a new way to think about ME/CFS. It is based (1) on the existence of common damaging mutations in human IDO2, (2) on the well-studied kinetic characteristics of IDO2 and IDO1 including substrate inhibition of IDO1, and (3) on the demonstrable bistability that results when these enzymes are expressed in cells that rely on the large neutral amino acid transporter, LAT1, to import tryptophan, which is their carbon-containing substrate. The model has considerable explanatory power because of the cell types expressing these enzymes, and a relatively straightforward experimental test based on tracer kinetics is proposed. If the IDO metabolic trap is found to be a feature of ME/CFS immune cells, a strong basis for the development of a specific ME/CFS diagnostic will have been discovered.

2. Materials and Methods

Public databases: Starting from the inference that predisposing damaging mutations must be common in order to account for the existence of ME/CFS outbreaks, a search of public (NCBI dbSNP) [28] and purpose-built ME/CFS (see Acknowledgments) databases for common damaging mutations in genes coding for proteins, particularly enzymes and transporters, involved in energy metabolism was undertaken. Results were displayed in standard genome browsers, IGV [29] and UCSC [30]. Allele frequencies for alternate alleles were obtained from dBSNP [28] and large-scale genome sequencing projects cited therein. Damaging mutations were identified based on standard prediction algorithms, PROVEAN [31], SIFT [32], and PolyPhen-2 [33] as well as published reports [34].

Bioinformatics: To generate a table of genes that are damaged in at least 85% of the severely ill ME/CFS patients, we first filtered all the variants found in the OMF END ME/CFS dataset (see Acknowledgments) considering only mutations that were not excluded by six standard criteria. (1) Indel genotypes from two or more loci conflict in at least one sample. (2) The site contains an overlapping indel call filter. (3) Locus GQX is less than 15 or not present. (4) The fraction of base calls filtered out at a site is greater than 0.4. (5) The sample SNV strand bias value exceeds 10. (6) The locus depth is greater than 3× the mean chromosome depth. Mutations were deemed damaging if the mutation received a score less than or equal to −1.82 by PROVEAN, less than or equal to 0.05 by SIFT, and greater than or equal to 0.95 by PolyPhen-2. Mutations were then grouped by gene, and a table was compiled of (82) genes such that at least 85% of the SIPS patients have one or more damaging mutations in that gene.

A second table containing all enzymes and transferases/transporters (208 total) damaged by common mutations (AF > 0.03) was generated by joining all the filtered non-synonymous mutations considered damaging by the above definition with the data extracted by BRENDA [35], KEGG [36], and TCDB [37].

Mechanistic kinetic modeling: Nonlinear kinetic models were formulated in the ProcessDB software (Integrative Bioinformatics, Inc, Mountain View, CA, USA) [38]. ProcessDB implements the CVODE algorithm [39] for a numerical solution of the differential equations. Steady-state solutions were graphed in the Origin 2019 software (OriginLab Corp., Northampton, MA, USA). Full equations and parameter values are provided in the text and can be implemented in any general-purpose differential equation solver. Parameters and some rate laws were obtained from expert reports on the recombinant human enzymes, IDO1 and IDO2 [17,18,40,41].

3. Results

Examination of the two tables of candidate genes described in Bioinformatics Methods revealed common mutations in 208 enzymes and transporters. Of these, eight had more than one common damaging mutation. Reasoning that multiple common damaging mutations would increase the probability of a damaged protein product, we turned our initial attention to this subset.

3.1. Common Mutations in IDO2

Given the hypometabolic phenotype of ME/CFS, our search for common damaging mutations began with genes coding for enzymes involved in energy metabolism. Of the eight enzymes with multiple common damaging mutations (allele frequency > 0.03) IDO2 stood out because it has four such mutations and because it is one of the enzymes catalyzing the first step in the kynurenine pathway. Classically, the kynurenine pathway is considered the "de novo" pathway for the synthesis of nicotinamide adenine dinucleotide (NAD^+), a molecule essential for transferring reducing equivalents from central carbon metabolism to the mitochondrial electron transport chain and thus powering oxidative phosphorylation. Table 1 lists both the common and rare mutations in IDO2 that are considered damaging by the PROVEAN, SIFT, and PolyPhen-2 prediction algorithms.

Table 1. Common and rare mutations in IDO2 identified as damaging [3].

Row Label	R248W	Y359STOP	I140V	S252T	N257K
dbSNP ID	rs10109853	rs4503083	rs4736794	rs35212142	rs774492001
Allele ref > alt	C > T	T > A	A > G	T > A	C > G
exon	9	11	5	9	10
Min pop AF [1]	0.418	0.220	0.0746	0.0100	0.000017
Max pop AF [2]	0.487	0.230	0.160	0.0390	0.000020
SIFT	damaging	nonsense	damaging	damaging	damaging
PROVEAN	deleterious	nonsense	neutral	deleterious	deleterious
POLYPHEN	probably damaging	nonsense	possibly damaging	probably damaging	probably damaging

[1] minimum alternate allele frequency (expressed as a fraction) reported [28] for any sampled population, [2] maximum alternate allele frequency reported for any sampled population, [3] 'damaging" means the enzyme encoded by the mutant protein is either known or predicted to be catalytically impaired.

The two most common damaging mutations, R248W and Y359STOP, are known to abolish enzyme activity in an in vitro cell kynurenine production assay [34]. While the corresponding experiments for I140V, S252T, and N257K have not been reported, the SIFT, PROVEAN, and POLYPHEN predictions are suggestive and could contribute compound heterozygosity for individuals who are merely heterozygous for R248W or Y359STOP. There are no such common mutations in IDO1 or in the remainder of the kynurenine pathway.

Importantly, the IDO metabolic trap hypothesis does *not* propose that these common damaging mutations in IDO2 are causal for ME/CFS. The only requirement for a predisposing mutation is that it is present in ME/CFS patients. On this hypothesis, population allele frequencies recorded in Table 1 should be statistically significantly different from the corresponding allele frequencies in ME/CFS patient populations. Considering the extremely high variant allele frequencies in the general population (Table 1), achieving statistical significance may require targeted sequencing of the IDO2 gene in a very large ME/CFS patient population.

3.2. Consequences of Non-Functional IDO2

Since IDO2 and IDO1 catalyze the same reaction at the beginning of the kynurenine pathway, we are obligated to ask how a non-functional IDO2 has any metabolic impact. After all, IDO1 is unimpaired by the IDO2 damaging mutations and is perfectly capable of converting tryptophan to N-formyl kynurenine (NFK). One possibility is that IDO2 can do something that IDO1 cannot, which leads to a more detailed consideration of IDO1 and IDO2 enzyme kinetics.

Figure 1 plots the flux of NFK production as a function of substrate concentration for IDO1 and IDO2. These graphs are calculated using kinetic parameters reported in the literature (see Methods) for the normal Michaelis-Menten behavior of human IDO2 and the substrate inhibited behavior of human IDO1.

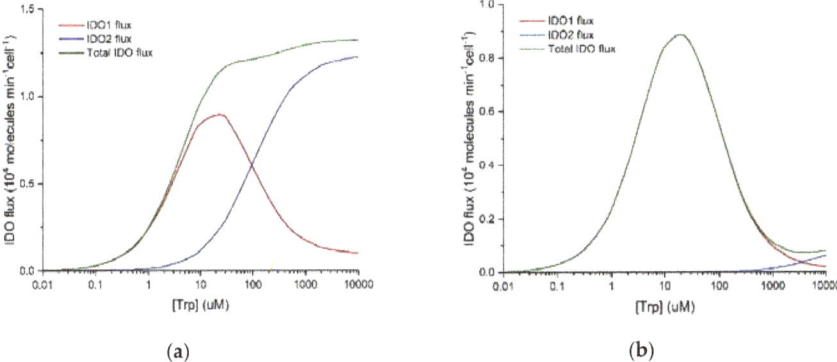

(a)   (b)

Figure 1. Differences in IDO1 (red) and IDO2 (blue) enzyme kinetics as functions of Trp concentration. Total IDO flux (green) is the sum of the IDO1 and IDO2 fluxes. (**a**) Wild type situation with IDO1 and IDO2 having comparable V_{max} values; (**b**) Fluxes when IDO2 flux is 90% reduced, for example, by the homozygous common damaging mutation, R248W.

Three important points emerge from examination of Figure 1. First, IDO1 is a substrate inhibited enzyme with $K_i(Trp)$ = ~50 µM and IDO2 is characterized by normal Michaelis-Menten kinetics. Second, IDO1 is a high-affinity enzyme with $K_M(Trp)$ = ~5 µM and IDO2 is a low-affinity enzyme with $K_M(Trp)$ = ~100 µM. Third, when both enzymes are functional, the total IDO-mediated conversion of Trp to NFK is monotonically increasing and approximately Michaelis-Menten in form over a wide range of substrate (Trp) concentration (panel a), but when IDO2 is functionally impaired by a common damaging mutation (panel b), total IDO flux decreases when substrate [Trp] increases above ~30 µM. Thus, what IDO2 can do that IDO1 cannot is to catalyze Trp + O_2 → NFK even when [Trp] > 200 µM.

These features of IDO kinetics can, when the supply of substrate Trp does not decrease when IDO1 is substrate inhibited, create an untoward metabolic situation that can be referred to as a metabolic trap. To provide a quantitative description of this IDO metabolic trap, we can consider the abbreviated metabolic model illustrated in Figure 2.

3.3. A Mechanistic Model of the IDO Metabolic Trap Reveals Bistability

Tryptophan is an essential amino acid; for humans, its only source is dietary. Transport across the intestinal epithelium is dominated by the LAT2 transporter while crossing the capillary endothelium, the blood-brain barrier, and the serotonergic neuronal plasma membrane is mediated by the heterodimeric transporter, LAT1. LAT1 is an obligate antiport; it transports a large neutral amino acid (often leucine) out of the cell each time it transports tryptophan in. An important feature of LAT1-mediated transport is that K_s values for amino acid uptake are in the 15 µM range, while K_s values for amino acid export are in the mM range [42,43].

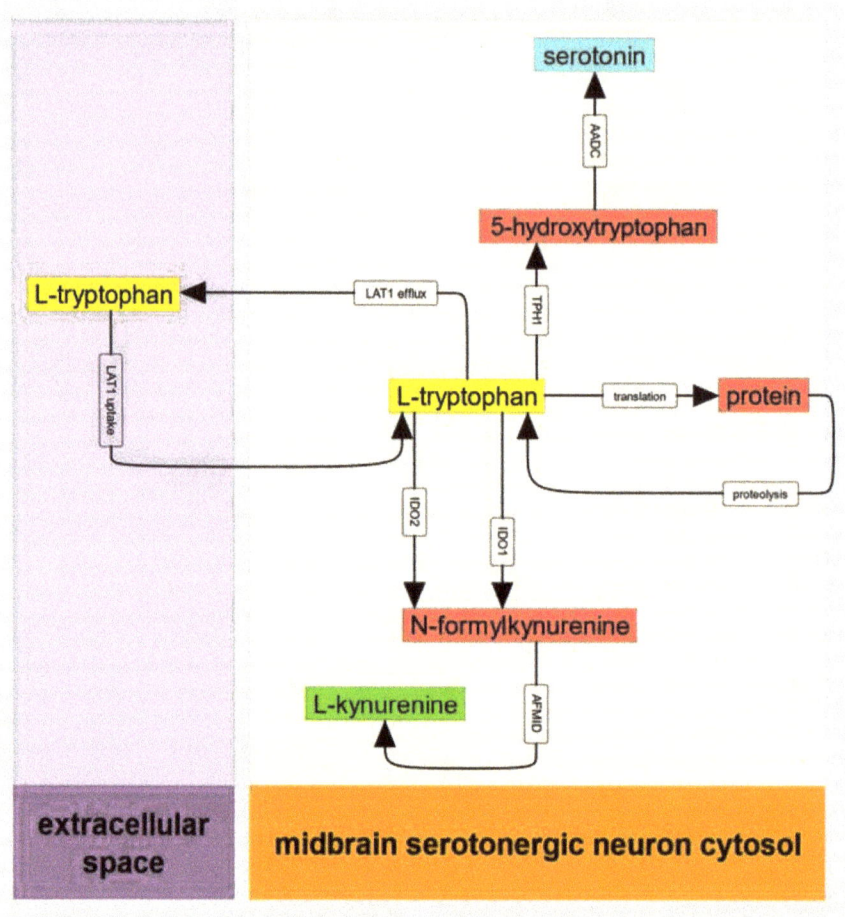

Figure 2. Diagram of the kinetic model of the IDO metabolic trap. Colored rectangles represent molecules in either extracellular space or serotonergic neuron cytosol. Arrows represent processes including transport and biochemical reactions. LAT1 = large neutral amino acid transporter (SLC7A5:SLC3A2), IDO = indoleamine-2,3-dioxygenase, AFMID = arylforamidase, TPH = tryptophan hydroxylase, AADC = aromatic amino acid decarboxylase.

To capture this kinetic asymmetry, a reversible Michaelis-Menten rate law [44] for the flux (molecules/min/cell) can be written as:

$$J_{LAT1} = \frac{V_{mf}\left(1 - \frac{T_{cyto}}{T_{ECF}K_{eq}}\right)\left(\frac{T_{ECF}}{K_s^{T_{ECF}}}\right)}{1 + \frac{T_{ECF}}{K_s^{T_{ECF}}} + \frac{T_{cyto}}{K_s^{T_{cyto}}} + \frac{A}{K_i^A}} \qquad (1)$$

where J_{LAT1} is the net flux of tryptophan (positive means the net flux is into the neuron cytosol from the extracellular space), V_{mf} is the maximal forward (into the neuron) velocity of LAT1 transport, T_{cyto} is the tryptophan abundance (molecules/cell) in the neuron cytosol, T_{ECF} is tryptophan abundance in the extracellular fluid, K_{eq} is the equilibrium constant for LAT1 transport, $K_s^{T_{ECF}}$ is the substrate constant for tryptophan uptake, $K_s^{T_{cyto}}$ is the substrate constant for tryptophan export, A is the abundance of other large neutral amino acids (either in ECF or cytosol) competing with tryptophan for transport via LAT1, and K_i^A is the inhibition constant for those competing amino acids.

Next, we need a quantitative expression for the flux through the substrate-inhibited enzyme, IDO1. This can be written using a standard substrate inhibition rate law:

$$J_{IDO1} = \frac{k_{cat}^{IDO1} IDO1_{cyto} T_{cyto}}{K_M^{Trp} + T_{cyto}\left(1 + \frac{T_{cyto}}{K_i^{Trp}}\right)} \quad (2)$$

where J_{IDO1} is the flux (molecules/min/cell) of Trp conversion to NFK catalyzed by IDO1, k_{cat}^{IDO1} is the catalytic constant for IDO1, $IDO1_{cyto}$ is the abundance (molecules/cell) of cytosolic IDO1, T_{cyto} is the abundance of cytosolic tryptophan, K_M^{Trp} is the IDO1 Michaelis constant for tryptophan, and K_i^{Trp} is the substrate-inhibition constant for Trp inhibition of IDO1.

A full kinetic model would also include rate laws for IDO2, for tryptophan hydroxylase (TPH1 or TPH2 depending on the cell type being modeled) and for protein translation and proteolysis. Here, we can consider the case where IDO2 is disabled by common damaging mutations, where serotonin production is negligible compared to the kynurenine pathway flux, and where (in a steady-state) the flux of protein synthesis is equal to the proteolytic flux and thus there is no net flux between cytosolic tryptophan and cellular protein. These must be relaxed when it comes time for data analysis, but to establish bistability only the principal input of Trp, J_{LAT1}, and the principal output, J_{IDO1}, need be considered.

Thus, we can write the differential equation for cytosolic tryptophan as:

$$\frac{dT_{cyto}}{dt} = J_{LAT1} - J_{IDO1} \quad (3)$$

where J_{LAT1} and J_{IDO1} are as defined above. This is the simplest possible mathematical model of the IDO metabolic trap. To obtain the steady-states of this model requires only that we set $\frac{dT_{cyto}}{dt} = 0$, and solve for T_{cyto}. This would require solving a cubic algebraic equation, which is entirely feasible, but a more straightforward approach is to solve for T_{cyto} graphically as illustrated in Figure 3.

In Figure 3 the horizontal axis represents the cytosolic Trp abundance on a logarithmic scale. This is why the LAT1 flux decreases as Trp increases. Indeed, at the largest values of T_{cyto}, the LAT1 flux becomes negative indicating that the net LAT1 flux is directed out of the cell. The increasing and then decreasing shape of the IDO1 flux curve will be familiar from Figure 1 and is caused by the substrate inhibition of IDO1 by tryptophan. Since setting $\frac{dT_{cyto}}{dt} = 0$ requires $J_{LAT1} = J_{IDO1}$, the three steady-states correspond to the intersections (labeled A, B, and C) of the blue and red curves in Figure 3.

Steady-states labeled A and C are stable, and the steady-state labeled B is unstable. These conclusions can be drawn directly from Figure 3. Consider the steady-state labeled A. If stochastic variation increases cytosolic Trp abundance then IDO1 outflux will be greater than LAT1 influx, and T_{cyto} will decrease until it returns to point A. If, instead, the initial variation decreases T_{cyto}, LAT1 influx will become greater than IDO1 outflux, and T_{cyto} will increase until it again returns to point A. The same is true for the steady-state labeled C.

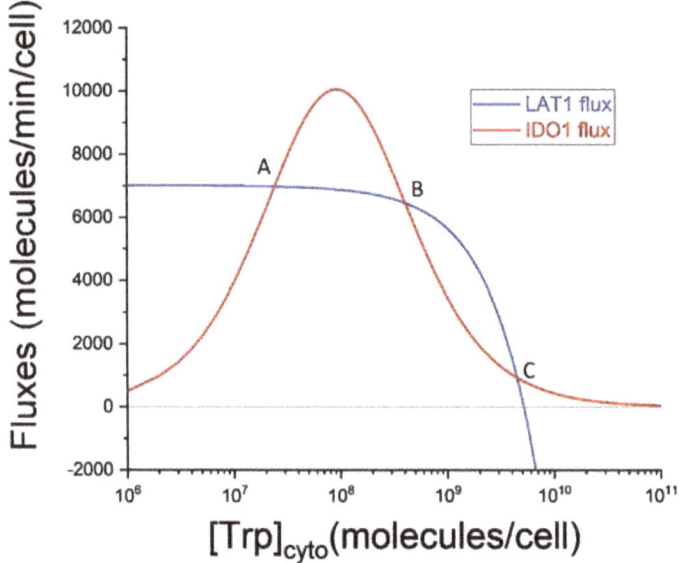

Figure 3. Multiple steady-states in the simplest model of LAT1 tryptophan (Trp) transport and IDO1-mediated Trp oxidation. Horizontal axis: cytosolic Trp abundance. Vertical axis: Fluxes (molecules·min^{-1}·cell^{-1}) cellular Trp influx (blue) carried by the LAT1 membrane transporter, and Trp removal (red) catalyzed by IDO1. Three possible steady-states are defined by the three points (A, B, and C) where the two fluxes are equal. Numerical parameter values are: k_{cat}^{IDO1} = 84 molecules·min^{-1} IDO1·molecule^{-1}, $IDO1_{cyto}$ = 208 IDO1 molecules/cell, K_M^{Trp} = 3.4 × 10^7 molecules/cell, K_i^{Trp} = 2.5 × 10^8 molecules/cell, V_{mf} = 1.2 × 10^8 molecules·min^{-1}·cell^{-1}, T_{ECF} = 1.5 × 10^9 molecules/cell, K_{eq} = 3.43, $K_S^{T_{ECF}}$ = 2.2 × 10^{10} molecules/cell, $K_S^{T_{cyto}}$ = 2 × 10^9 molecules/cell, A = 5 × 10^6 molecules/cell, and K_i^A = 4.3 × 10^3 molecules/cell.

But steady-state B is different. It is unstable because stochastic variation in T_{cyto} results in changes to influx and outflux that drive the system to either steady-state A or steady-state B. For this reason, point B defines what is called a *critical point*. If cytosolic tryptophan exceeds the value defined by this critical point, the system falls inexorably into steady-state C. This extremely simple model is thus *bistable*. It is capable of both a normal physiological steady-state (A) in which kynurenine production is supported by LAT1-mediated import of tryptophan and cytosolic tryptophan is ~2 × 10^7 molecules/cell, and a pathological steady-state (C) in which kynurenine production is nearly abolished and cytosolic tryptophan is ~5 × 10^9 molecules/cell, more than two orders of magnitude greater than normal for a cell expressing the kynurenine pathway.

3.4. An Experimental Design to Test the Trap Hypothesis

Every hypothesis needs an experimental test capable of rejecting or corroborating it. For the IDO metabolic trap hypothesis, the natural test is based on metabolic tracer kinetics [45] and the well-developed set of computational tools [46–49] for analysis of the resulting tracer data. Here, the natural tracer is tryptophan labeled with ^{14}C or ^{13}C in its indole ring and, optionally, in its alpha and carboxyl carbons as well. Tryptophan labeled with either isotope can be used in animal studies and freshly isolated or cultured cells, while the stable isotope, ^{13}C, is, today, widely preferred for human metabolic studies. For isolated cells, the choice usually depends on local expertise and training.

A useful test requires methods for isolating intracellular compounds after exposing the cells to ^{13}C-tryptophan for a specified loading period. At specified times thereafter multiple cold washes both stop the cellular reactions and remove the extracellular medium so that intracellular measurements are not contaminated with extracellular unlabeled or labeled tryptophan or secreted serotonin or kynurenine. It would then be possible to measure cytosolic ^{13}C-tryptophan as well as the incorporation of labeled tryptophan into cellular kynurenine and serotonin. If transients in ^{13}C-kynurenine and ^{13}C-serotonin are measured after removing the tryptophan tracer from the medium. A great advantage of stable isotope kinetics is that the corresponding endogenous ^{12}C compounds are measured simultaneously and quantified separately by the liquid chromatography-mass spectrometry workflow and thus further constrain the computational analysis of the data. The hypothesis will be corroborated if the flux through IDO to kynurenine is substantially reduced in cells from ME/CFS patients compared to healthy control subjects. The hypothesis will be rejected for the cell type tested if there is no difference in the IDO fluxes measured in the two experimental groups.

4. Discussion

The IDO metabolic trap hypothesis for ME/CFS thus suggests that four cell types are at risk of being driven into the pathological steady-state C (Figure 3): (1) antigen-presenting cells (such as dendritic cells and macrophages), (2) serotonergic neurons in the midbrain raphe nuclei, (3) serotonin-producing enterochromaffin cells in the intestinal mucosa, and (4) melatonin-producing pinealocytes. This risk, according to the hypothesis, is magnified by the absence or dysfunction of the backup enzyme, IDO2. A cell in the pathological steady-state C can be described as being in the IDO metabolic trap.

4.1. Consequences of the IDO Metabolic Trap

Consequences of being in this abnormal steady-state depend on many factors. For example, if the normal flux through the kynurenine pathway is the major route of tryptophan oxidation/removal, then cytosolic tryptophan will increase dramatically if IDO1 becomes substrate inhibited. In turn, increased cytosolic tryptophan will drive excessive serotonin production in cells, like serotonergic raphe neurons, that express TPH2 (human chromosome 12) [50] with its normal Michaelis-Menten kinetics [51], or may result in decreased serotonin and melatonin production in cells, such as antigen presenting cells, enterochromaffin cells, and pinealocytes that express the classical "peripheral" tryptophan hydroxylase, TPH1 (human chromosome 11) [50]. This is because TPH1 is, itself, substrate inhibited at high concentrations of its substrate, tryptophan [51,52].

Even if serotonin and melatonin production are unperturbed, the absence of kynurenine and its metabolites can have untoward effects. For example, kynurenine is spontaneously converted to trace condensation products called TEACOPs that are potent activators of the aryl hydrocarbon receptor (AHR), a transcription factor that controls the development of T_{reg} cells [53]. In addition, kynurenine is deaminated by kynurenine aminotransferase and the resulting kynurenate is a potent neuroprotective alpha 7-nicotinic acetylcholine receptor antagonist [54].

If instead we follow the main branch of the kynurenine pathway, additional consequences of insufficient kynurenine production appear. First, the spontaneous synthesis of quinolinate from 2-amino-3-carboxymuconate semialdehyde will decrease. Not only is quinolinate itself neuroexcitatory, but it is also the precursor of nicotinate mononucleotide, which is an important source of NAD$^+$, especially if dietary nicotinate is limited [55]. Second, the enzymatically catalyzed route from 2-amino-3-carboxymuconate semialdehyde leads to picolinate, which is widely described as a neuroprotectant. Perhaps importantly, picolinate production is potently inhibited by glycolytic triose phosphates [56]. Thus, if cytosolic NAD$^+$ is insufficient to maintain a high glycolytic flux through glyceraldehyde 3-phosphate dehydrogenase, the resulting increase in triose phosphates will divert the kynurenine pathway away from neuroprotective picolinate and toward quinolinate/NAD$^+$. This regulatory cross-talk between glycolysis and the kynurenine pathway will certainly fail in trapped cells.

4.2. IDO1-LAT1 Critical Point as the Threshold of Chronic Disease

In Figure 3, the unstable steady-state, B, is the critical point in cytosolic tryptophan concentration. Mathematically, it is the threshold above which the solution of the differential equation switches to the alternate attractor. Practically, the critical point marks the cytosolic tryptophan concentration above which the cell is destined for the pathological low-kynurenine steady-state.

It may be important to recognize that at some increased level of LAT1 expression, only one steady-state is possible. And that steady-state is the pathological one. Conversely, there are decreased levels of LAT1 expression that are only compatible with a normal physiological steady-state.

Another implication of the critical point is that therapeutic perturbations need only reduce cytosolic tryptophan below the critical point. Below that point a return to the normal physiological steady-state is inevitable. It must be kept in mind, however, that the trap persists, and subsequent triggers can cause relapse.

It remains to be determined whether this bistable system is also capable of limit cycle oscillations or deterministic chaos, which could explain relapsing-remitting forms of ME/CFS and the seeming impossibility of multiple metabalomics studies converging on the same plasma signature.

Again, we emphasize that all these points are based on a hypothesis. Without experimental corroboration of that hypothesis and, optimally, a clinical trial, these statements about therapy are not actionable. They are intended to provoke research.

4.3. Underlying Assumptions

Deficits in kynurenine production and decreases in the abundance of its downstream metabolites (kynurenate, anthranilate, picolinate, quinolinate, NAD^+, and others) will occur in any cell whose IDO1 becomes substrate inhibited. Implicit in this scenario is that IDO2 activity provides insufficient backup at high cytosolic tryptophan. This, of course, is the rationale for the attention paid to common damaging mutations in IDO2. Similarly, the IDO metabolic trap cannot occur in any cell type that also expresses tryptophan-2,3-dioxygenase (TDO).

Hypo- or hyper- synthesis of tryptophan-derived serotonin or melatonin depends on the extent to which cytosolic tryptophan abundance is increased relative to the K_M and K_i values of tryptophan hydroxylase. This, in turn, depends on the assumption that the normal kynurenine pathway flux is much greater than the normal tryptophan hydroxylase flux. This assumption can be tested in any given cell type with the tracer kinetic experiment proposed in Section 3.4.

A final assumption of the IDO metabolic trap model is that tryptophan uptake by LAT1 has the features described in the literature [42], namely its kinetic asymmetry. The K_M for tryptophan on the outside aspect of the transporter is reportedly in the uM range while the K_M on the cytosolic aspect is 1000-fold greater. Any other allosteric control of the transporter that maintains tryptophan transport despite decreased utilization by the kynurenine pathway would also satisfy this assumption. This feature of the model deserves further attention because all cytosolic large neutral amino acids (including kynurenine) can play both activator and inhibitor roles for LAT1-mediated tryptophan import.

4.4. Potential Role of Bistability and Substrate Inhibition in Chronic Disease

While it is possible that the IDO metabolic trap lays bare the etiology of ME/CFS, the probability that this is so is small. When we search for common damaging mutations in the human genome, we, by definition, find many. Consequently, the hypothesized increase in damaging alleles in ME/CFS will be difficult to demonstrate without a much larger population of carefully diagnosed ME/CFS patients whose genome sequences are available. For a given trap hypothesis, such as the IDO metabolic trap, it is likely that targeted sequencing of the relevant gene is a more efficient and cost-effective approach. Furthermore, one could question whether a classical genetic family study would be fruitful in this context because the presence of a predisposing mutation need not correlate with the presence of disease. If a common damaging mutation is predisposing (not causal), its allele frequency in a given population may be far greater than the prevalence of the disease for which it is predisposing. The mutation(s) will have low penetrance because it is one or more rare combinations of environmental circumstances that trigger the disease and determines its prevalence. If this is true, the fraction of the world's population at risk for ME/CFS may be vastly greater than its 2% estimated prevalence of the disease.

Another model of chronic disease is the comprehensive healing cycle (HC) model of Naviaux [57]. The HC model emphasizes that knowing the causes of ME/CFS (or other chronic diseases) will not point to a cure. Instead, ME/CFS is seen as a failure to pass the third and final checkpoint in the healing cycle [57]. On this theory, diseases like ME/CFS are characterized by abnormal cell-cell communication that, in turn, is caused by dysfunctional G-protein coupled receptors (especially purinergic receptors) and their regulatory metabokine networks. The result is the failure of the healing cycle and, thus, chronic disease. It is in this sense that the HC model views chronic disease as "a systems problem that maintains disease".

The IDO metabolic trap is a prototype for a different class of systems-level problems. Like the HC model, the trap model implies that chronic disease is not the result of chronic exposure to a pathogen or toxin. Unlike the HC model, the trap model does not suggest a failure of healing or, indeed, a failure of anything at all. Instead, the trap hypothesis identifies substrate inhibition, an inherent and well-studied feature of some enzymes that can, in response to pathogenic triggers, unmask metabolic bistability. Bistability is a phenomenon unique to nonlinear dynamics that has been studied for decades [23,24,58,59]. The essential fact of bistability is that it is possible for a bistable system to be driven into an alternative (e.g., pathological) steady-state and be maintained in that chronic disease state long after the trigger is removed and *without requiring a chronic infection or chronic exposure to a toxin*. Furthermore, nothing need be broken or dysfunctional. The possibility of this chronic disease state is inherent in the detailed molecular mechanism of substrate inhibition.

Because substrate inhibition is relatively common [10], the features of the IDO metabolic trap may appear in other pathways and constitute the mechanisms of other chronic diseases. As an example, tyrosine hydroxylase, the first and rate-determining step in dopamine synthesis, is also substrate inhibited and could provide an alternative explanation for low dopamine production in Parkinson disease or for insufficient production of catecholamines in other cell types.

To summarize, the IDO metabolic trap hypothesis for ME/CFS suggests that substrate inhibition of IDO1 creates the possibility of metabolic bistability in cells expressing the kynurenine pathway. Transition from the normal physiological steady-state to the alternative steady-state can be initiated by any trigger that increases cytosolic tryptophan concentration above the critical point (point B in Figure 3). The alternative, or pathological, steady-state is characterized by insufficient kynurenine production from tryptophan, and consequent impairments in the central nervous system, gastrointestinal, and immune function, as well as energy metabolism. Depending on the relative expression and kinetics of other tryptophan-dependent enzymes in enterochromaffin cells and pinealocytes, production of other tryptophan metabolites (e.g., serotonin and melatonin) may be pathogenically altered as well. For any given cell type, this hypothesis is testable using labelled tryptophan combined with standard tracer kinetic analysis [48].

Author Contributions: Conceptualization, R.D.P.; methodology, R.D.P.; software, A.A.K.; validation, R.W.D. and A.A.K.; formal analysis, R.D.P. and A.A.K.; investigation, R.D.P. and A.A.K.; resources, R.W.D. and R.D.P.; data curation, A.A.K.; writing—original draft preparation, R.D.P.; writing—review and editing, A.A.K., R.W.D., and R.D.P.; visualization, R.D.P.; supervision, R.D.P. and R.W.D.; project administration, R.D.P.; funding acquisition, R.D.P.

Funding: This research was funded by Open Medicine Foundation, Agoura Hills, CA, USA (EIN# 26-4712664), research grant numbers IDOMT-IB-1 and IDOMT-IB-2, to R.D.P. and Integrative Bioinformatics, Inc. The APC was funded in part by Integrative Bioinformatics, Inc., Mountain View, CA, USA.

Acknowledgments: Genome sequencing data used for bioinformatic analyses described in this publication were contributed by Investigators of the OMF END ME/CFS Project, and are available at http://endmecfs.stanford.edu/. The authors thank ME/CFS patients around the world, notably Paolo Maccallini, Mateusz (Matt) Kaczmarek, Jenny TipsforME, Cort Johnson, and other members of Phoenix Rising and S4ME for their insightful blog posts, thoughtful critiques, and public discussion of the IDO metabolic trap. We also thank Whitney Dafoe, Nina Khosla, and Moritz Ernst for their courage, for the inspiration they offer to all of us, and for their parents whose extraordinary generosity has made this work possible. Portions of this work were presented at the March 2019 eMerge International Research Symposium on ME/CFS, in Geelong, VIC, Australia. That presentation won the Day 2 MDPI-sponsored best presentation award.

Conflicts of Interest: The authors declare no conflict of interest. The funders had no role in the design of the study; in the collection, analyses, or interpretation of data; in the writing of the manuscript, or in the decision to publish the results. Disclosure: R.W.D. is on the Scientific Advisory Board of Open Medicine Foundation.

References

1. Straus, S.E.; Hickie, I.; Komaroff, A.; Fukuda, K.; Sharpe, M.C.; Dobbins, J.G. The Chronic Fatigue Syndrome: A Comprehensive Approach to Its Definition and Study. *Ann. Intern. Med.* **1994**, *121*, 953–959.
2. Committee on the Diagnostic Criteria for Myalgic Encephalomyelitis/Chronic Fatigue Syndrome; Board on the Health of Select Populations; Institute of Medicine. *Beyond Myalgic Encephalomyelitis/Chronic Fatigue Syndrome: Redefining an Illness*; The National Academies Collection: Reports Funded by National Institutes of Health; National Academies Press (US): Washington, DC, USA, 2015; ISBN 978-0-309-31689-7.
3. Naviaux, R.K.; Naviaux, J.C.; Li, K.; Bright, A.T.; Alaynick, W.A.; Wang, L.; Baxter, A.; Nathan, N.; Anderson, W.; Gordon, E. Metabolic features of chronic fatigue syndrome. *Proc. Natl. Acad. Sci. USA* **2016**, *113*, E5472–E5480. [CrossRef]
4. Germain, A.; Ruppert, D.; Levine, S.M.; Hanson, M.R. Metabolic profiling of a myalgic encephalomyelitis/chronic fatigue syndrome discovery cohort reveals disturbances in fatty acid and lipid metabolism. *Mol. BioSyst.* **2017**, *13*, 371–379. [CrossRef]
5. Hornig, M.; Montoya, J.G.; Klimas, N.G.; Levine, S.; Felsenstein, D.; Bateman, L.; Peterson, D.L.; Gottschalk, C.G.; Schultz, A.F.; Che, X.; et al. Distinct plasma immune signatures in ME/CFS are present early in the course of illness. *Sci. Adv.* **2015**, *1*, e1400121. [CrossRef]
6. Montoya, J.G.; Holmes, T.H.; Anderson, J.N.; Maecker, H.T.; Rosenberg-Hasson, Y.; Valencia, I.J.; Chu, L.; Younger, J.W.; Tato, C.M.; Davis, M.M. Cytokine signature associated with disease severity in chronic fatigue syndrome patients. *Proc. Natl. Acad. Sci. USA* **2017**, *114*, E7150–E7158. [CrossRef]
7. Esfandyarpour, R.; Kashi, A.; Nemat-Gorgani, M.; Wilhelmy, J.; Davis, R.W. A nanoelectronics-blood-based diagnostic biomarker for myalgic encephalomyelitis/chronic fatigue syndrome (ME/CFS). *Proc. Natl. Acad. Sci. USA* **2019**, *116*, 10250–10257. [CrossRef]
8. Bell, D.S. *The Doctor's Guide to Chronic Fatigue Syndrome: Understanding, Treating, and Living with CFIDS*; Addison Wesley Publishing Company: Boston, MA, USA, 1994; ISBN 978-0-201-62616-2.
9. Fisher, R.A. Gene Frequencies in a Cline Determined by Selection and Diffusion. *Biometrics* **1950**, *6*, 353. [CrossRef]
10. Kaiser, P.M. Substrate inhibition as a problem of non-linear steady state kinetics with monomeric enzymes. *J. Mol. Catal.* **1980**, *8*, 431–442. [CrossRef]
11. Kühl, P.W. Excess-substrate inhibition in enzymology and high-dose inhibition in pharmacology: A reinterpretation. *Biochem. J.* **1994**, *298*, 171–180. [CrossRef]
12. Yoshino, M.; Murakami, K. Analysis of the substrate inhibition of complete and partial types. *SpringerPlus* **2015**, *4*, 9. [CrossRef]
13. Cleland, W.W. Substrate inhibition. *Methods Enzym.* **1979**, *63*, 500–513.
14. Reed, M.C.; Lieb, A.; Nijhout, H.F. The biological significance of substrate inhibition: A mechanism with diverse functions. *BioEssays* **2010**, *32*, 422–429. [CrossRef]
15. Sono, M.; Taniguchi, T.; Watanabe, Y.; Hayaishi, O. Indoleamine 2,3-dioxygenase. Equilibrium studies of the tryptophan binding to the ferric, ferrous, and CO-bound enzymes. *J. Boil. Chem.* **1980**, *255*, 1339–1345.
16. Yamamoto, S.; Hayaishi, O. Tryptophan pyrrolase of rabbit intestine. D- and L-tryptophan-cleaving enzyme or enzymes. *J. Boil. Chem.* **1967**, *242*, 5260–5266.
17. Lu, C.; Lin, Y.; Yeh, S.-R. Inhibitory Substrate Binding Site of Human Indoleamine 2,3-Dioxygenase. *J. Am. Chem. Soc.* **2009**, *131*, 12866–12867. [CrossRef]
18. Efimov, I.; Basran, J.; Sun, X.; Chauhan, N.; Chapman, S.K.; Mowat, C.G.; Raven, E.L. The Mechanism of Substrate Inhibition in Human Indoleamine 2,3-Dioxygenase. *J. Am. Chem. Soc.* **2012**, *134*, 3034–3041. [CrossRef]
19. Nienhaus, K.; Nickel, E.; Nienhaus, G.U. Substrate binding in human indoleamine 2,3-dioxygenase 1: A spectroscopic analysis. *Biochim. Biophys. Acta (BBA) Proteins Proteom.* **2017**, *1865*, 453–463. [CrossRef]
20. Rapp, P.E. An atlas of cellular oscillators. *J. Exp. Biol.* **1979**, *81*, 281–306.

21. Degn, H.; Olsen, L.F.; Perram, J.W. Bistability, oscillation, and chaos in an enzyme reaction. *Ann. N. Y. Acad. Sci.* **1979**, *316*, 623–637. [CrossRef]
22. Kotte, O.; Volkmer, B.; Radzikowski, J.L.; Heinemann, M. Phenotypic bistability in Escherichia coli's central carbon metabolism. *Mol. Syst. Biol.* **2014**, *10*, 736. [CrossRef]
23. Bagowski, C.P.; Ferrell, J.E. Bistability in the JNK cascade. *Curr. Biol.* **2001**, *11*, 1–20. [CrossRef]
24. Mulukutla, B.C.; Yongky, A.; Daoutidis, P.; Hu, W.-S. Bistability in Glycolysis Pathway as a Physiological Switch in Energy Metabolism. *PLoS ONE* **2014**, *9*, e98756. [CrossRef]
25. Gupta, S.; Aslakson, E.; Gurbaxani, B.M.; Vernon, S.D. Inclusion of the glucocorticoid receptor in a hypothalamic pituitary adrenal axis model reveals bistability. *Theor. Boil. Med Model.* **2007**, *4*, 8. [CrossRef]
26. Craddock, T.J.A.; Fritsch, P.; Rice, M.A.; Del Rosario, R.M.; Miller, D.B.; Fletcher, M.A.; Klimas, N.G.; Broderick, G. A Role for Homeostatic Drive in the Perpetuation of Complex Chronic Illness: Gulf War Illness and Chronic Fatigue Syndrome. *PLoS ONE* **2014**, *9*, e84839. [CrossRef]
27. Robinson, C. *Diagnosis and Treatment of Chronic Fatigue Syndrome and Myalgic Encephalitis*; Chelsea Green Publishing: White River Junction, VT, USA, 2018; Catastrophe Theory and CFS/ME.
28. Sherry, S.T. dbSNP: The NCBI database of genetic variation. *Nucleic Acids Res.* **2001**, *29*, 308–311. [CrossRef]
29. Robinson, J.T.; Thorvaldsdóttir, H.; Wenger, A.M.; Zehir, A.; Mesirov, J.P. Variant Review with the Integrative Genomics Viewer (IGV). *Cancer Res.* **2017**, *77*, e31–e34. [CrossRef]
30. Kent, W.J.; Sugnet, C.W.; Furey, T.S.; Roskin, K.M.; Pringle, T.H.; Zahler, A.M.; Haussler, D. The Human Genome Browser at UCSC. *Genome Res.* **2002**, *12*, 996–1006. [CrossRef]
31. Choi, Y.; Chan, A.P. PROVEAN web server: A tool to predict the functional effect of amino acid substitutions and indels. *Bioinformatics* **2015**, *31*, 2745–2747. [CrossRef]
32. Vaser, R.; Adusumalli, S.; Leng, S.N.; Sikic, M.; Ng, P.C. SIFT missense predictions for genomes. *Nat. Protoc.* **2016**, *11*, 1–9. [CrossRef]
33. Adzhubei, I.; Jordan, D.M.; Sunyaev, S.R. Predicting Functional Effect of Human Missense Mutations Using PolyPhen-2. *Curr. Protoc. Hum. Genet.* **2013**, *76*. [CrossRef]
34. Metz, R.; DuHadaway, J.B.; Kamasani, U.; Laury-Kleintop, L.; Muller, A.J.; Prendergast, G.C. Novel Tryptophan Catabolic Enzyme IDO2 Is the Preferred Biochemical Target of the Antitumor Indoleamine 2,3-Dioxygenase Inhibitory Compound D-1-Methyl-Tryptophan. *Cancer Res.* **2007**, *67*, 7082–7087. [CrossRef]
35. Jeske, L.; Placzek, S.; Schomburg, I.; Chang, A.; Schomburg, D. BRENDA in 2019: A European ELIXIR core data resource. *Nucleic Acids Res.* **2019**, *47*, D542–D549. [CrossRef]
36. Kanehisa, M. KEGG: Kyoto Encyclopedia of Genes and Genomes. *Nucleic Acids Res.* **2000**, *28*, 27–30. [CrossRef]
37. Saier, M.H. TCDB: The Transporter Classification Database for membrane transport protein analyses and information. *Nucleic Acids Res.* **2006**, *34*, 181–186. [CrossRef]
38. Chasson, A.K.; Phair, R.D. ProcessDB: A cellular process database supporting large-scale integrative kinetic modeling in cell biology. In Proceedings of the 2nd International Conference on Systems Biology, Pasadena, CA, USA, 5–7 November 2001.
39. Cohen, S.D.; Hindmarsh, A.C. CVODE, A Stiff/Nonstiff ODE Solver in C. *Comput. Phys.* **1996**, *10*, 138–143. [CrossRef]
40. Meininger, D.; Zalameda, L.; Liu, Y.; Stepan, L.P.; Borges, L.; McCarter, J.D.; Sutherland, C.L. Purification and kinetic characterization of human indoleamine 2,3-dioxygenases 1 and 2 (IDO1 and IDO2) and discovery of selective IDO1 inhibitors. *Biochim. Biophys. Acta BBA Proteins Proteom.* **2011**, *1814*, 1947–1954. [CrossRef]
41. Pantouris, G.; Serys, M.; Yuasa, H.J.; Ball, H.J.; Mowat, C.G. Human indoleamine 2,3-dioxygenase-2 has substrate specificity and inhibition characteristics distinct from those of indoleamine 2,3-dioxygenase-1. *Amino Acids* **2014**, *46*, 2155–2163. [CrossRef]
42. Napolitano, L.; Scalise, M.; Galluccio, M.; Pochini, L.; Albanese, L.M.; Indiveri, C. LAT1 is the transport competent unit of the LAT1/CD98 heterodimeric amino acid transporter. *Int. J. Biochem. Cell Boil.* **2015**, *67*, 25–33. [CrossRef]
43. Yanagida, O.; Kanai, Y.; Chairoungdua, A.; Kim, D.K.; Segawa, H.; Nii, T.; Cha, S.H.; Matsuo, H.; Fukushima, J.-I.; Fukasawa, Y.; et al. Human L-type amino acid transporter 1 (LAT1): Characterization of function and expression in tumor cell lines. *Biochim. Biophys. Acta (BBA) Biomembr.* **2001**, *1514*, 291–302. [CrossRef]

44. Sauro, H.M. *Enzyme Kinetics for Systems Biology*, 2nd ed.; Sauro, H.M., Ed.; Ambrosius Publishing: San Bernardino, CA, USA, 2012.
45. Cobelli, C.; Foster, D.; Toffolo, G. *Tracer Kinetics in Biomedical Research: From Data to Model*; Kluwer Academic/Plenum: New York, NY, USA, 2000; ISBN 0-306-46427-6.
46. Berman, M. The formulation and testing of models. *Ann. N. Y. Acad. Sci.* **1963**, *108*, 182–194. [CrossRef]
47. Jacquez, J.A. *Compartmental Analysis in Biology and Medicine*, 2nd ed.; University of Michigan Press: Ann Arbor, MI, USA, 1985; ISBN 0472100637.
48. Phair, R.D. Differential equation methods for simulation of GFP kinetics in non-steady state experiments. *Mol. Boil. Cell* **2018**, *29*, 763–771. [CrossRef]
49. Buescher, J.M.; Antoniewicz, M.R.; Boros, L.G.; Burgess, S.C.; Brunengraber, H.; Clish, C.B.; DeBerardinis, R.J.; Feron, O.; Frezza, C.; Ghesquière, B.; et al. A roadmap for interpreting 13C metabolite labeling patterns from cells. *Curr. Opin. Biotechnol.* **2015**, *34*, 189–201. [CrossRef]
50. Walther, D.J.; Bader, M. A unique central tryptophan hydroxylase isoform. *Biochem. Pharmacol.* **2003**, *66*, 1673–1680. [CrossRef]
51. Windahl, M.S.; Boesen, J.; Karlsen, P.E.; Christensen, H.E.M.; Christensen, H.E.M. Expression, Purification and Enzymatic Characterization of the Catalytic Domains of Human Tryptophan Hydroxylase Isoforms. *Protein J.* **2009**, *28*, 400–406. [CrossRef]
52. McKinney, J.; Knappskog, P.M.; Haavik, J. Different properties of the central and peripheral forms of human tryptophan hydroxylase. *J. Neurochem.* **2005**, *92*, 311–320. [CrossRef]
53. Seok, S.-H.; Ma, Z.-X.; Feltenberger, J.B.; Chen, H.; Chen, H.; Scarlett, C.; Lin, Z.; Satyshur, K.A.; Cortopassi, M.; Jefcoate, C.R.; et al. Trace derivatives of kynurenine potently activate the aryl hydrocarbon receptor (AHR). *J. Biol. Chem.* **2018**, *293*, 1994–2005. [CrossRef]
54. Hilmas, C.; Pereira, E.F.R.; Alkondon, M.; Rassoulpour, A.; Schwarcz, R.; Albuquerque, E.X. The Brain Metabolite Kynurenic Acid Inhibits α7 Nicotinic Receptor Activity and Increases Non-α7 Nicotinic Receptor Expression: Physiopathological Implications. *J. Neurosci.* **2001**, *21*, 7463–7473. [CrossRef]
55. Minhas, P.S.; Liu, L.; Moon, P.K.; Joshi, A.U.; Dove, C.; Mhatre, S.; Contrepois, K.; Wang, Q.; Lee, B.A.; Coronado, M.; et al. Macrophage de novo NAD+ synthesis specifies immune function in aging and inflammation. *Nat. Immunol.* **2019**, *20*, 50–63. [CrossRef]
56. Garavaglia, S.; Perozzi, S.; Galeazzi, L.; Raffaelli, N.; Rizzi, M. The crystal structure of human α-amino-β-carboxymuconate-ε-semialdehyde decarboxylase in complex with 1,3-dihydroxyacetonephosphate suggests a regulatory link between NAD synthesis and glycolysis. *FEBS J.* **2009**, *276*, 6615–6623. [CrossRef]
57. Naviaux, R.K. Metabolic features and regulation of the healing cycle—A new model for chronic disease pathogenesis and treatment. *Mitochondrion* **2018**, *46*, 278–297. [CrossRef]
58. Geiseler, W.; Föllner, H. Three steady state situation in an open chemical reaction system. I. *Biophys. Chem.* **1977**, *6*, 107–115. [CrossRef]
59. Guidi, G.M.; Carlier, M.-F.; Goldbeter, A. Bistability in the isocitrate dehydrogenase reaction: An experimentally based theoretical study. *Biophys. J.* **1998**, *74*, 1229–1240. [CrossRef]

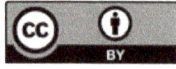 © 2019 by the authors. Licensee MDPI, Basel, Switzerland. This article is an open access article distributed under the terms and conditions of the Creative Commons Attribution (CC BY) license (http://creativecommons.org/licenses/by/4.0/).

MDPI
St. Alban-Anlage 66
4052 Basel
Switzerland
Tel. +41 61 683 77 34
Fax +41 61 302 89 18
www.mdpi.com

Diagnostics Editorial Office
E-mail: diagnostics@mdpi.com
www.mdpi.com/journal/diagnostics

www.ingramcontent.com/pod-product-compliance
Lightning Source LLC
LaVergne TN
LVHW071947080526
838202LV00064B/6694